Angst

Angst

Origins of Anxiety and Depression

Jeffrey P. Kahn, MD

Clinical Associate Professor of Psychiatry
Weill Cornell Medical College
New York, NY

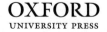

OXFORD
UNIVERSITY PRESS

OXFORD
UNIVERSITY PRESS

Oxford University Press is a department of the University of Oxford.
It furthers the University's objective of excellence in research, scholarship, and
education by publishing worldwide.

Oxford   New York
Auckland   Cape Town   Dar es Salaam   Hong Kong   Karachi
Kuala Lumpur   Madrid   Melbourne   Mexico City   Nairobi
New Delhi   Shanghai   Taipei   Toronto

With offices in
Argentina   Austria   Brazil   Chile   Czech Republic   France   Greece
Guatemala   Hungary   Italy   Japan   Poland   Portugal   Singapore
South Korea   Switzerland   Thailand   Turkey   Ukraine   Vietnam

Oxford is a registered trademark of Oxford University Press in the UK
and certain other countries.

Published by Oxford University Press, Inc.
198 Madison Avenue, New York, New York 10016
www.oup.com

© Jeffrey P. Kahn 2013

Library of Congress Cataloging-in-Publication Data
Kahn, Jeffrey P.
Angst : origins of anxiety and depression / Jeffrey P. Kahn.
p. ; cm.
Includes bibliographical references and index.
ISBN 978–0–19–979644–1 (alk. paper)
I. Title.
[DNLM: 1. Anxiety Disorders—etiology.   2. Depressive Disorder—etiology.
3. Instinct. WM 172]
616.85'22—dc23
2012014064

1 3 5 7 9 8 6 4 2
Printed in the United States of America
on acid-free paper

TABLE OF CONTENTS

PREFACE

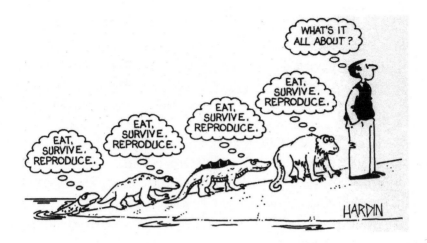

"The most beautiful thing we can experience is the mysterious. It is the source of all true art and all science. He to whom this emotion is a stranger, who can no longer pause to wonder and stand rapt in awe, is as good as dead: his eyes are closed."
—Albert Einstein (German physicist; 1879–1955)

Over the last 30 some years, I have had the pleasure of learning psychiatric diagnosis, psychotherapy, medication, and research. My travels have taken me into psychiatric aspects of heart disease, anxiety disorders, depressive disorders, schizophrenia, and workplace mental health. These experiences have come as a student, clinical practitioner, educator, researcher, author, and consultant. I have learned from teachers, colleagues, students, patients, friends, journals, and books.

Sometime in 2008, I realized I had seen some 2,500 patients, and I began to wonder if it was possible to step back and gain some larger perspective on their collective angst. This thought experiment was soon followed by a conversational introduction to social psychology and by reading books about beer. I soon found myself on a flight home, learning about the theory that humans domesticated grain in order to make beer, sometime near the dawn of civilization, and that bread was only an afterthought. As I drifted off, I wondered why beer was worth all that effort.

Waking up, I suddenly realized that our ancestors may well have used alcohol to quench the same anxiety and depressive disorders that we suffer from today. A mere five diagnostic subtypes account for the lion's share of my own patients' clinical distress, and each of these syndromes has social implications. Our primeval ancestors must have evolved these syndromes as instincts with social purposes. Later, they moved beyond these social instincts to civilization with the help of a few cold ones to quench the angst (more likely warm ones, but why quibble). So if our modern angst derives from evolved instincts, then the existing body of medical research should support that theory.

Though I had encountered a small amount about evolutionary psychiatry over the years, I was amazed to find that the topic had a long and illustrious history, and a more recent minor explosion of publication and theory. This present theory draws some on my predecessors' work; offers novel perspective on this discrete group of five core instinctive syndromes; and with some help from a sixth instinct, suggests an overarching social instinct synthesis. Much of the academic research cited in support of the 2008 theoretical synthesis was published after that date.

To my surprise, my great uncle Karl Landauer, on the occasion of Sigmund Freud's 80th birthday in 1936, said that we must ultimately find an evolutionary conception of psychiatry. "We shall follow Darwin," he said—in reconceiving emotions as instincts that may no longer serve their original purposes. With advances since then in diagnosis, medication, psychotherapy, and biological research, his dream may now come to pass.

At the same time, there is much work to be done, and evolutionary psychiatry will evolve with further understanding of genetics, psychopharmacology, physiology, social psychology, neuroscience, ethology, psychoanalytic theory, and clinical observation. Although the theory can help understand why current diagnoses make sense, and why current treatments can work so well, it offers only modest improvements to currently optimal treatment. We are already at the point where most patients can get better quickly and reliably if they receive the right diagnoses and treatment. Even for psychotic disorders, novel approaches using existing medications and psychotherapies can offer substantial and sometimes dramatic improvement.

Writing this book was an adventure in scientific literature review; discussion with colleagues, friends, and family; workplace observation; and clinical contemplation. Modern technology makes it possible to search vast amounts of research quickly and efficiently. The PubMed service of the National Library of Medicine was an invaluable tool, the Weill-Cornell Medical College Library allowed instant access to the world's medical literature, and the Internet offered up relevant books, cartoons, and quotations at the click of a mouse. Many years' research was accomplished in less than one, and although the speculative leaps may seem reasonable to many, they are no one's fault but mine. Further information, including information about the diagnoses in this book, can be found at TheOriginOfAngst.com.

Jeffrey P. Kahn, M.D.
New York, March 2012

ACKNOWLEDGMENTS

The list of those who have helped to teach, guide, support, advise, and assist me could go on forever. What follows is a selection of those who have been most helpful for this project, listed alphabetically.

I have been fortunate over the years to learn under the supervision of such luminaries in psychiatric research as Donald Klein, as well as Wagner Bridger and Edward Sachar. My psychiatric thinking has also been strongly shaped by many teachers including Roger MacKinnon, Alan McLean and David Peretz. Psychiatrists Eli Einbinder, Richard Frances, Richard Friedman, Eric Hollander, Thomas Kalman, Dolores Malaspina, Stefano Pallanti, Jonathan Polan, Michael Poyurovsky, Maurice Preter, Sally Satel, Adam Savitz, Margaret Spinelli, and Dan Stein have given valuable advice, assistance, and criticism, as have scientists and physicians Danielle Engler, Gus James, Steven Kucera, Karen Overall, Robert Sapolsky, Simeon Schwartz, Edward Shorter, and three anonymous peer reviewers who commented for Oxford on the initial manuscript proposal. Other readers who valuably commented, advised, or edited include Sharon Davison, Ronald Feiman, Jeremy Marks, Zarya Rathe, Curtis Roberts, Andrew Rooks, and Sophie Sun.

I am also indebted to Weill-Cornell Medical College and its faculty, to friends and colleagues, to corporate consultation clients, and especially to patients whose painful angst, although intellectually inspirational, is now hopefully diminished. This project would never have moved forward without the encouragement and expert guidance of Laura Yorke and Carol Mann of the Carol Mann Agency. David D'Addona and Craig Panner of Oxford offered wise and extensive editorial guidance, helped curb my excessive enthusiasm for musical lyrics, cartoons, and exclamation points, and made the manuscript far better than it could ever have been without them.

Curtis Roberts helped obtain reprint permissions for lyrics (listed below). Wayne Goodman (mountsinaiocd.org) gave permission to partially reprint the FOCI scale, Cartoonstock (cartoonstock.com) licensed the cartoons, and the American Psychiatric Association licensed selections from the *DSM-IV*.

Finally, I am especially indebted to my home herd of family and friends, whose unwavering encouragement, support, and editorial guidance have made this project possible. This book is lovingly dedicated to my wife and children, whose affection and wisdom give life meaning, purpose, and joy.

MEDICAL, LEGAL, AND CONFLICT
OF INTEREST DISCLAIMER

This volume contains general information about mental health and medical diagnosis, treatment, and prognosis intended for both a general audience and clinical professionals. Every effort has been made to ensure accuracy; however, the field is evolving, and new information may later emerge. Neither the author nor the publisher is responsible for any remaining errors. This book is not intended as a layperson's manual of mental health or medical care. The accurate diagnosis and effective treatment of any distressed individual requires careful attention by a professional in the field, with comprehensive and appropriate training, and with full knowledge of the specific case.

This book includes fictional case presentations set off in italics. They are based on composite clinical and nonclinical experience, academic findings, supposition, and invention. Some brief one- and two-sentence anecdotes in text are fictionalized from clinical and nonclinical experience, and without identifying information. Similarity of characters in any case to any person living or dead is coincidental. No efforts were made to hide the identities of Cassidy and Bonnie.

Medications named are merely examples from specific classes of medication, all of them off-patent, and some mentioned for common off-label uses. This project was not financially supported in any way by pharmaceutical or health-care companies, the American Psychiatric Association, Cornell University, or any source other than the publisher. The author has no financial ties to pharmaceutical or health-care companies, no role in the *DSM-5* development process, and no conflicts of interest to disclose.

Angst

1

LIONS AND TIGERS AND BEARS ARE NOT WHY: ANGST IS THE MODERN ECHO OF EVOLVED SOCIAL INSTINCTS

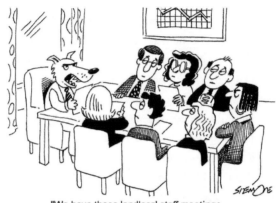

"We have these 'endless' staff meetings Shirley, because I enjoy working in a pack."

"Democratic man, as I have remarked, is quite unable to think of himself as a free individual; he must belong to a group, or shake with fear and loneliness."
—Henry Louis Mencken (American author; 1880–1956)

"No society has been able to abolish human sadness, no political system can deliver us from the pain of living, from our fear of death, our thirst for the absolute. It is the human condition that directs the social condition, not vice versa."
—Eugene Ionesco (French playwright; 1909–1994)

FEELING THE PAIN

These days it seems that nearly everyone is nervous or sad. Unhappiness has many causes, but psychiatrists know that when unhappiness is persistent or intense, there is usually an underlying anxiety or depressive disorder. Even though circumstances may be difficult, the pain of serious or ongoing unhappiness often means that there's more going on than just a really bad situation. The commonplace anxiety and depressive disorders are very commonplace indeed. They are mostly chronic, and they affect at least 20% of the United States at any one time. That's about 60 million people. So why is that? Nobody likes anxiety and depression, but we end up with them anyway, and it's probably always been that way. If they are so common, they must have served some kind of purpose for us in our evolutionary past.

It is more than possible that these common problems were not born as "disorders." Instead, they evolved biologically as social adaptations in ancient tribal societies. How's that again? Well, here are some examples: The severe anxiety and phobias of "Panic Disorder" prevent many people now from flying and driving, yet they may have kept our tribal ancestors from traveling dangerously far from tribe, family, home or Mom. Extreme emotional sensitivity to minor social rejection causes ongoing episodes of mild "Atypical Depression" for many of us, but may have helped maintain social harmony and coherence in our ancestors. Although the biology of "Social Anxiety" makes people feel quite shy in our modern Western world, it may have started as a biological instinct that helped our ancestors feel more at home as tribal followers, rather than top-dog tribal leaders. Since too many chefs spoil the broth, it can be a bottom dog's life, indeed. Just to whet your appetite, we'll soon introduce six specific instincts that evolved to help us get along together, with five of them corresponding to clinical syndromes.

Clearly, these sorts of biological adaptation to ancestral society are still present, and still sometimes helpful, in modern humans. Amazingly, those instinctive biological sensations that told our primeval ancestors how to comport themselves in society can today turn up as conscious emotional pain. So when you feel the pain of angst, you are actually feeling the unrecognized call of ancient social instincts. These days we don't always obey these painful instincts blindly. They become especially unpleasant when they conflict with our rational choices—that is, when we experience them as anxiety and depressive disorders. So, in our modern context, these social instincts can become so intense that they backfire, certainly not providing just the socially adaptive benefits that evolution had in mind. Maybe we have a better life today than our ancestors long ago, but for some of us it can still be a dog's life.

SO WHERE DOES ALL THIS SUFFERING COME FROM?

As we try to understand this evolutionary theory, it is important to know some central evolutionary concepts. First of all, the "mind" of evolution is not a deliberate or conscious process. However, the results of evolutionary adaptation do reflect the kinds of problems that were encountered and overcome during eons past. Charles Darwin (English naturalist, 1809–1882) is considered the father of modern evolutionary theory. He proposed that natural selection had the effect of increasing the reproductive advantage of more adaptive trait variations Above all, Darwin showed us the way that certain physical traits are biologically determined and evolve over time. The genetic inheritance of every species is different, and each species has developed its own paths to greater survival, and to more reproductive success. So different finches, on the different Galapagos Islands, have different beaks to feed from different foods. However, it isn't that evolution favors happily fat birds; rather, it favors well-fed birds that are better able to pass on their genes through reproduction. Thanks to James Watson and Francis Crick, we now know the chemical make-up of the DNA that encodes the instructions for our biological blueprint.

Darwin also pointed out that evolution rewards altruism within a society. In other words, a genetically strong and brave mouse may altruistically die childless to defend its family, but its genes for strength and bravery will live on through family members similarly endowed. A childless bird that is exceptional at locating food for its extended family will have its genes passed on through nieces, nephews and other collateral descendants. Latter-day evolutionary theorists have focused on evolutionary altruism as a seemingly novel notion, but Darwin (if not others before him) was there first.

Darwin also pioneered the notion of psychological evolution (prompted perhaps by his own struggles with anxiety). In *The Descent of Man* in 1871,[1] he emphasized the importance of certain inherited social instincts for the practical and thus evolutionary success of social groups. Three of those same instincts are among the six that are central to our present theory of evolutionary psychopathology: "All animals living in a body…must indeed be in some degree faithful to one another." Second, "those that follow a leader must be in some degree obedient." And third, they must also stick together, "as lions are always on the lookout for the individuals which wander from the herd." Evolution would punish the genes of any who disregarded these three instincts because "…those that cared least for their comrades, and lived solitary, would perish in greater numbers."

Inspired by the importance of communicating emotion within social groups, and maybe by his earlier self-professed lack of expertise, he moved on to *The Expression of Emotions in Man and Animals* (1872).[2] The facial expression of emotions, he proposed, is an evolved mechanism for communicating social instinct and behavior. Additionally, it is similar across species. Humans, along with all other animals, have biologically based behaviors like eating, breathing and walking, but also smiling, romancing, imagining, and moralizing. Charles Darwin knew that social communication is important enough for evolution to pay attention (through natural selection, of course), and that there had to be some underlying biological instinct. He also knew that there was a potential conflict between these instincts and conscious thought: "The very essence of instinct is that it's followed independently of reason," he said. Darwin, wondrous scientist and prodigious autodidact though he was, was not a psychiatrist, though in any case there was precious little psychiatric knowledge around in his time.

Some people are afraid that evolution means we are descended from apes. We are not. We and apes (and all other creatures) are actually descended from bacteria, if you go really far back. Modern apes, though, are our closest cousins, and so we do feel more kinship with them than with modern bacteria, ferns, earthworms, iguanas or mice. Still others are concerned that evolution suggests that there is no higher power, but natural law, it seems, has designed evolution intelligently enough that from humble bacteria *homo sapiens* have evolved. This fortunate occurrence happened, to repurpose the words of Albert Einstein (German physicist; 1879–1955), because "God does not play dice with the world."

SO IS ANGST GENETIC?

If this angst came to us through this evolution by natural selection, then there must be something genetic about it somewhere. There has been a huge amount of research on the genetics of different emotional conditions. What we know now is that a great many of these syndromes run in families, and may indeed be at least partly inherited through genes. Meanwhile, though, there has been only limited progress in identifying specific genes (or groups of genes) for various emotional conditions. This is because those conditions are not simple genetic "flaws," but rather the consequences of highly complex processes that have gradually evolved since primeval times. So, those social instincts that trigger anxiety and depression may have many different genetic influences. When you think about it, it is also doubtful that our physical abilities to sneeze, yawn, smile and laugh are enabled by single genes or even by simple genetic mechanisms.

DOES GENETIC MEAN STRICTLY WRITTEN IN OUR DNA?

Recent research has focused on how inherited factors interact with the environment, especially in childhood, before a problematic condition turns up. (It is called "gene-by-environment" interaction, or GxE). For example, aggressive rhesus monkey mothers can cause changes in the activity of a serotonin-regulating gene of rhesus monkey infants (more later on about how serotonin is the "social director" among brain chemicals). If that gene-activity level then goes down, the young monkeys become more impulsive; they are more likely to push around a newly presented white cylinder.[3] Of course, this study was in New York, where some people even like to push each other around.

But doesn't DNA pretty much set our genes at conception? Well, yes, but not completely. The genes can be chemically modified (through "epigenetics," if you want to be technical, in which a chemical process called methylation can turn off certain genes). If you ever thought about it, you might have wondered how female bees with identical DNA can turn either into small overstressed worker bees or else into majestic queens of the nest. The answer, according to one research group is that the queen bees have a different set of functioning genes.[4] That happens because their genes are modified by the methyl group containing royal jelly that they are fed early on. Clearly, bees are what they eat. The epigenetic methylation of mouse DNA, by the way, can be affected even by social stress as adults. For those mice that responded to social defeats with mousey social avoidance, some of the methylation of one particular gene (part of the stress-related "cortisol" system) fades away.[5] More methyl, anyone?

HAS ANYONE THOUGHT THIS WAY ABOUT HUMAN DISTRESS BEFORE?

There is a long history of work on evolution and psychiatric syndromes. Some of it goes way back, more of it has been written lately, and there is much room for improvement. Sigmund Freud (Austrian psychiatrist; 1856–1939), the self-defined founder of scientific inquiry into the unconscious, is a good place to start. Keep in mind, though, that although Freud started modern psychotherapy on its way, he is far from the last word. Modern theory and practice has moved well beyond his starting place, and he was well aware that there were biological factors unknowable to the science of his time. As Freud put it, "Our provisional ideas on psychology will one day be explained on the basis of organic substrates."[6]

As early as 1915, he drafted a manuscript (*A Phylogenetic Fantasy*, first published only in 1987),[7] that postulated a human nature that evolved to meet the needs of a hyperaggressive Ice Age man (Freud has this preoccupation with aggression and sex). He also tried to apply the then-current concept that "ontogeny recapitulates phylogeny." People used to think that if you look at the stages of anatomical development in the human fetus, the sequence of stages mirrored the evolutionary history of our species. So if the fetus has something that looks like gills, then sometime in the past we were fish. There is actually some evidence that we are descended from electricity-sensing fish,[8] though our fish ancestors must have lived a very, very long time ago. Freud didn't get very far trying to apply "ontogeny recapitulates phylogeny" to human emotional problems, but he did make a serious effort to examine evolutionary psychiatry from that perspective.

CIVILIZATION AND ITS DISCONTENTS

Some of his later thoughts on the role of evolution in human angst are in his book *Civilization and Its Discontents*.[9] This classic work doesn't dwell much on those controversial "Freudian" theories that are largely disused today. Instead, Freud's main point here is about a clash between man's basic nature and the modern civilization in which he lives. Indeed, a more accurate translation of his German title (*Das Unbehagen in der Kultur*) would be "The Uneasiness in Culture." As he saw it, civilization causes unhappiness in man because it requires us to contain primitive sexual and aggressive instincts, and to mute our independent natures in order to maintain a civilized society. In Freud's own words, "It is impossible to overlook the extent to which civilization is built upon a renunciation of instinct." He even wrote an essay called "Instinct and Its Vicissitudes."[10]

If you read carefully, Freud, like Charles Darwin before him, even seems to touch glancingly on four of the instinct-related syndromes we'll get to shortly: Panic Anxiety (adolescents separated from family), Social Anxiety (guilty dread of authority), Atypical Depression (guilty dread of the conscience—known to Freud as the "superego"), Obsessive-Compulsive Disorder (cleanliness, orderliness, thriftiness, and control of aggressive instincts through sublimation—the same four traits nowadays considered OCD subtypes), as well as on Consciousness (Freud's "ego"). He sees these largely as culturally and developmentally determined individual traits that socialize us by controlling our aggressive and sexual instincts. Our present theory, though, sees it a different way. Those traits are inborn social instincts, and much of the discontentedness in modern society springs from our rational independence prevailing over those painful social instincts that were more adaptive in earlier human society.

CARL JUNG

Carl Jung (Swiss psychiatrist: 1875–1961) was a student of Freud's, with an independent streak that led to a serious break with his teacher. Jung had the thought that human emotion is guided by the Collective Unconscious—an inherited set of experiences and associated emotional structures that derive from the long history of human kind. In other words, we have a set of evolved instincts ("Archetypes") that are sometimes painfully aroused by incompatibility with modern society: "A man is ill, but the illness is Nature's attempt to heal him," says Jung.[11] A sample Archetype for some of us might be the Anima—a man's instinctual inner view of women.

Although the structure of Jung's Archetypes varies considerably from the social instincts at the heart of our discussion, his work does include attention to core issues of social attachment and social hierarchy.[12] Clearly, Jung's notion of unconscious inherited Archetypes resonates with the unconscious biological social instincts that we plan to explore. His ancient Archetypal Unconscious is supplemented in every person by a Personal Unconscious of individual experiences: each person's uniquely personal method of adapting their evolved instincts to their modern environment. In the same way, every human has re-fashioned his or her social instincts through personal experience and conscious modification. Jung points out that:

> In studying the history of the human mind one is impressed again and again by the fact that the growth of the mind is the widening of the range of consciousness, and that each step forward has been a most painful and laborious achievement. One could almost say that nothing is more hateful to man than to give up even a particle of his unconsciousness. Ask those who have tried to introduce a new idea![13]

So adapting our instincts through consciousness and reason is not so simple. We face the intransigence of our own hidden instincts.

EVOLVING BEYOND SIGMUND AND CARL

It is worth noting that there has been growing interest in evolutionary psychopathology, including a steady emergence of hypotheses, books and textbooks over the last 15 years (some of which are cited in these chapters or noted in the bibliography). Much of the existing work on evolutionary psychopathology focuses on complex and dramatic problems like Schizophrenia (which occurs in only about 0.5% of the population), even though there is general consensus that there are at least several biologically different Schizophrenia subtypes. Some of the theories look at symptoms such as paranoia, or at certain pieces of complex behavior, including psychoanalytic constructs such as the "oedipal conflict." More importantly, much of the theorizing has been on benefits to affected individuals, rather than to the interaction of individuals within their social groups.

There are many evolutionary ideas that have been floated on depression.[14] For example, one Australian group has proposed that clinical depression is a means to avoid social exclusion.[15] That isn't too far from what we'll be talking about. Another paper proposed that depression makes people "ruminate" in a way that helps them solve problems better, but then again, depressed people don't often find better solutions for paying the bills or getting work done.[16] Even so, it could be that rumination about social problems is a very helpful part of some depressions,[17] at least for those who ponder their social blunders.

Maybe depression in the face of failure makes people inactive in a way that allows them to recuperate; however, depressed people don't actually think about returning to the fray, and are usually tentative when they do. There is more, of course, though little work has focused on subtypes such as Atypical Depression and Melancholic Depression.

There are also theories concerning anxiety disorders, including evolutionary psychiatrist Dan Stein's (South African psychiatrist, 1962–) work on Social Anxiety, which is pretty close to what we'll talk about ahead. There is only limited work on Panic Anxiety and Obsessive Impulsive Disorder, and less still on a linking theory for an overarching evolutionary perspective on the origin of anxiety and depressive disorders. All in all, there are many theories, little yet that we can be sure about, and much room for logical synthesis that is consistent with clinical experience and scientific research.

THE PSYCHO-NORMALITY OF EVERYDAY EMOTION

Commonplace anxiety and depressive disorders are qualitatively quite different from the more everyday and generalized experience of emotions such as nervousness, sadness, joy and pleasure. Those ordinary emotions are generated as reactions to circumstances, and we have words for many different types. For example, the list of everyday "anxieties" can include fear, worry, hurt, fight/flight reaction, deadline pressure, financial distress, and just plain ordinary anxiety. They are all exceedingly important evolved instincts themselves, and they are essential for specific social and environmental interaction, as Charles Darwin pointed out. They can be increased by an emotional disorder, but they are not emotional disorders when they are all by themselves.

Everyday nervousness and sadness can be prompts to leave unhappiness or danger behind by finding more effective solutions, better circumstances, or more empathic companions. However, the more specific anxiety and depressive disorders are not at all the same as everyday nervousness and sadness. The commonplace anxiety and depressive disorders are instinctive primeval "solutions" that use emotional distress as prompts to stay in evolutionarily fixed social roles. They provide socially instinctive angst that tells us to know our place in the social neighborhood. We have many other instincts, social and otherwise, that don't now seem central to common emotional problems. Our everyday feelings are for everyday problems, and it may well be that every single one of our emotions is an evolutionary adaptation to safeguard the perpetuation of our human DNA.[18] Emotion allows people and animals to cooperate, survive, prosper, and procreate.

A HEARTY APPETITE IS A DIFFERENT KIND OF PROBLEM

One more thing. Instinctive behaviors that lead to happy positive emotions are not usually problems themselves. Most people like to eat, drink water, imbibe alcohol, play, speak, feel affection and love, have sex, have faith, and even wonder about their world. Problems arise only when people are deprived and thus hungry for appetitive satisfaction, when they indulge in these things in excessive or inappropriate ways, or when these appetitive instincts are seriously diminished by illness or distress.

Frustration of appetitive instincts in keeping with cultural or religious requirements can be a bit unpleasant on purpose; religious fasts are mandated for both theological and ethical reasons. Frustration because of actual scarcity or deprivation takes away even that moral consolation for the suffering. These appetitive instincts can also be decreased or increased by anxiety and depressive disorders. Concerns about appetitive fulfillment are sometimes even disguised concerns about other people. Sibling rivalry about toys is mostly about desire for parental affection and attention. BMW and jewelry envy among adults may be a later manifestation of that same social focus displaced to more expensive appetites. Some people, in a desperate and incautious attempt to overcome social angst, will try to quell that distress by having as much fun as possible. For those with long musical memories, Commander Cody and his Lost Planet Airmen were on to that long ago in their song "Too Much Fun."

Among these appetites are social instincts that our genes promote through pleasurable reinforcement. For example, affection, bonding, play, sex—all of these provide positive reinforcement through conscious thought, and through automatic self-medication when our brains release endorphins (morphine-like substances) and oxytocin (the "trust hormone"). Maternal-infant bonding is helped along by endorphin- and opiate-like chemicals that are digestive products of human breast milk proteins ("casomorphins"). Breast-feeding makes babies feel good around Mom, and maybe high on Mom as well. Why do some people bond over chili peppers? They trigger endorphin release, too. Okay, so that one isn't actually a social instinct.

The primeval social instincts of our present theory are not appetitive instincts about seeking food, sex and positive feelings. These social instincts involve unpleasant negative feelings that shape our social behaviors, and those very behaviors may have fundamental conflicts with our rational wishes and with our modern society. Even so, our social instincts are sometimes re-adapted to serve newer purposes. Either way, some of us are exposed to way too much angst and find ourselves looking for some kind of relief.

BECAUSE IT TAKES A COMMUNITY

Robert Benchley (American humorist, 1889–1945) famously said: "There are two kinds of people in the world: those who divide the world into two kinds of people, and those who don't." It isn't that people are either basically all good or basically all bad. Deep down inside, we are basically social animals. Self-esteem is not nearly so important to us as the social esteem of others. Few of us can live truly alone as hermits. Even Henry David Thoreau (American author, 1817–1862), who wrote about his self-sufficiency at Walden Pond, in reality lived quite close to civilization. He often had meals brought to him. Faced with lesser technology and knowledge, more limited resources, and more exposure to predator species and environmental dangers, any primeval human living alone would have had quite a challenge on his or her hands. Young humans or animals that stray from the pack are more likely to die than those who stay close. The challenge of solitary survival resonates with us today—witness the television shows and movies that glorify people taking on the wilderness alone (and where most are accompanied more by nylon tents than by tense lions). Even now, the ultimate punishment is often solitary confinement ("now go to your room").

Long after the solitary bacterial days, the social instincts of our primeval ancestors evolved so that they could all live more effectively in ancient communities, and so that they could more successfully pass on their DNA. Life back then was about harmonious collaboration for communal living and basic survival. Those social instincts weren't about office etiquette, Emily Post, Miss Manners, working the room, cocktail party chatter, individualism, or even about the urge to merge. Indeed, an amazing statistical analysis of primate behaviors suggests that our ancestors evolved biologically from solitary survival to group living some 52 million years ago, and then on to pair living (or male-led harems) some 16 million years ago. Most primate groups are similar even today, but modern human social groups have been enhanced by our more recent developments of Consciousness and civilization.[19]

Group cohesion, teamwork, the Golden Rule, altruism, and more were and are essential for our survival. There has, indeed, been a flurry of writing on evolutionary altruism. Since families and tribes share a common gene pool, then altruistic behaviors protect your shared familial genes, even if you don't yourself reproduce. To be sure, altruism is also influenced by rational thought and external circumstance. Altruism takes many forms, from the humble and sterile worker bees who keep a bee hive running, to noble warriors who risk all for country, to self-sacrificing humanitarians like Mother Theresa, to those who share food and treasure with others, and to those who make humble widgets for the common good.

THE ESTEEM OF OTHERS

Looking only to the individual for evolutionary benefit of social instincts is looking in the wrong place. To adapt a famous query about trees from George Berkeley (Anglican philosopher, 1685–1753), "If a human cries out in the forest, and no person hears him, is he still in emotional pain?" The esteem and attention of others is what matters most to people, much more than self-esteem. There have even been studies of "self-esteem" interventions.[20] For example, telling schoolchildren that they are smart impairs their future performance, whereas telling them that they work hard or not praising them at all leads them to better work in the future.[21] Therefore, attempting to convince people to be impressed with themselves can actually make people do worse, which isn't all that surprising really.[22] Convincing people to rely mostly on their self-esteem is really telling them that they can't count on other people, and that is a mighty unhappy thought indeed. Worse still, some probably hear the message that they should think and act like they are better and more important than other people, or even that ordinary rules don't apply to them. Real "self-esteem" derives from the esteem of others. Why shout out your victories if no one hears you?

It is worth mentioning the growth of psychoanalytic "object relations" in recent decades. (Time passes slowly in psychoanalysis. If a human year is seven dog years, then perhaps a "psychoanalytic year" is five human years, or about the length of an orthodox formal psychoanalysis). "Objects" are those people who are the objects of our emotions. Following the work of some earlier researchers and theorists, Otto Kernberg (American psychiatrist, 1928–) has advanced and expanded this work, and he writes eloquently about patients with severe Borderline and Narcissistic Personalities. The object-relations approach, more so than the work of Freud himself, focuses on problematic social interactions, even for patients who have problems not notably severe.

We can really see people's social focus at work, (not to mention sometimes at home). That's how the "field observations" of a psychiatrist in the workplace help us understand where our modern syndromes come from. It sometimes feels a bit like a scientist observing primates in the wild. Even though every worker behaves differently, those people with particular anxiety and depressive syndromes interact and socialize in particular ways. So if we listen carefully about work behavior, we can hear the echoes of evolved social instincts.

LET'S BE DIAGNOSTICALLY SPECIFIC!

In order to formulate an evolutionary model of understanding, we need to figure out just what entities we are trying to explain. That brings us to some basic psychiatric notions. There is a difference between symptoms, signs and syndromes. A sign is something a physician observes—say a limp, or a tense face. A symptom is something a patient describes—painful walking or sudden bursts of anxiety. A syndrome is a group of signs and symptoms that tend to cluster together—a broken ankle or Panic Anxiety, for these two examples. When these syndromes cause problems, they are called disorders (or illnesses).

From a treatment point of view it is very important to diagnose the syndromes, rather than just listing signs or symptoms. You wouldn't want your broken ankle treated just with painkillers (yes, this does actually happen). Physicians use patient history, physical examination and laboratory tests to provide signs, symptoms and data that allow diagnosis of physical illness syndromes. Likewise, psychiatrists are physicians that use patient history, mental-status examination and laboratory tests to provide syndromal diagnosis of psychiatric disorders (or related physical illnesses). It's not just sadness and nervousness—good psychiatrists look for very specific depressive and anxiety syndromes. Even though they may look similar on the surface, they have different unhappy thoughts, different behaviors, different treatments, and different biologies. You wouldn't want your Panic Attacks treated with just painkillers (yes, this happens too).

These syndrome subtypes are essential to understanding evolutionary perspective. Psychiatric syndromes are defined (more or less well) in a standard book called *DSM-IV-TR*.[23] The *DSM-IV* was composed by exhaustive analysis of how certain signs and symptoms cluster together into recognizable and problem-causing syndromes. Use of these syndromal diagnoses makes for more specific and more effective treatment of disorders. Trying to treat ill-defined and nonspecific sadness or nervousness doesn't work so well. Likewise, treating "foot pain" without knowing the underlying diagnosis is a bad idea.

BUT WHICH ONES?

DSM-IV has a whole bunch of syndromes (way too many, some think). However it is that that came to pass, this book will focus on just five common subtypes of anxiety and depression. The five that we will look at are Panic Anxiety, Social Anxiety, Obsessive-Compulsive Disorder, Atypical Depression and Melancholic Depression. We'll describe them as we go along. So why focus on just these five syndromes? The first answer is that they are among the most common ones in the general population, and among the most common by far among generally successful people who walk into a psychiatrist's office.

This reductionist observation depends, though, on a very careful diagnostic interview process, and leads us to our second answer: broader syndromes, although quite widely used and recognized, can be overinclusive. For example, Major Depressive Disorder (MDD), Generalized Anxiety Disorder (GAD), and an ostensibly mild form of Bipolar Disorder (Bipolar II) are all commonly used diagnoses. However, when you look closely enough, you can nearly always find a more specific subtype or alternate diagnosis, and sometimes more than one. Our own unpublished consulting data (on corporate employees) suggest that nearly all people with a history of MDD also have a history of Panic Anxiety, Atypical Depression, Melancholic Depression and/ or Social Anxiety. This goes along with the idea that more specific syndromes are usually there when you look at Major Depression more closely.[24,25,26]

In the case of PostTraumatic Stress Disorder (PTSD), it could be that childhood adversity and a serotonin genetic marker sensitize people to anxiety and depressive disorders, and also help cause PTSD in response to adult traumatic events.[27] So, childhood memories, as well as existing anxiety or depressive disorders, could intensify the memory and recall of traumatic events. A Panic Attack can definitely focus the mind on bad memories,[28] and some research suggests that PTSD is largely a form of Panic Anxiety.[29,30,31] Drugs that increase focus on distressing events can also cause a similar sort of postevent memory enhancement.[32,33,34]

The third reason for focusing on these five syndromes is that they also explain many of the other subtypes. Panic Anxiety may lie beneath rage attacks ("Intermittent Explosive Disorder") and Social Anxiety may present as seeing oneself embarrassingly ugly ("Body Dysmorphic Disorder"). So if just five syndromes can do the heavy lifting of a far larger number, then it is a more parsimonious solution. That would conform with Occam's Razor, the principle that says the simplest explanation is usually the best one (although someone failed to apply this Razor when borrowing the name of Sir William of Ockham).

DOES ANYONE ELSE THINK SO, TOO?

Many psychiatrists have likewise called for more specific syndromes than broadly defined Major Depressive Disorder (MDD). Although our selection of five commonplace and accepted syndromes as predominant is far from a universal standard, it is pretty much in keeping with some research. When researchers look at large groups of people with MDD, they find that a huge number have at least one of our five syndromes. What hasn't been done in recent studies is to show that those syndromes can replace MDD as the explanatory construct for most afflicted folks. This is a shame, because more specific syndromes make for simpler and more effective treatment. They also make for more precise and focused research. While evolutionary psychiatry is not new, a coherent theory can only emerge from a correct set of diagnoses. Otherwise we are shooting in the dark.

Let's look at a few examples. In a Boston study, at least half of patients with MDD also have an anxiety disorder.[35] At least some psychiatrists have suggested that "depression" with Panic Anxiety is really just an elaboration of Panic symptoms.[36] Social Anxiety in Munich predicts a high rate of MDD later on.[37] At least 39% of people with MDD have the Atypical Depression subtype.[38] Melancholic Depression is a different and distinct form of MDD.[39] So we can do the math. It is not hard to imagine Major Depression as largely accounted for by these other syndromes. The same kind of math applies just as well to GAD, Bipolar II, and PTSD.

There is another way to look at this notion. For example, Panic Attacks predict a variety of later syndromes.[40,41] This could mean that either they trigger other syndromes, that they are part of the other syndromes, that they occur together with the other syndromes, or that they actually are just confused with the other syndromes. So this diagnostic reductionism, although not yet mainstream, is hardly far-fetched. Moreover, it has the potential to improve treatment—and to target exactly those traits most needing evolutionary exploration.

Of course, there is the opposing point of view that the broader syndromes such as MDD, GAD, Bipolar II and PTSD make more sense clinically than more specific subtypes. That view suggests that GAD is GAD even if someone has recognizable Panic Anxiety or Social Anxiety, and that the more specific symptoms, even if noted, should be overlooked in favor of treating the more global diagnosis of GAD. This approach doesn't fit as well with careful clinical perspective nor does it lead to maximum treatment responsiveness. Ockham would turn over in his grave.

This raises the question: Why aren't the subtypes more often diagnosed? The subtypes are well known, officially sanctioned and you just have to look for them. Part of the problem is that some clinicians don't think that they matter, or don't routinely ask about them. However, there is something more: Patients follow these social instincts without any awareness of their purpose—only with some awareness of feeling bad from anxiety or depression, and of the life problems that they see. Clinicians (even the most well-trained and knowledgeable ones) have an instinctive reluctance to probe too deeply, especially into those sacrosanct core instincts that are the very glue that helps hold human society together. Although this would improve treatment, patients and clinicians alike are instinctively fearful that exposing that glue to the light of reason would be like opening Pandora's box.

INSTINCTS INSIDE AND OUTSIDE

Just because many people have the same emotional syndromes (the exaggerated social instincts that we've been discussing), doesn't mean that their behaviors all appear in the same way. Many things shape the outward appearance of that syndrome: Culture, family, religion, gender, social rank, social role, education, economic status, treatment history, self-improvement history, other instinctive influences, self-presentation, and other factors all influence the appearance of any given syndrome. One more factor that will be a major focus of our discussion is counter-instinctive behavior ("reaction formation" in psychoanalytic parlance)—the tendency to do the opposite of one's instincts. With so many factors influencing the appearance of our instincts, it is easy to miss the forest of instinct for the trees of our complex behaviors in the larger world. Our main focus here is on those herd-like instincts that define our core selves.

BUT DON'T PEOPLE GO TO PSYCHIATRISTS FOR LIFE, LOVE, AND WORK PROBLEMS?

In psychiatric office practice, most patients are active and functional members of society. Sometimes they turn up just because of serious anxiety or depression, but mostly they come for help because they are unhappy for reasons of circumstance, relationships, career and emotional distress. While they may focus on a financial setback, a problem boss or a difficult spouse, their concern about those very real problems is typically amplified by the presence of an equally real underlying anxiety or depressive syndrome. Unhappy circumstances vary tremendously, but unhappy syndromes are much more alike. People without unhappy syndromes are less likely to seek help for unhappy circumstances.

After an initial evaluation, ongoing medication and diagnostic issues are only a small percentage of session time. Most, by far, of what takes place in the office from then on is psychotherapy. There are always those emotional issues of family, career, finances, circumstances and more. Through that psychotherapeutic process you can further see the world-views of diagnosable syndromes now treated with medication. The overt symptoms may be gone, but the patterns of thinking linger on in sometimes counter-productive ways.

Perhaps not by accident, our five instinctive syndromes are the very ones that most permit evolutionary perspective. Because they are so common, they may have served some essential evolutionary purpose, and facilitation of social harmony and communal life seems to be a common thread. We'll see that, although anxiety and depression were instinctual prompts to primeval humans on how to play their roles in a successful tribal society, they can cause unhappiness and disadvantage today. At the same time, they can still have some evolved social advantages, and even modern paradoxical advantages.

ARE THERE OTHER SYNDROMES BESIDES THIS GANG OF FIVE?

Of course there are. Though some are uncommon or little known, there are also such important syndromes as Schizophrenia, Bipolar Disorder I (old school "manic-depressive" disorder), personality disorders, and substance abuse. Schizophrenia, for one, has long been considered a collection of different syndromes that have a similar clinical appearance. Although some syndromes have been removed from the Schizophrenia group over the decades (Psychotic Melancholia, Psychotic Mania, Neuro-Syphilis), there are other subtypes that have been suggested, and that may now be on the path to fuller documentation. Indeed, recently proposed subtypes include psychotic forms of Panic Anxiety, Social Anxiety and OCD. So it may be that an eventual question will be: How did evolution lead us to psychotic versions of anxiety or depressive disorders? It may well be that our six core social instincts also play a central role in Schizophrenia subtypes (with our human Consciousness instinct playing one of those roles). We'll cover that, too.

Likewise for personality disorders, some are clearly related to our social instincts, many are related to incapacity for emotional closeness (impaired "object relations"), and a couple are related to psychosis-proneness. There is a growing interest in something called the Five-Factor Personality Model (also known as: OCEAN, CANOE, NEO, Big Five). As we shall see in chapter 8, if we lump all sorts of personality measures together and stir them together in a computer, there are only five major ingredients of personality. The Five Factors in that model correspond to five of our six social instincts, and provide an alternate way of understanding personality—as well as an alternate take on the well-verified standard personality disorders that we already know. In addition, our six instincts correspond nicely to work on categories of moral character, the basics of kindergarten culture, core social instincts in other species, and the essential flight instructions for flocks of birds. We'll get to all this when we address the human herd as a whole. Then there is substance abuse. We'll touch on that for its role as an over-the-top attempt at self-medication for problematic social instincts.

OKAY, SO THEN WHAT ARE THESE SIX INSTINCTS?

Just by way of brief introduction, here is the short version of what these instincts once did for our primeval selves and tribes so long ago:

Panic Anxiety
Purpose: Kept us close enough to home and group that we could find our way back.
Motto: Catastrophes await if you can't find your way home.

Social Anxiety
Purpose: Kept us in line in our tribal social hierarchies to keep the peace at home.
Motto: Shame and embarrassment come from not knowing your primeval rank.

Obsessive Compulsive Disorder:
Purpose: Kept us on track for the work needed to let people live together safely.
Motto: Clean, arrange, save and behave for a sure and tidy nest.

Atypical Depression:
Purpose: Kept us well-enough behaved for a cooperative society.
Motto: Behave yourself to avoid rejection, remorse and exile.

Melancholic Depression:
Purpose: Kept us from using scarce resources when no longer useful to the group.
Motto: Take one for the team if you are too old or too ill.

Consciousness:
Purpose: Kept us responsive to our companions and environment.
Motto: Thoughtful understanding leads to better solutions.

The titles of the gang-of-six chapters link both the instinct and the syndromes, just to keep track. Remember, even though our ancestors obeyed these instincts more fully back then (as most other modern species do even now), that certainly doesn't mean we are inflexibly stuck with their edicts today.

I THINK I THINK, THEREFORE I THINK I FEEL MY INSTINCT

The last of these six instincts is worth special mention here. Rene Descartes (French philosopher; 1596–1650) famously answered the philosophical question of existence with an appeal to Consciousness: "I think, therefore I am" ("Je pense donc je suis"). Plato (Greek philosopher, 424 BC–348 BC) and Aristotle (Greek philosopher, 384 BC–322 BC) were there first (of course), and self-effacing Augustine of Hippo (Algerian theologian, 354–430) even mused "If I am mistaken, I am."

We humans, more than any other species, are aware of ourselves, of each other, and of the world around us. This conscious awareness allows us to understand nature and people, and drives us to understand how everything works. Two of those things (and maybe they are the same thing) are our biological social instincts, and the unpleasant emotions that can make us so unhappy. Our ability to go our own conscious way, despite awareness of the anxiety and depression that push us to obey social instincts, differentiates us humans from other species. Unlike the other instincts in our theory, Consciousness does not itself correspond to some sort of psychopathology, but consciously overriding our social instincts can inadvertently lead to angst, while too little consciousness can also cause yet other problems (more on this in chapter 7).

HAVE WE HEARD ABOUT THESE
CENTRAL INSTINCTS BEFORE?

If these syndromes are so common and instinctive, then why haven't we heard something about them before? Well, maybe we have. Charles Darwin and Sigmund Freud dropped some hints, and the instincts are in the culture everywhere (as reflected in small part by the cartoon and quotes at the top of each chapter). As Albert Einstein pointed out, "The whole of science is nothing more than a refinement of everyday thinking." From one angle or another, you'll find similar themes in Shakespeare, classical literature and myth, psychotherapy theory, religious texts, and music of all kinds.

Music is a special part of culture. The combination of lyric, rhyme, rhythm and tonality is ideal for communicating emotional concepts, and music has carried messages of human feeling for millennia. Music touches our very soul, and it's hard to believe that music hasn't always served central social functions. Nowhere are core emotional syndromes better expressed than in American blues music, as the very name would suggest. Originally written under circumstances often dire and deprived, blues lyrics focus on such elemental human themes as leaving home and losing mother, the pain of second-class status, the need for perseverance in the face of adversity, the hurt of rejection, and the inevitability of death. As we'll see, these five themes are not far at all from the instincts underlying our five syndromes, and some well-known lyrics offer strikingly precise awareness of commonplace anxiety and depressive disorders. It's not easy being blue.

ISN'T THERE BIOLOGY IN HERE SOMEWHERE?

Most people have heard of serotonin these days (one of many natural chemical "neurotransmitters" that send messages from one nerve cell to another), and serotonin is a central scientific theme for our five social instinct syndromes. Popular medications like fluoxetine (notably described in Peter Kramer's *Listening to Prozac*)[42] are selective serotonin reuptake inhibitors (SSRIs) that indirectly increase serotonin activity, and have greater or lesser benefits for all five of our biological syndromes. That's probably because serotonin plays a central oversight role in moderating social behavior, and despite the fact that each diagnosis has a different biology. We can think of serotonin as the "social director" of the brain. (In a later chapter we'll also get to the idea that the neurotransmitter dopamine is the "appetitive director.")

When locusts are crowded together, their serotonin goes up and they become oh-so-gregarious.[43] Now, they can swarm together instead of feeding as loners. So from that perspective, serotonin deficiency promotes loners who can have their own solitary turf and also expand the range of the tribe. Increased serotonin promotes group cohesion. What triggers the move from loners to groupies? Other locusts. It turns out that it isn't the just the sight or smell of nearby locusts—it is the physical feeling of other locusts on a rear leg. This can even be mimicked by researchers throwing grain—The serotonin just flows. With all those other locusts crowding you from behind, it is better to be social about it, and to look together for newer opportunities.[44] The increased serotonin level somehow promotes group behavior, and a swarming search for proverbial greener pastures. On the other hand, locust swarms are not so good for human farmers. When you look at photos of locusts, the loner phase uniform is camouflage green (to blend into the background), whereas the social phase outfit is brightly colored yellow or red (to stand out at the party).

Mammals can have similar sentiments. Benjamin Franklin (American politician and polymath; 1706–1790) punningly advised prudent interdependence at the signing of the Declaration of Independence: "We must all hang together, or assuredly we shall all hang separately." Surely, his enthusiasm for togetherness reflected his high serotonin level as much as his fear of the British response.[45] Somehow, over the eons, ancient social serotonin mechanisms evolved to influence a variety of types and levels of social behavior. The serotonin system is still susceptible to evolutionary change, even during a human lifetime, as we are about to see.

SIBERIAN FARM FOXES

Speaking of mammals, let's talk about foxes. In a famous and ongoing Russian study, silver foxes have been bred for tameness for more than 50 years. Using only that single selection criterion, the foxes have become as people friendly and tame as pet dogs. However, that is not all: The tame foxes have developed noncamouflage patterns in their coats: white patches and bits of brown, even chestnut color, thus developing a more social appearance—"party clothes" perhaps (genetically linked traits are known as "pleiotropy"). Additionally, they have more serotonin in their brains—there is a pattern here[46,47,48].

Some wild animals have naturally domesticated over the past 15,000 years or so. Domesticated animals tend to trust humans and mostly have floppy ears, in contrast to their more attentive and fearful wild cousins. Darwin noticed the floppy ears, as one of several changes in the appearance of domesticated animals. This suggests a biological link between lowered ears and lowered fears. For what it is worth, wild elephants also have floppy ears, perhaps because they evolved without much to be afraid of. But as we humans do not have floppy ears, this does raise the question of how truly domesticated humans really are.

Curiously, some people have a rare genetic condition called Williams-Beuren syndrome. These folks have characteristic elf-like bodily features, so that they retain childlike features into adulthood ("neoteny"), as do our pet dogs and foxes (with their large eyes and friendly playful behavior). They may be quite musical, and they often do have enlarged earlobes. Additionally, they have an unusual personality: They are uncommonly friendly and gregariously sociable. They may even be the very inspiration for the notion of elves. Although the genetic basis of the syndrome is known, no one has yet looked at their serotonin systems. Perhaps someone will.[49]

SIMPLISTIC SEROTONIN

So we start our thought experiment with an oversimplification: more serotonin activity makes people feel closer, or at least makes them more comfortable being close.[50] When romantically involved couples were given a selective serotonin reuptake inhibitor (SSRI) instead of a placebo, both men and women (in their own particular ways), felt closer and more secure in their romance (and women additionally felt less preoccupied with the relationship).[51] That makes it easier to get along. And the closer you feel, the less you are concerned about the social fine points and niceties that our social instincts help us produce. Not surprisingly, when people fall in love, their level of serotonin activity increases—and this could even be an evolutionary adaptation for attaching to each other.[52]

On the other hand, an absence of serotonin makes people feisty. When a group of research subjects were given food that depletes serotonin (a protein drink without the amino acid tryptophan—the "tryptophan-depletion test"), they became more impulsive, and also more likely to reject others for their transgressions.[53] They played a game in which one player proposes how to divide a sum of money, and the other decides whether to accept. With depleted serotonin, the deciders were more likely to reject an unfair division, even if it meant they received nothing at all themselves. In Oxford, they used the same dietary depletion method, and then asked men and women to rate photographs of couples. The largest change after serotonin depletion was that the couples in the photos were seen as less close and intimate.[45] Be careful about your protein shakes.

From another point of view, certain life stresses can decrease serotonin, and in a nonspecific way thus increase expression of psychopathology (such as anxiety and depressive disorders).[54] You can even do this in the lab, where the tryptophan-depletion test causes nonspecific increases in common psychiatric symptoms.[55] This reinforces the idea that serotonin plays a general role in fostering social comfort.

Indeed, researchers have recently been intrigued by a genetic variant that changes how serotonin behaves in the nerve cells of people, monkeys and rats. People with this genetic variation (we are talking about the short-allele version of the 5-HTT serotonin transporter gene) are more prone to various psychiatric symptoms after stressful events in childhood, adolescence or adulthood. This gene plays an important role in some of our social instincts, with modification by gene-by-experience interactions.[56] Because it is one common underlying factor, it may help explain why the diagnosable versions of the five instincts so often occur together ("co-morbidity") in the same angst-prone people. Likewise, there could be environmental factors, like early parental loss, that aggravate multiple genetic factors.[57] From here on, we'll refer to this genetic variation as "genetically reduced serotonin activity." Keeping this stuff in everyday language feels more civilized, not to mention more social.

SEROTONIN IS COMPLICATED STUFF, WITH COMPLICATED COMPANIONS

To be sure, serotonin isn't everything biologically social in our brains. There are many other compounds known to be involved in social behaviors, including oxytocin (a hormone that increases feelings of trust), endorphins (opiate-like chemicals that increase feelings of well-being and reduce pain), vasopressin, dopamine, and many others. However, we do know the most about serotonin, and it does seem to play a particularly important social role. We should add, too, that we have distinct serotonin systems that may vary in their purposes and effects. In particular, there are at least fifteen different serotonin receptors (the proteins on nerve-cell walls that receive the serotonin "message"), as well as different areas of the brain that have serotonin activity, and emerging work has already begun to spell out some of the details.

For now, we'll focus on serotonin in general, and look forward to more refined explanations that emerge soon. Occam's Razor also applies where the facts aren't all known. Indeed, as philosopher Bertrand Russell (Welsh philosopher, 1872–1970 pointed out: "Whenever possible, substitute constructions out of known entities for inferences to unknown entities." Or, as more clearly framed by James Taranto (American journalist; 1966 –): "When all you have is a hammer, it is hard to wield Occam's Razor." Simplified serotonin is our hammer, a starting point if you will, and future science may spell out more detail about serotonin sub-systems and the other compounds. Although future research will allow simple theories that are more detailed and precise, we have enough now for a pretty good start.

WHAT HATH CIVILIZATION BROUGHT?

The origin of civilization is a whole nother subject. As human civilization developed over the last 10,000–100,000 years (give or take), there was less reliance on the

instinctual social roles essential to primeval tribes, and there was greater opportunity and need for independent thought and behavior. Civilization brought more
social opportunity to Everyman. An everyday member of the tribe could decide to
play a more prominent or successful role—that is if he or she was willing to tolerate a bit of angst. Real civilization takes more than a village—it needs free-thinking
individuals. As we will see, the most free thinking of all are often troubled by anxiety
and depression.

WHAT HATH CIVILIZATION WROUGHT?

Civilization has its discontents, perhaps because our inbuilt social instincts are still
there. So, civilization has developed correctives such as government, laws, democracy, religion, beer, and healers to help us. More later about beer. Even so, disobey-
ing our instincts can still make us more anxious and sad. Yet at another level, the
instinctual pain can have real paradoxical advantages when used in another way.
Ancient warning cues can become modern self-improvement prompts. For example,
top salespeople and performers are often outwardly extroverted, yet when you listen carefully, and ask the right questions, they are inwardly Socially Anxious. Their
exquisite sensitivity to the possibility of self-embarrassment allows them to achieve
excellence at managing the complex interactions of sales negotiations and audience
engagement. Counter-instinctive behavior, you could say.

SHOULD WE DO SOMETHING?

Modern treatment can modify the effects of these syndromes and social instincts.
So, we'll also look at treatment from an evolutionary perspective. Modern medication can relieve these syndromes, but does that affect a patient's social interactions
and career in a good way, a bad way, or both? Evolutionary perspective doesn't actually suggest some newfangled sort of psychotherapy, but it can explain (and maybe
enhance) those psychotherapeutic techniques that are already effective. Beer, as
a treatment, has been replaced by much safer, much more effective and far less tasty
alternatives.

A THEORY ABOUT THEORIES

This book is about the theory that common anxiety and depressive disorders are
descended from ancient social instincts. The theory offers an overarching view of
common syndromes, and a new synthesis of established mental-health knowledge. Occam's Razor dictates that we aim for the simplest possible explanations for

available data. We know what some of you may be thinking: This book has missing details, unsupported assumptions, overlooked studies, some notions that have gone astray, and that it isn't the last word. Moreover, you might point out, some of the research noted is recent and not yet replicated by other scientists. Scientific fact relies on compulsive and logical attention to all details. But, at the end of the day, there is far more than enough detail to propose and support this scientific model of evolved social instincts, and there are fascinating new questions to address.

Scientific theory draws on known facts to derive broader perspective and greater explanatory power. Albert Einstein said, "Logic will get you from A to B. Imagination will take you everywhere." When all is said and done, though, imagined theory must be supported by fact. As Richard Feynman (American physicist, 1918–1988) said: "It doesn't matter how beautiful your theory is, it doesn't matter how smart you are. If it doesn't agree with experiment, it's wrong." Feynman also pointed out that one test of a theory's accuracy is that it should be explainable in simply understood language ("Feynman's Razor" perhaps). We will follow his advice.

How can we test our theory of anxiety, depression and social instincts? One way to start is to look at what we already know about the syndromes and the instincts. Some parts of the theory are already described, and they are directly supported by at least some research. To test our theory, we should ask: Does this theory do a good job of explaining what we already know? Does it provide a better way to organize seemingly unconnected facts? These first questions are about reasonableness and "face validity." From there we ask: Does the theory lead to more research questions, or to better treatment? If that new research is done, then do the results continue to support the theory? New theories offer new answers, and many offer new questions. So, feel free to gauge the overall plausibility of this theoretical perspective.

SO ARE WE GOING TO LOOK AT SYNDROMES, OR AT SOCIAL INSTINCTS, OR WHAT?

How has each instinctive syndrome evolved with the development of *Homo sapiens* and of our human civilization? How do they resemble behavior in other species? How do they correspond to the five clinical syndromes? What do we know about their biology, genetics and epigenetics? Let's start with a look at six social instincts. Each one dates from our distant past, and each one corresponds to a distressing subtype of anxiety or depression, or worse.

Shall we begin?

PART ONE

Six Social Instincts and Five Usual Suspects

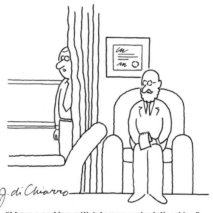

"I have a problem with interpersonal relationships."

"Though our conduct seems so very different from that of the higher animals, the primary [social] instincts are much alike in them and in us. The most evident difference springs from the important part which is played in man by a relatively strong power of imagination and by the capacity to think... [as] servants of the primary instincts."*
—Albert Einstein (German Physicist; 1879–1955)

* Commencement Address, Swarthmore College, 1938

2

DON'T STRAY FROM FAMILY, HOME, OR SAFETY: PANIC ANXIETY

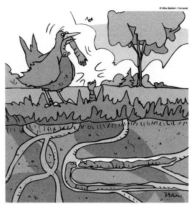

"He didn't want to go. Probably suffering from a little separation anxiety."

"We experience moments absolutely free from worry. These brief respites are called panic."
—Cullen Hightower (American author; 1923–2008)

"Offer them what they secretly want and they of course immediately become panic-stricken."
—Jack Kerouac (American novelist; 1922–1969)

THE SOCIAL INSTINCT

If we can't all stick together, then there is no one around to be social with. So maybe we should start with that most basic and urgent need of social animals to stay close enough together to be social. Let's not forget, there is safety in numbers, and comfort at home. Some instinct had better tell us when we stray too far from the fold. As it happens, that ancient separation alarm may trouble us today as Panic Anxiety.

BACK IN THE DAY: THE SYNDROME IN PRIMEVAL HUMAN SOCIETY

Case Study: How It Might Have Helped Long Ago

Once upon a time, a very very long time ago, there lived a little boy in a troop of humans on the African savanna. He wasn't much different from anyone else. When he was a baby, he stayed close to his mother. When she went off to grab some food or take some time off, he would notice pretty quickly. He was rather alarmed, actually. Where would he be without his mother to feed and protect him? With a surging activation of his nervous system, his heart would race, he would breathe faster, and he would be extra alert to his surroundings. Revving up his system was a good thing, for separation from Mom meant he was in real danger (Mom was more of a stay-near-home gatherer, but business-minded Dad was often away on hunting trips). It isn't likely that he thought to himself that he was in a Panic, but that's what someone looking at him would have seen.

More importantly, he called out as best he could, and soon cried out in a desperate tone for his mother. He probably wasn't aware of his purpose in crying out, but cry out he did, and she responded, time and again. Sometimes it took her a little longer than other times, but she knew she was needed, (and no doubt quite aware of that). Although it wasn't exactly the same, occasionally it was Dad or some other relative who would help comfort him. The troop worked together when separation Panic called. Everyone protected one another—especially when it came to protecting the kids. If they didn't, the troop would lose kids to lions, hyenas, dehydration, injury and who knows what else. Helping everyone stick together was a top priority.

Over time, our little boy became better at tolerating Mom's absences. He could play, be with others, and even be alone for a while. Not so scary anymore, no need to Panic if Mom went off somewhere. She would be back, and she would be there when needed. Meanwhile, there was much to learn about getting along, hunting, gathering, tools and so much else.

More than a decade later, though, there was a new problem. Now the boy wanted to move away from Mom, Dad, hearth and home. Maybe not far, maybe not even geographically away, but it was time to start thinking about setting up his own home, starting his own family, taking responsibility for his own food and hand-hewn gadgets. He was eager to be a man, and to have his own family, but this was an alarming concern. Had he learned to lead a zebra or wildebeest hunt? Could he manage without Mom and Dad and the others at his side? Would they be angry if he moved on? Would they ever let him come back? Some of these fears he could think about, but others merely passed through the back of his mind. And often, when these thoughts happened, he would have that startled, Panicky feeling again. His heart and breathing would race, and he'd think twice about leaving the safety of the nest.

When Lucy turned up, they were inseparable from the start. With her help and companionship he gradually gained the knowledge, confidence, calm and determination to start his own life and family. He pictured themselves in a hut by the river, with baobab trees and more mellow lives. Lucy and her guy, with strong minds. Panic? Not so much anymore.

BASIC PRINCIPLE: HOME IS WHERE THE HERD IS

In one way or another, Panic Anxiety is about not wanting to leave home and family. In primeval human society, Panic served as an alarm mechanism. It warned people not to wander too far from their mother or from the tribe, not to get trapped in caves, and not to unduly incur the wrath of authority or of the community (what we and the ancient Greeks called hubris). The tribal member who built the bigger cave might incur the envy and wrath of others. So, one or two Panicky feelings would warn him off his big plans. If only Icarus had Panic instead of hubris, he would have avoided flying so close to the sun that his wings melted away.

AMONG THE ANIMALS

Now, if these are actually evolved social instincts, then our animal relatives should have something similar going on, and they do.[1] For example, our ornery baboon friends probably know something about Panic, or at least about separation anxiety. When young baboons are separated from their mothers, or older ones are separated from the troop, they let out very specific "contact barks," as if to call for a reunion.[2] To human eyes, these separated baboons (and their mommies) can look pretty Panicky or even agitated when they can't quickly find their way back to each other. It is hard to know what baboons actually think, but it certainly seems like they have an instinctive way of keeping the family together.

Dogs are friendlier than your average baboon, and much closer at hand. When our own Bonnie was a young puppy, she wanted to have someone nearby at all times.

If no one was in sight, she let out quiet yips—contact yips, perhaps, until someone found her. Staying close was so important to her at first that she would only eat from her bowl while being held.

Some dog breeds are known as lap dogs, because, well, they like to just hang around in our laps. At least one dog expert has pointed out that Pomeranians (a lap dog par excellence), are also prone to separation anxiety. Maybe they like being with people, but then again maybe they are just trying to stop the angst of separation anxiety.[3] Dogs with separation anxiety tend to be calm and relaxed when they are in a room with their owners, but when their owner leaves they rise to the occasion and jump on the door.[4]

Of course there is another reason for any social animal to stick with the group. If you've ever seen movies of predatory animals, you know that lions, coyotes, wolves and the rest tend to attack the prey animals that stray from the group. Isolated animals are easier prey to catch—easier still if they are inexperienced, young, or slowed by age or illness—and they are less likely to be defended by their companions. Lions and their ilk know this. They work together to split off their target from the group, and then move in. This is another reason we humans feel instinctive Panic about separation from our group.

TIMES HAVE CHANGED

Well, so far so good—separation anxiety, Panic, and contact barks keep the family together and the lions at bay. How could that evolved instinct ever be a problem? Well, it becomes a problem when things change. We don't live the same lives as our primeval ancestors. Kids today go off to nursery school, and maybe off to college. Nowadays, we don't physically stick around like we used to. More symbolically, we don't feel bound to the same family success levels in sports, career, education, income, and who knows what else. Being on top of the world can be a terrifying height. So for some people, moving on from family triggers Panic and causes whole bunches of angst.

HOW INSTINCT BECOMES SYNDROME
IN MODERN HUMAN SOCIETY

Instinct and Worldview

What do Panicky thoughts tell us about this instinct? For one, they tell us to stick close to home. When people have an actual Panic Attack, they often want to flee from where they are, and get to someplace safer. That usually means home or the company of a trusted companion. However, they also tend to worry about catastrophic events. When our ancient ancestors strayed too far afield, they had to worry about getting physically trapped, cornered by predators, geographically lost, and dying if left on their own. Kind of like what Panic patients worry about—trapped in an airplane or elevator, lost in an open field or shopping mall, or dying in some catastrophic way. On the other hand, patients in Panic worry far less about modern-day dangers like electrical shocks, oncoming trucks or radiation hazards. Those aren't built-in ancient fears, nor are we protected from them by staying close to home. They are newer concerns that we must learn from others, or from painful experience.

In addition, we are faced today with amplified situations that our primeval ancestors never even imagined. Deirdre Barrett (American psychologist) calls these "Supernormal Stimuli"[5]—new kinds of real and symbolic separations (college away, planes, trains and automobiles) and entrapments. For someone instinctually afraid of straying too far from home, a thousand mile journey can be dramatic. For someone instinctually afraid of being trapped in a cave (or cornered by a predator), a thousand mile journey in the closed metal can of an airplane can be terrifying.

Case Study: Instinctive Syndromes in Modern Society

Not very long ago, there lived another little boy in a family of humans in a downtown Saõ Paulo apartment. He was a little cranky and a little clingy as an infant, but going to school was when bigger problems arose. He didn't want to go. When his Mom or Dad tried to drop him off at nursery school, he would hold desperately onto their legs. He would cry miserably. This would come on suddenly, with racing heart and great fear. He probably felt he was being abandoned (though who knows what impending catastrophe he thought about), and his parents felt like they were doing something dreadful, (and found themselves actually thinking so). They knew that school was the right thing, but the agony! One parent or the other would stay outside the classroom, and that would help a bit. Gradually his desperation lessened to the point that his parents could safely leave him there. Even so, the boy still felt a bit lonely, abandoned, anxious and even angry on the inside. Getting home at the end of the day was always a big relief.

This boy's life then moved along more quietly for more than a decade. He learned to get along with others, to read, to write, and to calculate, and to master the electronic gadgets that he loved so much. When he finished high school, he and some classmates went to a college many miles from home. He was eager for this more adult phase of his life, for the independence, challenge and accomplishment, and for the chance to meet new people. It was very exciting at first. However, after two months, he was miserable. He missed classes and stayed in his room. Actually, he was apprehensive even about leaving his room. Every time he tried, his system would suddenly remind him of his Panic. At least when he forced himself out for a party he could look forward to large quantities of alcohol to ease his fear. Classes and the library didn't offer that consolation. More and more he ate meals in his room. Although his frequent calls home let his parents know of his distress, he didn't mention any of the problems he had.

The semester did not go well. The boy failed his courses, dropped out of college, and moved back home with his parents. He panicked less there, but was dismayed at the turn of events, to say the least. His parents had been worried, and were relieved to have him safely at home. After some months of recuperation, and under pressure from his parents, he eventually found a job. After a few months it felt so stressful that he quit. Over time, he held on to jobs longer and longer, and even won promotions at one. After a few years, he found a steady girl, and was able to move into his own apartment, just down the road. The first thing he brought in was a supply of cachaça (Brazilian rum). He thought he was just drinking to celebrate his new home that night, but the cachaça also drowned out the Panic. It was those thoughts of independence, accomplishment and adulthood again. Could he make it on his own? Would it be okay with everyone if he did?

Working at his best job ever, he made some mistakes and started to have the old anxieties about not cutting the mustard. His girlfriend urged him get help before he quit. When vitamins didn't help, he tried capoeira (Brazilian martial arts), and drowned his anxiety at the bar. He even made some drinking buddies in the process. Things didn't work out, though. He'd sometimes sleep in, and sometimes take a drink to get himself to work. Eventually he lost that job too, along with his pickup truck and even his girl. He joked at the bar that he was just living out the standard storyline of American country music. Inside, though, he couldn't figure out what went wrong.

Maybe If Things Had Been Different...

When the vitamin and exercise treatments didn't help (and with good cachaça costing what it does), his girlfriend made him see the psychiatrist who had helped her cousin. On the right medication (imipramine, a tricyclic antidepressant), the Panics stopped, and the anxiety diminished enough that he didn't quit after all. With much persuasion, he stopped drinking and went to Alcoholics Anonymous (AA). Talking things through, this man eventually realized that the reason he wasn't doing well enough was because of his Panic and anxiety, rather than the other way around. Much later, he started to understand how much his aspirations frightened him, how much he thought manhood meant leaving the fold, and how much he feared the envy of others.

After a while, with a pay raise in hand, he married and settled down. Some years later, still at the same job, the Panics and the pattern started again. This time he could tell when he panicked, and his wife sent him back for help. Solutions came quite quickly this time. He never fully understood exactly what the medication and therapy did, but life did seem to go better.

HOW DOES THAT MAKE YOU FEEL?

Panic Anxiety doesn't feel good. It is the raw primal sensation of your instincts telling you painfully that you are straying dangerously far from the nest. It makes you think that some catastrophe is about to happen, if it hasn't started already. It is an overwhelming sensation of, well, Panic. The evolutionary advantage of this is that you know there is some urgent imperative to do something fast. Our ancestors wouldn't want to find themselves separated from the tribe, where they might be on their own and exposed to all sorts of dangers. The sudden and intense symptoms get that message across clearly. When we have recurring Panic Attacks, though, we do get a bit used to them. They still affect us, but they may seem milder, more ordinary or less urgent. Sometimes they get to the point where people hardly notice them.

Being human, we try to ignore the warnings of this instinctual Panic signal. Don't get on an airplane? How silly, planes don't crash (much). However, our instincts don't understand reason—they are more responsive to concerns about traveling far from the home nest, or of being trapped in that small metal box. So, our human reason can lead us to longer, more frequent, or more intense Panic when we do get on that plane. Panic also causes another anxiety. "Anticipatory anxiety" is really worry about when the next Panic will happen, and just one Panic can be enough to start that off. It is a warning to avoid thoughts and situations that might trigger Panic, and, while heightened worry makes us more aware of dangers generally, it can also focus our attention in the wrong direction. That leaves us at home instead of on a flight to a warm sunny beach resort somewhere.

WHAT THIS SYNDROME IS

How long have we known about Panic Anxiety? There are actually two Old Testament mentions of sudden fear. Proverbs 3:25–26 (King James Version) says, "Be not afraid of sudden fear, neither of the desolation of the wicked, when it comes. For the LORD shall be thy confidence, and shall keep thy foot from being taken." Job 22:10 also says, "Therefore snares are round about thee, and sudden fear troubleth thee." Both mentions link the sudden fear of Panic to the risk of being trapped in place. This is not too different from those who fear being trapped in airplanes, elevators, and enclosed CAT scans. Indeed, Panic can be of biblical proportions.

The modern history of Panic Disorder is usually dated to Jacob Mendes Da Costa's 1871 description of "soldier's heart" afflicting soldiers in the American Civil War. In 1894, Freud labeled similar symptoms as "anxiety neurosis." Although a topic of ongoing interest, the next major advance was not until 1964, when Donald Klein (American psychiatrist, 1928–) published research showing that Panic Anxiety responds to different medication (tricyclic antidepressants) than other anxiety, and thus must be a separate disease entity.[6] This research logic has come to be known as "pharmacologic dissection." In 1980, the official *DSM-III* diagnostic manual formalized diagnostic criteria for Panic. Even then, it was sometime before Panic Anxiety even began to be widely diagnosed and treated.

Panic Disorder may be the most common, if often unrecognized, syndrome in clinical practice, and frequently occurs together with other syndromes. Panic Attacks are not just an extreme version of ordinary anxiety: They are a special kind of anxiety, and only some people are even physically capable of having one. In addition to its physical symptoms (racing heart, shortness of breath, chest pain and dizziness are just some examples), the abrupt onset of Panic Anxiety is often associated with thoughts of catastrophe (syndrome details are in the appendix). So, people with Panic Disorder instinctively avoid situations that they associate with catastrophe—that ancient alarm mechanism for situations that seem dangerous.

Phobias of flying, driving, leaving the house, and closed spaces are a few modern examples. Most of these phobias have to do with staying close to home, access to home, or at least not feeling trapped somewhere else. Then there are folks who are afraid of being trapped in small spaces, or lost on the trackless wide open spaces. Back in the old days, both of these would present a risk of being separated from the hearth and home, facing the difficult task of fending for oneself, or maybe subject to the unwanted attentions of any predator who might be nearby. Either way, Panic is a reminder to get back to the safety of the home and tribe.

Panic Attacks often seem to come out of the blue, for no apparent reason. Here, too, if you look carefully enough, there are often environmental cues or passing thoughts that may actually trigger the Panics. One study even suggests that there are subtle changes in heart rate and respiration that precede out-of-the-blue Panics by as long as 10–60 minutes.[7]

Some of those passing thoughts may be related to fears of emotional intimacy or of societal advancement. Even though these are sought-after goals, they can leave some people feeling trapped, exposed to danger, or isolated from the group. Working in a graduate-school mental-health service many years ago, the director pointed out that most of the students who turned up would ask for help in dealing with their fear of impending utter failure in graduate school. Not only that, but they would likely be at the top of their programs, and on the verge of some yet vaster accomplishment. Sure enough, that story fit nearly everyone, and most of them had Panic Anxiety triggered by their anticipated successes. How to deal with that anxiety? It felt safer to them to think of themselves as mere failures. Because this could be readily figured out and treated, they all stayed in school, and some of them have gone on to do things wonderful enough to turn up in the news.

Panic is an alert about where the limits of safety are for all sorts of risks. How successful can we safely be in career and in emotional life? How far away can we travel; how separated from our loved ones? It is important to remember that not everyone is even able to have a Panic Attack. Depending on which study you read, the rate of full Panic Disorder as 1–5% of the population.[8] If you look at the looser category of everyone who has ever had one Panic Attack, then that number is about 22%[8] (about 15% in our own data on employed people[9]). Considering the angst and disruption of Panic, how come evolution left even that many of us afflicted? This minority may be the only people who are even biologically able to have a Panic Attack. That leaves most adults not panicking even when faced with plane rides, stuck elevators, or crowded stores. Panic causes phobias, and *agoraphobia* translates from the Greek as "fear of the market." Later on, we'll also look at whether increased Panic in some adults has newer advantages for individuals and for societies. So then, if you think about the essential advantages of Panic, how come it isn't even more common?

Most people with Panic Disorder don't realize at first that they are having Panic Attacks. Instead, they think that they are trapped, or in danger, or that they are miserably angst ridden in some nonspecific way. That's only natural, of course, because, although people are prompted by the instinctive biological message, they are not consciously aware of what that message is about. Instincts are like that. Once people understand the symptoms, though, they can recognize Panic Attacks. This usually happens after a diagnosis is made, or by learning about the syndrome through reading or television.

Early on, our ancestors developed innate fears of spiders, snakes, and heights, and stayed away from them. Some people today Panic at even seeing photos of those dangers. We call that a simple phobia. It stands to reason that our ancestors didn't want to be bitten, and they didn't want to fall down. Monkeys and crows, to give two other examples, also have reactions to a few particular dangers and distinct vocal calls for each one. For example, monkeys react to snakes, eagles, and lions, and each reaction pattern is different and specific. They jump into a tree for snakes and look up to spot eagles. Are these some sorts of ingrained monkey phobias linked to self-protective behaviors? They haven't told us yet, but you have to wonder. The impending catastrophes that trigger most human Panic are not about specific dangers—they are about issues of real and symbolic separation, abandonment and loss, which expose people to other dangers.

Our beta dog Cassidy, left by his lonesome in the house, would get frantic and Panicky at the sound of dangerous rainstorms and thunder (he didn't actually tell us this, but it was written all over his face when we arrived home). Over the course of a few storms, he actually managed to dig his way through a hollow door into a closed room, though this did not really get him very far. When a solid new door was put in, he learned to turn the round doorknob, despite his lack of opposable thumbs. He needed to escape into a larger space no matter what. Ever seen someone run desperately out of a restaurant, classroom or movie?

When people have Panic Anxiety, (and sometimes after just one attack) they can stay nervous most of the time. This "Anticipatory anxiety" used to be known as "free floating anxiety," but is actually a state of readiness for the next Panic Attack. For some people, the ongoing anxiety is more distressing than the Panics themselves. Curiously, this Anticipatory anxiety can also be counter-productive in other ways. In an Australian study, researchers wanted to figure out how to prevent falls in the elderly. It turned out that the presence of a fear of falling or of anxiety were better predictors of actually falling down than was a standard physical limitations assessment. Fear of falling led to severe anxiety and more falls, even in people with no physical risk. Actually, since Panic is associated with very real changes in balance, the anxious elderly might also have another physical fall risk that doesn't show up on standard screening methods.[10]

WORST CASE SCENARIO

At the clinical extreme, Panic Disorder leads to agoraphobia—people who try not to leave their homes at all. People have less Panic at home, but what a price to pay.

This doesn't always mean that they have more frequent or more severe Panics, but it does mean that they have a more pronounced self-protective response. Agoraphobia without Panic is somewhere between rare and nonexistent. Most people don't usually notice when someone else is having a Panic Attack (except maybe in the movies). Intimates, at least, sometimes do sense the intense distress, and respond by trying to reassure the Panicky person that he or she is safe and not alone. Even agoraphobics can leave home with a close companion, if their instincts are calmed by that "phobic partner." We all know couples, relatives and friendly companions who seem to be "attached at the hip," and for some of them, fear of Panic Anxiety is the glue that holds them together. That brings us back to lap dogs, those canine companions that stay especially close to us.

Perhaps the two most symptomatically severe cases of Panic Anxiety ever to arrive in the psychiatric office were successful men, newly promoted in the midst of corporate layoffs that left them with many newly unemployed friends. It was nice to have a better job and a raise, but awful to see the suffering of friends and to be afraid of their envy and anger. Catastrophic envy and abandonment could lie ahead.

There may also be another kind of severe Panic. Agitated Depression is, as it sounds, a syndrome of severe unhappiness, anxiety, pacing, and restlessness. There is often a history of Panic Anxiety, and these episodes are highly prolonged Panic Attacks, lasting for days or weeks at a time, rather than for only minutes.[11]

SUBTLE AND CLOAKED SYNDROMES

Some people have only very mild or infrequent Panics, but the effects can be very much the same:—Anticipatory anxiety, work impairment and disability, and relationship problems.[12] Panic can turn up in so many different ways that it has been called the "Great Imposter" of modern medical practice (the "Great Imposter" of long ago was syphilis). Chest pain, dizziness, seizures, asthma, anxiety, Mania and depression are just a few common medical misdiagnoses for Panic, although all of these can also occur together with Panic Disorder.[13] Less well studied are Panic subtypes that have a different look. There are "nonfear" Panics that mimic the chest pain of heart disease.[14] Maurizio Fava (Italian psychiatrist) has described anger attacks that seem like Panic, but with an added feeling of inner rage. What is with that? Well, for some people, in some situations, it may have been adaptive to face danger with head-on attack. Either fight your way back into the tribe or be ready to fight off the predators outside. Because Panic is part of how we process social interactions, it isn't surprising that some people Panic in their dreams. These nocturnal Panics wake them from sleep feeling startled, terrified, or sweaty.

Post Traumatic Stress Disorder (PTSD) is often a form of Panic Anxiety.[15] If a Panic Attack occurs during or soon after a traumatic event, it intensifies memory of the circumstances. You Panic when you can't find your way home or when you witness a horror, and you also learn not to end up in that situation again. Post Traumatic Stress Disorder occurs when those intensified memories get out of control as a result of ongoing Panics. This could be studied by looking at the effects of induced Panic just after laboratory memory formation (to coincide with the process of transforming new memory into biological form), and then testing recall later, both during induced Panic and also while at rest.

WHAT THE SYNDROME ISN'T

It is important to remember that fear, anxiety, and Panic are all different things (we'll get to some biology later on). It is fear (and the "fight or flight response") that protected people who were face-to-face with lions and other predators then and now. If someone today (with or without Panic Disorder) were in front of a bus that was bearing down on them, they'd probably be terrified (and that would be a very good thing). They might even be anxious later on about when they'd next have to confront an oncoming bus. However, for those people with Panic Disorder, Panic Attacks don't actually happen when a dangerous oncoming bus looms ever closer. Instead, they might suddenly occur while they are sitting inside a perfectly safe and comfortable bus, and traveling in that closed box to somewhere far away from home.

People can have intense fear or intense anxiety that has nothing to do with Panic, and everyone feels at least some fear or anxiety sometimes. The "fight-or-flight" reaction is one example. It happens to everyone, and is not at all about separation or Panic Anxiety. It is about what to do if you encounter a hungry mountain lion looking for lunch (actually, look it in the eye, try to seem as large and imposing as you can, and back away slowly), or a turf- or cub-conscious bear (look down, look small, and back away slowly) or an angry hamster (fight it off, but gently).

THE AGES OF PANIC ANGST

Separation anxiety in young children seems pretty logical at first glance. Why leave parents behind for the uncertainties and dangers of nursery school? But then how come only some children have it? It is partly genetic, and it is a little bit environmental. However, it is not only having Mom (or Dad) around that reduces early separation anxiety, it is also about those casomorphins (natural opiates) from Mom's breast milk. We also know this from experimental work with baby chickens.[16] A little casomorphin to ease the pain, and those baby chickens don't complain so much about separation. Feel good, feel close, feel less Panicky.

Early separation anxiety predicts Panic Disorder later on and maybe other problems as well. Panic usually reappears in late adolescence, often triggered by the physical separation of leaving home for college, and the emotional separation of becoming an adult (or trying to, anyway). The same biological social instinct kicks in its painful warning at two different stages of life. In some people, it is an ongoing problem. Maybe we humans have somehow evolved with a form of childhood separation anxiety that persists through adulthood ("behavioral neoteny"), and maybe that's because angst can have its advantages.

There is at least one more particular time for increased Panic. A new mother needs to take special care of her infant—if it crawled away all sorts of bad things could happen. Sure enough, Panic Disorder gets worse in women after childbirth, just when they need to keep track of the little one.[17] When new mothers today have an exaggerated Panic response, this is a mixed blessing for the child: He or she is less likely to get lost, but Mom is a bit too distracted by her Panic and anxiety. Sometimes, the postpartum Panic can intensify to the point that it looks like what we now call postpartum depression.[18,19,20] So, we have come full circle to the other side of infancy and the importance of Mom feeling close to her newborn child.[21] Mothers who Panic after delivery may keep that baby close by and safe.

HOLDING US BACK

Alas, people with Panic Disorder tend to be less successful in society.[22] For one thing, many unwittingly avoid career and social advancements that might trigger Panic—their instincts tell them to stop. It is hard to go to school if your instincts say no, and harder still if school is far away. It is hard to move up the economic ladder if your instincts tell you to stay within your family's socioeconomic tribe. One patient had a first onset of Panic in middle age, triggered by a happy promotion from a blue-collar to a white-collar job. It wasn't that he couldn't do it; the pay increase wasn't all that much and otherwise he was doing just fine. He just had the unwitting notion that his family expected blue-collar jobs, and taking an office job felt like he was breaking ranks. In our own studies of corporate employees, the rate of Panic Disorder is over 50% in the bottom-most rank of employees; it steadily decreases with each step up the corporate totem pole, and is near zero among the highest-ranking employees.[9]

Lack of assertiveness is a common trait among the Panic-prone,[23] and they may be held back by the non-specific emotional disruptions of their Panic symptoms. Panic Attacks are painful, but the "Anticipatory anxiety," can also be crippling, and sometimes more intense than the Panic Attacks themselves. People with "nervous breakdowns" often have a combination of Panic and Anticipatory anxiety. It gets worse. Panic also puts people at higher risk for serious depressions and many other emotional problems. As the life problems and emotional symptoms pile up, it is hard to get ahead. On the silver lining side, Panic may be especially common in creative people, and may even feed that creativity (see chapter 9). Both Charles Darwin and Sigmund Freud wrote about their own anxiety symptoms, and both may have had Panic Disorder themselves.

THE INSTINCT IS WITH US STILL

So does this particular social instinct still serve its original purpose today? All of us have at least some sense of the need to stay close to home and following society's rules. All of us have some awareness of the literal and symbolic dangers of straying from the nest, of being trapped and of being alone. No man (or woman) is an island. Many of us get a bit nervous going off to college, getting married, or trapped in a stuck elevator. However, only some people have actual Panic. To the extent that those folks follow the instinctive Panic message, Panic may help them stay closer to home, help keep family groups together, but keep a lower profile in love and work (Freud's two life essentials). However, it pans out differently for different people.

Romance

So if Panic is about keeping the tribe together, then how come it can interfere with basic stuff like romantic closeness and sex? There are some people who avoid sex (and serious relationships) because it makes them Panic.[24] Remember how some people Panic about leaving the family nest? Well, finding a romantic partner is a symbolic and very real way of feeling adult. Sex, of course, is part of that, at least in theory. Marriage is less common among those with Panic Anxiety.[25]

People with Panic Anxiety do get married anyway, although it can take many years for some to get up the nerve to endure the Panic. Most don't think of it as Panic Anxiety about closeness. They just think it took a long time to find the right partner, or to accept that a perfect mate didn't actually exist. When they do settle down, the Panic persists, and this can affect their relationship in a bad way. In fact, the more anxiety a partner has, the lower the level of emotional closeness in the relationship.[26]

That presents a dilemma. A stable relationship is reassuring, but stability without closeness is disturbing. Alas, many people with Panic Anxiety end up feeling trapped in this kind of claustrophobic relationship. They think of it in terms of real relationship problems and real lack of closeness. They look for useful solutions (more date nights, more flowers, more communication attempts), but they can't easily recognize the roles of their own Panic, phobia, and emotional distancing.

On the other hand, there are some couples who are able to feel so close to each other that it feels almost like home. These "phobic partners" have a reassuring effect on each other that keeps Panic at a minimum, and makes the couple want to spend as much time together as possible. Somehow, they have found relationships that don't feel too close, or that don't feel too adult.

Workplace

Panic is no picnic at work either.[27] People with higher anxiety levels (and mostly that would be Panic related), tend to perform less well at work, and are less likely to be promoted.[28] This isn't surprising, because anxiety can interfere with concentration, motivation and more. However, there is also our evolutionary angst perspective. In the workplace, that instinct to stay close to home is reinforced by Panic Attacks, and wreaks havoc on a job performance and career advancement. Doing too well would again run the risk of feeling isolated from home, and raise fears of catastrophe. Remember the heights reached by Icarus? Some people Panic about work altogether, and just stay home instead.[29] The workplace makes them want to go home to Mom. Okay, maybe there is a little of that in all of us, but with all that anxiety about work, people with Panic Anxiety have significantly lower average incomes.[25]

SYNDROME AND SOCIAL STIGMA

If someone Panics, other people usually don't notice. At least they don't think about it. However, they often feel a little bothered by people with serious anxiety, and a bit put off as a result. When they do think consciously about people whose life paths have been diminished by Panic, they respond to the struggles and failures. On the one hand, those people can be looked at as unmotivated, confused, or underachieving. On the other hand, they can be seen as lost souls in need of help and care. Either way, their career, social and emotional statuses are major parts of how they are seen, often with pessimism and concern about their prospects and character.

That is what we call stigma. Stigma may also derive from an intuitive notion that other people's adult Panic is a natural social instinct, and not to be messed with. Their own instincts silently tell them "Well, maybe they *should* just go home if they feel that way."

INSTINCT AND SYNDROME TURN UP IN CULTURE

So how does Panic Anxiety play out in human culture? For one thing, people are well aware when someone is seriously anxious, even if they don't know about any Panic Anxiety that lies beneath. Most people, most of the time, will see anxiety as a kind of call for help in a friend or relative. They offer comfort and do try to point out when there is rather little real danger about. The anxiety ridden are encouraged to ignore "irrational" anxiety in making decisions, and "tough it out." Being consciously aware of anxiety (and Panic) does indeed help, but the problems are not all solved.

Then there is self-medication. Too much alcohol is one approach, and other street drugs can also take the edge off. These days some people buy illegal clonazepam (a Valium-class benzodiazepine) on the street because it helps them, (even though it doesn't cause much of a high). However, without the right psychotherapy, guidance and dosing it doesn't work right and can cause some real problems.

There are more practical accommodations as well. Airline staffs are trained to handle the flying phobic. Some people are phobic about the enclosed spaces of an MRI scanner (magnetic resonance imaging), so now there are "open MRI" machines that feel more comfortable. For those so agoraphobic as to fear leaving home at all, there is home delivery of almost everything, and even the possibility of working from home by Internet and phone.

The thematic concerns of Panic Disorder play out in societal concerns as well. Catastrophe awaits if you stray from home, so attention to potential catastrophe can be primed by Panic Anxiety. Those who are overly alert to catastrophe play a vital role for society. As Walter Wriston (American banker and Citibank chairman, 1919–2005) pointed out, "The Doomsayers have always had their uses, since they trigger the coping mechanism that often prevents the events they forecast." If only the mortgage bankers had listened to the doomsayers before the Great Recession began.

Sometimes, however, the doomsayers have exaggerated concerns about issues of little real risk or little potential impact. That can be a distraction from more serious or pressing issues, but it can be very hard to know which catastrophes are really upon us and which are really not. Most likely, the end of the world is not at hand. The band R.E.M. made fun of these concerns in a song. The lyrics list an impressive collection of catastrophe theories, but while the title points out sarcastically that: "It's the end of the world as we know it," the chorus chimes in that everything is actually okay.

Separation from home and loved ones can certainly give you the catastrophe blues. Stevie Ray Vaughn (American bluesman; 1954–1990) sang in his classic "Texas Flood" about dark clouds and floods occurring when separated from his lover and home. No problem, just be reassured that "Well—back home are no floods or tornados. Baby—and the sun shines every day."

Panic afflicts people's lives, but at least in a democracy, even those limited by their angst get the vote, and they are equal under the law. They are also encouraged to leave the nest, go to college, succeed at love and work, and even to do better than their parents. This is good advice, but can worsen Panic Anxiety in those who have it. To their dismay, their comfort zone is home. There is a whole style of movies that grab our attention because they capture this conflict. Horror movies prime our underlying fears before springing a terrifying image on us. In teen slasher movies, the evil doer inevitably pounces just as the movie approaches an erotic peak. Yikes! Those adult desires can trigger terrifying fears in the teen audience.

TURN THE SYNDROME AROUND: ADVANTAGES OF COUNTER-INSTINCTIVE BEHAVIOR

Case Study: Counter-Instinctive Behavior

Not very long ago, there was a little girl who lived in a family of humans in a rural Scottish town. When the time came, she went bravely to nursery school, and there wasn't any problem. When she went to college, she rarely called home at all. Moving away from home was something to tough out by her lonesome. Her stoic response to anxiety and Panic was both a blessing and a curse. No matter how bad she felt, she just gritted her teeth, and put her nose to the grindstone. She was well known as a grind (we can safely think of this as a pun) in her smallish social circle, but she did make all of her classes and did very well in her economics courses. Some of the worst Panics were during public presentations, so she minored in drama, and plunged ahead. Few suspected how she felt inside, and she tried not to think about it herself, trapped onstage in front of all those people.

Naturally, her inclination after graduation was to overcome the performance Panic that had so long plagued her. Acting school, auditions, and small parts led her to larger parts and paying work. She never understood how no one saw the Panic that so often welled up inside her on stage, and why the Panic Attacks still continued despite her experience. Actually, the more experience and success she had, the longer the on-stage Panics became. One- or 2-minute episodes in college were often 10 or 15 minutes now. However, the money was enough, the reviews were great, and the waitressing job went by the wayside. Her biggest concern was that she would forget her lines completely during a Panic.

During the Edinburgh Fringe Festival one day, the theater lights went out. She froze just like everyone else, but she alone had the presence of mind to run off the stage and check the master circuit breaker and turn the lights back on. Running back on stage, she picked up her lines, and even threw in a quip in character about the brief blackout. Afterwards, she was flabbergasted to realize that she hadn't panicked. Her worst fear had come true, and yet there was no anxiety at all!

Now with Angus as her first serious boyfriend and the possibility of a major film role, she was overwhelmed by Panic. "Damn the torpedoes, full speed ahead" she gamely reminded herself, but press on she could not. She holed up in her apartment, twirling her hair as she paced back and forth for hours and thought about her impending failures. The film role fell through, Angus became frustrated by the fighting, and it took her months to recover herself. Eventually, she got back on her feet and resumed her success on stage. Creative people are known for their angst, so the episode was even a useful credential.

Maybe If Things Had Been Different...

While pacing in her apartment, she somehow remembered the theater blackout and her lack of Panic then. So, maybe there was another explanation. The good news was that she had had a rewardingly successful and creative career, but the bad news was that the emotional pain was only getting worse. She went for psychiatric help, and clonazepam every 12 hours soon relieved her Panic and agitation. Only then did she realize how long she had been enduring Panic and anxiety, and how she had focused her life on her attempts to overcome it. Continuing in psychotherapy, the Panic was gone, and a new romance began. She talked her way back into the film role, which led to more, and more varied, opportunities. Even in cloudy Scotland, the sun can shine every day.

SOCIAL ALARMS PROMPT SELF-IMPROVEMENT

We humans have an advantage over the other animals. We are much more able to use our reason and Consciousness to make decisions that conflict with our instincts. Other species would know enough to overcome their fear if they have to jump from the second story window of a burning building, but not many would respond to the separation alarm of Panic by actually increasing their separation. Some of us can do that, but why do we? For one thing, our reason tells us that going to our jobs and having close relationships are actually good things, so we try to ignore whatever Panic and phobia we might feel. This might actually make the distress continue and even intensify, but some of us just try harder to cope.

Some people take that another step further. If they sense Panic, they see a chance for challenge and self-improvement. As one patient put it, "skiing terrifies me, so I go for the steepest runs to get past that fear." Or as one woman eventually noted, "I chose you for my treatment because I panic at the thought of men, and you are a man." Both of these highly successful people used this same kind of "counter-instinctive" approach to their careers as well. One of them achieved success by consoling a string of scary (but needy) clients. Looking around, counter-instinctive reactions to Panic are pretty common among extreme sports fans. Although there aren't good studies, the literature on scuba diving, for example, suggests that Panic is a major concern. Some people just dive right in to their claustrophobia.

This sort of counter-instinctive response can be very helpful. It leads Panicky people to become popular performers, attentive airline pilots, skillful skiers, and creative creatures. As the horror filmmaker Alfred Hitchcock (English director and producer, 1899–1980) said, "The only way to get rid of my fears is to make films about them."

UNINTENDED CONSEQUENCES

There are many downsides to counter-instinctive behavior, of course, not the least of which is ongoing anxiety, stress, and less-than-fulfilling relationships. In addition, this approach drives people toward choices that they fear most. Maybe the skier would rather be lying on a beach. Maybe the stage performer would have done well as the economist she first thought to be. And maybe, as we will see later, there are untoward effects on our health.

WHERE DOES THIS COME FROM, ANYWAY?

The Genetic Root of All Instinct

If Panic is an evolutionary adaptation, is it genetic? Well, yes and maybe. Panic Disorder clearly runs in families, and studies do suggest that it is an inherited tendency. However, years of research have yet to identify a "smoking gene" specifically responsible for its causation. Instead, there is probably a complex web of interacting genes underlying Panic Anxiety, just as there might be for such other complex behavioral instincts as smiling or sneezing.[30]

Gene/Environment Interactions

Whatever the underlying mechanisms are, not everyone with the genetic tendency (the "genotype," to be technical) gets Panic Disorder (that would be the "phenotype").

Environment and early development play a role in determining who actually Panics. In fact, studies in Italy, Norway and the United States suggest that factors such as early loss of a parent are important determinants of later Panic Disorder, but only have about 10% as much effect as do genetic factors.[31,32,33,34] Childhood maltreatment is another factor that increases risk of later Panic Anxiety.[35]

How can environmental factors work their magic? One way they might increase or decrease the effects of genetic factors would be by altering other biological systems that influence Panic. For example, there are laboratory techniques that use natural chemicals to trigger Panic Anxiety in people with Panic Disorder. However, if you try to chemically trigger Panic Anxiety in subjects who do not Panic on their own, nothing happens; they do not Panic. But, if you first give these Panic-free subjects medicine that blocks the effects of opiates (which include natural morphine, synthetic codeine, and the endorphins and breast milk casomorphins that are homemade in our own bodies), then they do have respiratory changes that vaguely resemble Panic.[36,37] So maybe people who lose a parent in childhood have a reduction in the amount of naturally occurring opiates ("endorphins") they make later on, and are, therefore, at even greater Panic risk if they already have the genes for Panic Anxiety. This could also be a matter of "epigenetics." Basically, some genes in our DNA are activated and deactivated by methyl groups that latch on to the DNA. In addition to the presence or absence of Panic genes, it could be that parental loss triggers a process that turns those genes on or off. If only we could figure out a way to turn off the Panic switch, or prevent it from ever being turned on.

The Primeval Origin of Instinct

Donald Klein has suggested that Panic may have started out as a "false suffocation alarm" that warned individuals about reduced amounts of the oxygen we breathe in, or excessive accumulation of the carbon dioxide we breathe out.[38] We know that breathing high-concentration carbon dioxide is one way to set off Panic in susceptible people. This sort of alarm could also be useful in a small crowded cave (especially in one with a campfire), underwater, in a forest fire, or if Mom accidentally rolled over on her infant kids—all situations in which carbon dioxide can increase to dangerous levels while vital oxygen disappears. From that original biological alarm mechanism, Panic evolved to provide yet other warnings of impending catastrophe. No doubt this mechanism existed long before our ancestors looked even vaguely mammalian. Of course, it is also possible that the same primeval instinct for staying close to Mom also helps in sensing dangers, even in primitive creatures.

Inner Workings

There are many known chemical triggers for Panic, including carbon dioxide (which we produce and exhale), sodium lactate (which naturally increases with exercise), and something called cholecystokinin (CCK, which helps digestion). It turns out that any of these can chemically trigger Panic —it occurs about two thirds of the time when you study volunteer Panic patients. However, when you use the same "challenge tests" in normal control subjects, virtually none of them Panic. All this is not nearly as ghoulish as it might sound. These tests are useful for many reasons. They let scientists look at the physiology and biology of Panic, hint at underlying mechanisms, demonstrate the beneficial effects of antipanic medications, provide more accurate research diagnosis of Panic (including of those with subtle symptoms), and much more.

Challenge tests may also help explore a common biology between human syndrome and animal instinct. There is already a suggestion that a lactate challenge can be used to trigger Fido's separation anxiety.[39] Something similar happens in laboratory mice. If they are taken at one day of age from their natural mothers and then raised by mice foster mothers, they are more sensitive to the effects of increased carbon dioxide,[40] Maybe someday, these tests will even be used to help human clinical diagnosis.

HOW TO FIX IT: EVOLUTIONARY PERSPECTIVE EXPLAINS MODERN TREATMENT

Coping and Self-Improvement

Well, if someone is stuck with Panic Anxiety, what can they do? Many people learn to endure. Over time, they just get used to the Panics, although the direct distress and indirect effects never go away. They are also at greater risk for serious depression, suicide and heart disease. Meanwhile, they often suffer serious consequences for their personal and work lives. Some people, as we saw in the case of the actress, take a more active approach, and deliberately learn to conquer their Panic and phobias. Having trusted people to talk to and family, social, and religious resources for support and guidance also helps coping. Some turn to alcohol,[41] but the benefits are far outweighed by the risks. Until very recently that was about all there was.

Evolved Treatment

Modern treatment typically includes antipanic medications. The selective serotonin reuptake inhibitor antidepressants (SSRIs) are often used, and they may work through a nonspecific enhancement of social closeness or a feeling of well-being. The more socially close you feel, the less historical evolutionary need you have to Panic about becoming an adult or about venturing out for a short trip to the store. The family and tribe will still want you around. Indeed, people with genetically higher serotonin levels not only feel a greater closeness, but they are less likely to respond to a Panic challenge.[42]

Serotonin-induced closeness is helpful, but SSRIs are not always fully effective for Panic. Some Panic often continues, though of diminished intensity and frequency. Not surprisingly, SSRI treatment only reduces Panic induced by Panic challenge tests; it doesn't completely prevent it.[43,44] In addition, there is often tolerance to SSRI benefits over time.[45] Panic often get somewhat worse after 6–12 months on SSRIs. Ever heard how depression treatment can fade into "Prozac Poop-Out?" This is often the re-emergence of Panic symptoms that were never properly diagnosed at the start.

The tricyclic antidepressants can be fully effective for Panic, though they are more likely to have uncomfortable side effects. Not surprisingly, treatment with these medicines will prevent challenge-test-induced Panic.[46] Anxiety, in general, is regulated by a neurotransmitter called gamma-amino-butyric acid ("GABA"). Benzodiazepine class drugs (such as diazepam, brand named Valium) reduce ordinary anxiety and work by increasing GABA activity. Although most of the benzodiazepines treat ordinary anxiety, they do not treat Panic Anxiety. For example, when you give diazepam before a challenge test, Panic still happens.[47] However, there are two benzodiazepines (clonazepam and alprazolam; brand names Klonopin and Xanax) that can be fully effective for Panic. Maybe these two have more effect on certain GABA sub-systems (just as with the serotonin neurotransmitter system, we are only now learning the complexities of the GABA system). Sure enough, if alprazolam or clonazepam are given before a challenge test, there is a major reduction in induced Panic, even with doses that are too low.[48] There is something unique in our evolutionary history about the biology of Panic Anxiety, and these two medications seem to find it. Indeed, some work suggests that clonazepam may be more effective and less problematic than some other medications for Panic.[49]

Medications work best when they prevent Panic from happening. Once Panic Attacks do happen, they are not only upsetting but they also feed ongoing ordinary anxiety levels and make it harder to overcome phobias of all kinds. Taking any kind of benzodiazepine only as needed after a Panic starts is not a great idea. For one thing, that Panic will likely be over before the medicine even starts to work.

All the medications work better when they are combined with formal psychotherapy. Real psychotherapy is a deliberate process; it is not just hand-holding or friendliness. Therapy focuses on relief of phobias, as well as on issues of real and symbolic separation anxiety in relationships and unwarranted fears that success has adverse consequences. Unwinding instinctive and learned fears and self-protections ("defenses") from the back of your mind is a modern variation of a "psychoanalytic" process. Not surprisingly, controlled research show that this kind of therapy used alone is helpful for Panic patients in many ways, even though Panic may not stop completely without medication.[50] Understanding the evolutionary role of Panic helps guide psychotherapy toward understanding that catastrophic fears may come from ancient dangers. It may even be helpful to remind patients that there is usually little physical danger today in leaving home, and that the emotional fear of symbolically leaving home by acting more adult is a solvable problem.

Cognitive behavior therapy (CBT) has become increasingly popular for treatment of Panic Disorder. While many studies show that it is clearly helpful, it may be helpful in a different way. Cognitive behavior therapy involves helping patients adjust their thoughts ("cognitions") and behaviors (such as phobias). For Panic, they learn that catastrophic events are not actually at hand, that there is no actual reason for Panic, that the physical symptoms of Panic are sensations of little importance, and that buses are perfectly safe (though late at times). In other words, they learn to better cope with Panic symptoms. However, this doesn't mean the Panics end.

Looking to challenge tests again, we find that although CBT reduces the odds that someone will report Panic in response to a Panic challenge, it doesn't actually have much effect on the biological evidence for Panic.[51] So maybe CBT teaches people to believe they are not panicking, even when they are. It is a bit like those counter-instinctive folks, who have their own internal CBT approach to life. Before there was any other treatment, people had to cope as best they could, (or else just stay phobically at home). Coping is better than not coping, but better still not to have any Panic that needs to be ignored. Not only that, but ongoing Panic may cause other emotional, relationship, and physical problems. Cognitive behavior therapy and relationship psychotherapies work best when combined with the right medications.

FOLLOW THE LEADER OF THE PACK:
SOCIAL ANXIETY

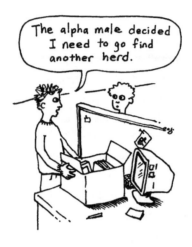

"Too Many Cooks Spoil the Broth."
—Old English Proverb

"It is a base thing for a man among the people not to obey those in command. Never in a state can the laws be well administered when fear does not stand firm."
—Sophocles (Greek philosopher; 497–406 BCE)

THE SOCIAL INSTINCT

Get enough people together, and pretty soon they'll be fighting over things—big things, little things, almost anything. Somebody could get hurt. Disagreement also makes it harder to get things done. Since this chaos makes most folks unhappy, we usually find a way to set up a hierarchy. When there is a pecking order, we are less inclined to pick fights, and we are more likely to work collaboratively. At work there is a boss selected by the higher-ups, and in private groups there are leaders chosen by the crowd. Sometimes we like to think there are no leaders, but in the end there is someone that people regard or treat as the leader anyway. Endless bickering and turf battles are not a good thing.

Animals and our ancient ancestors had less access to imposed or democratic hierarchies, or to rational rules of behavior. They did not have Robert's Rules of Order (the standard guide to parliamentary procedures). Their calming hierarchies were biologically determined. Social Anxiety today may reflect the biology of low social rank. Indeed, people with Social Anxiety may think or act as if they have a lower ranking in the hierarchy, not to mention having more submissive behavior and less closeness among peers, friends and romantic partners.[1]

BACK IN THE DAY: THE SYNDROME IN PRIMEVAL HUMAN SOCIETY

Case Study: How It Might Have Helped Long Ago

Eons ago, in a cave in southern France, there lived a boy in a troop of humans. He was shy as a child, speaking mostly to members of his immediate family. When other members of the troop tried to talk to him, he would hide behind his parents. As he grew into adolescence, he was paired with a girl his age. Gradually over time he became more comfortable with her. He was a dutiful child, a dutiful mate, and a dutiful member of the troop. In fact, he was the quintessential worker bee. He didn't look for a wide circle of friends, he never challenged troop leadership, and he always did what he was expected to do. Indeed, most of the troop was at least a bit like him. People moved up and down the hierarchy over time, but the hierarchy was pretty well known by all, and that helped keep things calm.

On the inside, the boy was terrified that he might somehow embarrass himself should he try to advance above his station. By keeping a low profile, he had a safe place in the troop, and he kept that anxiety at bay. Troop leaders always had first dibs on the meat from hunting trips. He always ate later and ate less, but he could count on getting something. When he did feel mistreated, there were a few people even lower on the totem pole than him, and that gave him a bit of an outlet. His troop wasn't exactly a democracy, but sometimes a consensus would build about when to move camp, or harvest crops early. He just went with the flow. Because he at least seemed content with his place, he was neither a threat nor a target for anyone.

BASIC PRINCIPLE: FOLLOW THE HERD

Presumably, biologically determined social ranking kept everyone in line, and reduced hostile competition within the tribe. Evolved instinct encouraged the lower-ranked members to forgo the culinary and romantic advantages of leadership, and instead accept the smaller but safer benefits of a lesser role. Beyond being an actual acceptance of lower rank, it also appeased the tribal "powers that be."[2] Remarkably, monkeys (and maybe people, too) who are given less food to eat actually live longer lives, and all is not lost on the romantic front either. So if "the meek shall inherit the earth" (Matthew 5:5), meekness must have some advantages.

AMONG THE ANIMALS

Then there are those baboons again. There is some wonderful work about baboon social behavior observed in the wild. It seems that social rank is extremely important to baboons. They pay close attention to where they stand in the pecking order, where everyone else stands, and even to where #7 stands in relation to #8. Because they know each other by voice, scientists can play tricks with doctored voice recordings. The baboons actually get visibly perturbed when audiotapes fool them into thinking that #8 is acting superior to #7![3] This careful ranking mechanism presumably reduces hostile competition within the troop, but it gives baboons a lot to keep track of, and may even be a major reason that their brains have evolved to a larger size.

Dogs, too, are very sensitive to social rank. They aren't called alpha dogs for nothing. Cesar Millan (American television's Dog Whisperer; 1969–) emphasizes the central importance of being the "pack leader" to your pet dog. That way, the dog knows to obey, and it is content to do so. That approach actually worked fine for our beta dog Cassidy, who quickly and cheerfully adopted his beta dog role. When alpha dog Bonnie arrived, though, she had other ideas. Any attempt by humans to impress her with her low social rank was met with a wagging tail while lying down in seeming submission, and was then quickly followed by jumping up for more play. Canine biology trumps human dominance displays? This has social consequences in the house, and, for now, anything chewable seems to be fair game. Cesar—are you listening?

TIMES HAVE CHANGED

Biologically determined social hierarchies may be fine for apes and primal humans, but they don't always go over well in human circles today. People can make conscious decisions about where on the social ladder they want to stand. If there is an unwitting conflict between their rational choices and their biological instincts, we encourage them to follow their conscious wishes. However, they may be in for way more anxiety than they had bargained for—and that anxiety may prevent them from pursuing their goals.

Social rank at play in modern society presents other issues. Afraid of embarrassment? Wait 'til word of your *faux pas* gets around by telephone, or Internet, or

Facebook—a supernormal potential embarrassment that is way beyond the normal circumstances that our evolutionary past knew about. And that's just for the bad stuff. These same technologies present new avenues of communication for high status levels and notable achievements that can make some feel exposed and embarrassed.

At the same time, higher status is available to a broader group of us than in our ancestors, and there are new heights of power, wealth, and gadgets to display or hide. A Ferrari is a Supernormal Stimuli for others to admire, along with Ivy League degrees, fancy publishers, plastic surgerized bodies, foreign travel, gourmet food, and heroic athleticism.

HOW INSTINCT BECOMES SYNDROME IN MODERN HUMAN SOCIETY

Instinct and Worldview

Mostly, people with Social Anxiety are afraid of embarrassing themselves. This crops up at times when they feel under scrutiny—public speaking, meeting new people, performance evaluations, or meeting with a boss. You get the picture. There are tremendous variations in fears about what can go wrong, but all these fears are about eventual self-embarrassment. People worry that their appearance, their knowledge, their performance, and even their anxiety itself might be embarrassing. The scrutiny of others risks the embarrassment of showing that they don't actually have the right stuff to be where they are. So, it's safer to keep a low profile. Better to be a socially accepted beta dog, than to worry about the powers that be. Indeed, one research study showed that people who are more easily embarrassed were deemed more likeable and trustworthy by other people—just what we would expect this instinct to do.[4]

Case study: Instinctive Syndromes in Modern Society

Not so long ago, on a suburban cul-de-sac in Virginia, there lived a girl in a human family who kept mostly to herself. She did speak to her family, but awkwardly and reluctantly. When she went to school, she stayed in the back of the classroom, and tried not to be seen. When the teacher started going around the room, the girl's anxiety would gradually build. So when the teacher called on her, she would first pretend not to notice. When that didn't work, she pulled herself together and spoke as bravely and briefly as she could. She usually got the answers right, but always quaked with fear inside. This was even obvious to some of the students closer to her. Mostly she was afraid of feeling embarrassed. That could happen with a wrong answer, but could also happen when people noticed her anxiety, or that pesky pimple on her nose. The girl particularly disliked those teachers who "democratically" called on students alphabetically or randomly. This felt malicious to her. Somewhere deep inside, she felt an urge to remain unobtrusively low in the classroom pecking order. The embarrassment she felt was powered by that hidden need to keep a low profile.

In fact, the better her answer, and the more recognition she got, the more she stood out, and the more anxiety she felt. Once, a teacher asked students to find a new hydroelectric plant on a state map. One after another, the more confident students pointed to spots in the wrong part of the state. Frustrated, the teacher was about to give up, when the girl walked to the front and pointed to the project, just ten miles from her old family farm. "Wonderful!" said the teacher, as the girl raced back to her seat, and hid her bright red face. Actually, her success didn't make the mistaken students happy. They felt a bit upstaged by this quiet nobody. Although she did well enough on tests, her usual lack of classroom participation always lowered her grades, but didn't threaten others.

At college, she was still too shy to make many friends. Even when she went to parties, she would keep to herself, and she always shied away from boys who tried to meet her. She felt trapped by her loneliness, but could not figure out a comfortable solution. There was no easy way for her to be socially active while still feeling low on the social pecking order. Eventually, she fell in with some equally shy people, who of course also kept to themselves.

After graduation, she moved into a low-level job at a large company. Managers noticed the quality of her work, but whenever she was offered a special assignment or a chance at promotion she would find an excuse. Just meeting with bosses made her nervous. A few times she procrastinated on projects, and turned them in late enough to make her look bad. She preserved her status as a low-level high achiever, and she came to wonder if she would ever move up the ladder.

The crisis came when the girl was assigned to a project team working on an urgent company problem. Long hours, close teamwork, team support, and real urgency let her overcome the anxiety and make essential contributions. She was proud of herself, and so were her managers and team. However, at the end of the day, the girl felt more anxiety than ever. Had she overstepped, asked the instinct inside? Her next two assignments on project teams were late, and one of them was by then unusable. The girl *took this as proof that she was only marginally competent, and should not have so much responsibility (or potential for credit). Off the project team after a few months, she returned to her lower level job, and stayed there for many years.*

Maybe If Things Had Been Different...

After her late-projects fiasco, she called in sick, and was asked to seek help. On medication for Social Anxiety and in psychotherapy, she felt a new sense of confidence and calmness. She talked about her loneliness, anxiety, and fears of embarrassment. On a whim, she went to a holiday party and found herself far less of a wallflower. Indeed, when a man approached her, she spoke with him for an hour and a half. She was surprised, though apprehensive, about this newfound comfort level. Back at work, people couldn't quite put their fingers on how she had changed. When she asked (asked!) for another team assignment, her boss tried to talk her out of it. However, she felt less anxiety during the project, came through again, and afterwards had only passing concerns about embarrassment and lack of competence. It took a while, but eventually she was promoted, and she found a boyfriend who was more than a bit shy himself.

HOW DOES THAT MAKE US FEEL?

Social Anxiety is unnerving. It is the raw primal sensation of our instincts telling us painfully that we are rising above our station. It makes us think that we will embarrass ourselves, be found out, and be put back in our place if we don't do it to ourselves first. The evolutionary advantage of this is that we know not to challenge a ruthless hierarchy. Our ancestors wouldn't want to find themselves beaten down, or thrown out of the tribe—another way they'd be on their own and exposed to all sorts of dangers. The chronic Social Anxiety symptoms are an ongoing reminder of our social status, increasing gradually to a crescendo when we feel ourselves stepping across the line. Although we can adapt some to Social Anxiety, inner fears and an outward intensity may never completely go away.

Being human, we try to ignore this instinctual social hierarchy. Too shy to meet new people? How silly; people are friendly (well, most of them). However, our instincts don't understand reason—they are more responsive to the thought of overstepping. So, just as with Panic Anxiety, our human reason can lead us to longer, more frequent, or more intense Social Anxiety. That can leave us feeling alone and lonely in the bar at that sunny beach resort.

WHAT THE SYNDROME IS

Social Anxiety Disorder (formerly "social phobia") is one particular kind of anxiety. Extreme shyness is one way to think of it, though we are all on a continuum of shyness severity. The core cognitive feature is the fear of embarrassing oneself. Thus, to avoid self-embarrassment, people with Social Anxiety shy away from public speaking, meeting new people, and situations that involve public scrutiny. (Syndrome details are in the appendix).

Diagnosable Social Anxiety Disorder occurs during the lifetime of about 12.1% of Americans, and in the past year in 7.1%,[5] not counting those with milder shyness. A German study put the one-year prevalence rate at 2.0%, but when they threw in detectable but milder forms, the total reached 12.5%.[6] Keep in mind that even these milder forms can still have major effects on happiness and social success.

People with Social Anxiety are alert to situations where they might be evaluated, and are keenly aware that they are afraid of looking bad. Less obvious to them is that deep inside, they are far more worried about looking far too good.[7] Too many cooks (culinary or societal "alpha dogs") would spoil the tribal effectiveness. In primeval times, followers lacked the confidence to challenge the tribe leaders, and were natural and effective followers instead. In other words, Social Anxiety created the followers in ancient human society.

Hippocrates (Greek physician; 460–377 BCE) knew about Social Anxiety: "He dare not come in company for fear he should be misused, disgraced, overshoot himself in gesture or speech or be sick; he thinks every man observes him." However, in modern times it wasn't seen as a distinct kind of anxiety until the early work of Isaac Marks (South African psychiatrist, 1935–) and other observers. This lead to a more modern definition in *DSM-III-Revised* (in 1987), at which point it returned to what Hippocrates described some 2,400 years ago. With the wheel newly reinvented, there was a call to arms,[8] and a new blossoming of Social Anxiety research.

WORST CASE SCENARIOS

People with Social Anxiety are among the wallflowers who hang around the fringes of social events. They observe, but participate little. When invited to dance or into conversation, they are uneasy and perhaps awkward. Some people are so shy that they hardly socialize at all. So-called "avoidant" personality is probably just a severe form of Social Anxiety. Sad as this social withdrawal might make them, some people are often more comfortable avoiding people as much as possible.

Some have their worst symptoms on stage. This sort of public performance is especially terrifying, and occasionally we read about actors and musicians who talk publicly about this fear. The Band's song "Stage Fright" spells out that situation pretty darn well. It makes you realize how hard some people are driven by their fears, and how glad we should be for some of their efforts. On the other hand, while many people are scared to perform, only a few of them will actually sing well if they drag themselves on stage.

That the syndrome of Social Anxiety can even become a worst case is very important to note. There are some who dismiss Social Anxiety as mere shyness or as something that drug companies foist off as illness; if only they were right.[9] They should take a closer look.[10] The instinct behind Social Anxiety makes people linger as low-level worker bees with a high risk for suicide,[11] and they have even more social and economic limitations than people with other anxiety disorders.[12] Those effects become worse still when there are yet other anxiety problems also present.[13]

SUBTLE AND CLOAKED SYNDROMES

Technically speaking, Social Anxiety is diagnosed when people reach a certain level of symptom intensity and problematic behavior. It is at that point that it is considered a medical "illness." However, some of the same symptoms can exist below the cut-off level for diagnosis. There is a spectrum of shyness that ranges from none at all, to modest amounts, to diagnosable Social Anxiety, up to serious social withdrawal.[14] This spectrum logically corresponds to the biological social hierarchy that regimented our primal ancestors and other species today. Even so, it is important not to confuse common shyness with Social Anxiety. Though they may be on the same biological spectrum of severity, only when symptoms reach a certain level do we call them an illness. Otherwise, nearly everyone would be suddenly ill with shyness.

Interestingly, when an SSRI antidepressant (which effectively boosts serotonin activity) is given to a group of healthy control students without diagnosable Social Anxiety, they look and act more dominant to their roommates.[15] Of course, these "normal" folks didn't need any simultenous psychotherapy to undo those psychological effects that can result from long-term Social Anxiety.

Social Anxiety disorder can also appear in different costume. Body Dysmorphic Disorder (BDD) is a condition in which people have highly exaggerated concerns for their appearance. Small physical flaws look to them like disfigurements, and major blemishes are seen where no one else sees anything amiss. This notion is tied to a fear of embarrassment, and it ties in with the perception that others see them (or ought to see them) in a negative way. Some believe that BDD often occurs together with Social Anxiety, responds to the same medicines, and may well be the same thing through a different cultural filter.[16,17,18]

When scientists observe apes in the wild, lower-ranked males will sometimes sneak in a quick bout of sex when no one is looking. Quick is important, because a more dominant male might soon be back, so they had better wrap things up fast. There is some kind of primate connection here, and indeed, The Who (British Blues band) sang "A Quick One While He's Away" a generation ago. It turns out that premature ejaculation is a fairly common problem among adolescent and some adult humans (the men, of course). If you take a careful look, many of these adult men do have diagnosable Social Anxiety,[19] not to mention some who have milder shyness. Not surprisingly, the same SSRIs that treat Social Anxiety also treat premature ejaculation. Curiously, some men would rather get a prescription from their urologist (their sex doctor) than the same prescription from their psychiatrist (their social-coping doctor).

There is also shy bladder syndrome ("paruresis") where men and some women can't urinate in the presence of others. They, too, are limited by their fears of embarrassment, may respond to SSRIs, and come from families in which Social Anxiety is common.[20] Dogs, and many other creatures, use the personal scent of their urine to mark the territory where they declare their dominance. A beta dog in Uruguay waited for a passing alpha dog to go away before re-marking his turf on a nearby tree (Jeremy Marks; American filmmaker, 1985–). Socially Anxious humans may similarly try to avoid the ancient (not to mention symbolic) confrontation of public urination. In an old joke, two Texans stopped on a bridge to urinate. "River sure is cold" said one man. "Deep, too" said the other. Of course, we hear tell that there are no beta dogs in Texas.

There are yet more syndromes that may come in handy in the face of human top dogs. They include, in obscure medical lingo: Erythrophobia (fear of blushing), Hyperhidrosis (excessive sweating), and Craniofacial Erythema (exaggerated blushing). Once you've made sure there are no other physical causes, these syndromes are commonly embarrassingly felt manifestations of Social Anxiety. Exaggerated blushing actually has a surgical treatment, perfected in Sweden, but although the blushing improves, the Social Anxiety still remains. For some people, it may feel less embarrassing to have surgery than to take an SSRI. After successful surgery, one woman even became seriously embarrassed that she wasn't blushing.[21]

WHAT THE SYNDROME ISN'T

Then there are other conditions. Severe "shyness" can also happen in people with psychotic disorders or with a form of Panic Anxiety. In "Speaking Social Phobia," people are uneasy because some performance situations trigger Panic Anxiety (also called "Secondary Social Phobia"), which is not at all the same thing as ordinary

Social Anxiety. Finally, there are cultural differences that can be mistaken for shyness. In some Asian cultures, for example, it is customary to be socially restrained, even if you are not following some biological instinct.

THE AGES OF SOCIAL ANXIETY ANGST

Diagnosable Social Anxiety tends to begin early in adolescence, exactly when evolution expects us to start taking on adult social roles.[22] Even so, some shyness and Social Anxiety symptoms can begin early in childhood.[23] The earlier the onset and the more severe the symptoms, the worse people do in their social and work lives.[24] Indeed, infants have a native awareness of social hierarchy even before they can speak. In one remarkable study, infants viewed images of two animated squares with eyes and mouths as they faced off against each other. By the age of 10 months, the infants could reliably tell that if a large square gave way to a small square, then something odd was going on. That social dominance hierarchy was not what their instincts expected.

HOLDING US BACK

Social Anxiety Disorder today is associated with fewer friends and lower hierarchical ranks in Western society. People with Social Anxiety are still, today, more followers than leaders. With so much shyness, they may be less likely to visit doctors, including psychiatrists.[25] They have trouble seeking and seeing positive experiences, and their social curiosity is restrained by shyness (no surprise there).[26] In an Israeli study, people with Social Anxiety perceived themselves as having lower social rank, more submissiveness and a smaller social network. [27] It's not that they are depressed but, rather, that they are uncomfortable with positive events, even though they might want them.

Indeed, most people today don't like to be lower on the totem pole. To the rational mind, it just doesn't seem fair, and it makes some of them envious and angry.[28] Do not feel alone: this happens in gorillas, too. Lower-ranked gorillas have a habit of hitting ("tagging") their superiors and then running away. Maybe they are trying to make a point.[29]

Social Anxiety, even when mild, is costly for those who have it, and costly for society as well. Social and communication comfort and skills are root causes of many problems for the Socially Anxious. As the prison guard in "Cool Hand Luke" mockingly said to inmate Paul Newman, "What we have here is a failure to communicate." Those with Social Anxiety are the most in need of improved communication skills, yet they are hardest to teach. Think about how doctors should communicate warmly, openly and confidently with their patients. Medical students with Social Anxiety find it much harder to learn those skills.[30] Humans amongst us with this biologically shy "worker bee" inclination have lower work productivity, more health-care costs, and many more deprivations and limitations.[31,32]

THE INSTINCT IS WITH US STILL

Other people sense the presence of Social Anxiety, and followers who have greater fear of self-embarrassment seem less threatening to the self-determined powers that be. One physician had this especially well figured out. He wore inexpensive suits to the hospital to appear meekly nonthreatening there, but each day he then changed into expensive suits in his office to look authoritative to his patients.

Since Social Anxiety is associated with more attention to other people's emotions, it is also associated with more accurate facial-expression identification—a good way to judge if one is being threatened.[33] With all that apprehension, the Socially Anxious are also more easily startled by both positive and negative social signals.[34] Direct eye gaze is one kind of threatening signal. Ever been stared down? As we'd expect, fear of direct eye contact is more common in people with Social Anxiety,[35] and they even widen their field of vision when more than one person is in view.[36] When you look them straight in the eye during a special brain scan ("fMRI"), certain areas of their brain light up with extra activity.[37] Avoiding direct eye contact is one way creatures show submission. So when you come upon that bear protecting its cubs and turf, be humble. Just like Darwin said, facial expressions are social communications even between people and bears.

It turns out that Social Anxiety is also associated with submissive body posture and increased vocal pitch, at least when men are in the presence of an attractive woman. If you look and sound small, you have less to worry about from that big guy across the room.[38] These physical behaviors were captured with extraordinary skill in the character of George McFly (father of time-traveler Marty McFly in the movie *Back to the Future)*: gaze avoidance, submissive posture, high-pitched voice, submission to bullies and other threatening figures, and extreme shyness with women.

Japanese culture and the cultures of some other countries are more hierarchical and less individualistic than the United States. There are many reasons for this, but Japan also has a high prevalence of Social Anxiety. One study suggests that this cultural difference could be partly mediated by serotonin differences.[39] If everyone's biological instincts tell them to honor hierarchies, then the culture as a whole may reflect, and encourage, that predilection. Of course, it could also be that Social Anxiety is caused by cultural influences.[40] Clinically diagnosable Social Anxiety is more common in Japan and other countries than in the United States. The Japanese even have their own name for Social Anxiety: *taijin kyofusho* ("interpersonal relation fear disorder"). Just because you live in a hierarchical society doesn't mean that hierarchical fears can't be a problem for you.

Romance

So how do really shy people find romance? This is truly a question for the ages. One recent study suggested that people lower in social rank may avoid competition for mates by using different criteria for evaluating prospects. By seeking mates whom the more confident might pass over, they are not competing against those who have a higher "instinctual" rank. In the laboratory, the Socially Anxious not only select photos of ostensibly less-attractive partners, but they also say that their choices are less likely to be the same as others'.[41] In the real world, this means that not everyone focuses on the same women and men. The diversity of tastes in physical appearance and personality reduces direct competition.

Once a relationship happens, the Socially Anxious are more likely to have a failure to communicate with their romantic partners.[42] They tend to show more negative behaviors and fewer positive ones. Among Socially Anxious college students, sex is less physically enjoyable, and it feels less emotionally intimate. The women (though not the men) tend to have less sex.[43] We've already talked about premature ejaculation, and it doesn't help romance. Young Socially Anxious adults are less likely to be married, but more likely to be divorced,[1] so you have to wonder, is this all merely lack of experience or knowledge? Or is there some ancient compunction to keep a low emotional profile and limit the appearance of social success? On the brighter side, some may have more lasting marriages. Perhaps they are overjoyed to find a socially comfortable marriage, or maybe they are too shy to find someone else, or to switch partners if they do.[44]

Workplace

The prospect of success can be terrifying (as we saw earlier with Panic). Social Anxiety instincts will say that if we rise too high above our station we had better watch out, because we could be in for big trouble. The higher we go, the more aware we are of the status of what we do, and the more stress we feel.[45] So faced with "too much" success, some people will inadvertently shoot themselves in the foot to undermine their success.

Others will provide themselves with a symbolic reduction in rank. A work promotion can be diminished by redefining it as a mere formality—or by defining oneself as incompetent in that elevated position. Some people demote themselves with the thought that they are mere "imposters," on the verge of public exposure. Actual praise is frightening, and leads some to think that it is false praise at best.[46] Not a few people have turned up in psychiatric offices after their bosses refused to let them quit—yet failed to convince them that they were actually top performers, and so in desperation their bosses told the subordinates to get help. This is not what happens with those people with limited skills who are really, truly in over their heads.

Then there are all those dreams about how we actually flunked that college exam so many years ago. Depressing is the thought that we didn't really earn our college degree, but it is a mental way of cutting ourselves down to size in the face of frightening new successes. These dreams reflect an attempt to demote ourselves in our own eyes, prove our imposter status, and thus reduce our anxiety.

People with Social Anxiety are relentlessly self-critical, especially when they have less to criticize themselves about.[47] They are much less bothered by their deliberate social transgressions (spitting out food that doesn't taste good) than they are by some unintentional transgression that might reveal them as the imposters they think they are (choking on food and coughing it out).[48]

So at the end of the workday, Social Anxiety leads to lower levels of career success. For example, in the Canadian military, 8.2% have a lifetime history of Social Anxiety.[49] About 70% of those soldiers say that Social Anxiety impairs their work performance; they are less likely to be officers, and yet they are unlikely to seek treatment.

SYNDROME AND SOCIAL STIGMA

People do notice. Social Anxiety is easier for other people to notice than Panic Anxiety. Maybe that is because it evolved to be a social cue that was obvious to others. It isn't always that people with Social Anxiety look outwardly anxious, but rather that they might come across as having a lower rank. Other people may sense this and react, without even realizing it. Shy, retiring, nonconfrontational, not openly competitive—you know the type. All of us are a bit that way at least sometimes. One man, without an ounce of Social Anxiety in his past, became very afraid of embarrassing himself when he knew that he could excel in front a large audience of powerful people who could determine his career. Stand out? Stand down? Tough call.

Then there are physical signs of Social Anxiety. People blush, sweat (especially their palms), and their hearts race. Keen observers know that this is a sign of Social Anxiety and shyness, and they respond. That flushed red face evolved as a sign of embarrassed subservience in the face of one's overlords. Blushing works the way evolution intended it to. Many of us enjoy the company of shy people, so a blush can be an endearing trait. Blushing also helps you get away with things you shouldn't. In one study, people played a trust game ("the Prisoner's Dilemma") on a computer, against what they thought were other players. Their opponents (who weren't real) betrayed them early on, and then showed either a blushing or nonblushing face. Blushing won hands down. Embarrassed subservience after betrayal won higher ratings of reliability and trustworthiness.[50] Perhaps blushing is a face-saving face. However, remember that hungry mountain lion. Not someone you would want to act subservient to. It's the same thing with malevolent people. Showing submission, fear, or blushing tells them that they have the upper hand, and that they should feel free to lower the boom.

Oh, and by the way, there is an actual smell of fear, at least for fear of the powers that be. If you have people smell sweat samples taken either from students awaiting an exam or alternately, from students who have just exercised, they can't tell the difference between the two. However, an effect is there nonetheless. Only the exam sample activates brain centers for social emotions,[51] increases awareness of facial expressions,[52] and increases the startle response to noise.[53] As we might expect, this awareness is more pronounced in the Socially Anxious. Visual perception, language, voice tone, smell—they are many ways to be alert to the higher-ups.

INSTINCT AND SYNDROME TURN UP IN CULTURE

Human civilization has ways of leveling out the social hierarchy, though it hardly disappears. In a democracy, even those at the lowest ranks get the vote, though it was not so long ago that the vote was restricted to landowners or the upper classes. Of course, in some settings, everyone is expected to participate, and this is painful if they are shy. Remember our classroom with the Socially Anxious child fearful of her turn to speak?

Japanese culture tells us something more about difficulties of social leveling. Not long ago, when Japan decided to adopt a more Western-style criminal jury system, its citizens wanting nothing to do with it.[54] In an attempt to overcome reluctance to stand out and to challenge authority, mock trials were staged to educate future jurors. Even when directly prompted, they were little able to express their opinions in a group, much less with a judge present, and they did not like the experience at all. Even when the classic jury room movie *Twelve Angry Men* showed the Japanese jurors the kind of outspoken behavior required, it did little to ease their hesitation.

A more acceptable cultural import to Japan is *kaizen* ("change for the better"). This business model, modified from American productivity methods, manages to mute some of the hierarchical issues. The focus is on a continuous critique of one's own work and work habits. Self-criticism comes easily for the Socially Anxious. Decisions are made by consensus rather than by individual action. In the less hierarchical United States ("the land of opportunity" for the individualist), on the other hand, workers find it difficult to self-criticize in front of their colleagues. As one Japanese team leader finally chided a reluctant American worker, "No problem to report is a problem."

Most of us are taught to overcome shyness. We have performance lessons, speech coaches, and romantic advice all built into our culture and education. There are expectations about proper etiquette at gatherings, office behavior, social networking, and marriage. Being aware of our shyness helps us follow those rules and be more extroverted, but does little for the instinctive biology beneath.

The name of Dale Carnegie (American self-improvement expert; 1888–1955) is still familiar to us. In his book *How to Win Friends and Influence People,* he lays out a self-help program for Social Anxiety that is as good as anything written today. A basic premise is that readers should avoid thinking about status, hierarchy and anxiety: "Did you ever see an unhappy horse? Did you ever see a bird that has the blues? One reason why birds and horses are not unhappy is because they are not trying to impress other birds and horses." Those Socially Anxious readers who followed his dictates could excel as salespeople, and become counter-instinctive in their adaptation. Carnegie probably pondered his own status in the hierarchy: He changed his last name from Carnagey, so as to appear related to steel tycoon and philanthropist Andrew Carnegie.

So status and hierarchy remain. The counter-instinctive may be the most outwardly extroverted and status-conscious of all. Thorstein Veblen (American economist, 1857–1929) was inspired by Darwin to take an evolutionary view of economic forces. He focused on the role of status-seeking behavior in this country in *The Theory of the Leisure Class,* and pointed out that "conspicuous consumption" of material goods was a waste of economic resources, unless, of course, you are trying to look like a leisurely alpha dog despite having a low-status biology.

So we have Ferraris, mega-yachts, mansions, and private jets for those who have lots of money to buy happiness by improving their place in the hierarchy. We also have name brand clothing, used luxury cars, travel and late-model electronics for most everyone else who wants to be happier about their perceived status in society. The issue isn't the practical or monetary value of these things; it is why people think they need them. Because luxury items reassure them that they have higher status in the eyes of others, Social Anxiety can contribute to what we call Narcissism (more on this in chapter 5). One patient with Social Anxiety was uncomfortable acknowledging his financial success. Instead, he was more focused on describing his plan to double his already six-figure income, largely so that he could have fancier vacations and larger gambling losses to show off to friends. Vacations and gambling losses are less anxiety provoking, because they don't stick around as evidence that you exceeded your self-perceived station in life. As Carnegie points out, birds and horses don't need luxurious things to be happy (even if horses do appreciate the odd carrot now and then). Money does not buy happiness, but if you are going to be unhappy, you might as well have a flat-screen television and all the best toys.

When we do transgress against our instinctual station, the culture provides ways for us to imitate the embarrassment of Social Anxiety. We are encouraged to repent (in court and out), be humble, and keep a low profile. We are supposed to "eat crow" (so distasteful a food that it is biblically forbidden, and that eating it is a sign of humiliation) or maybe consume "humble pie" (this was the meat pie of the English lower classes, not to mention that it was made from Magpie, itself a kind of crow). All these are deliberate efforts to look smaller in status.

There are other times when people mimic evolved subservience signals. Women's make-up serves many purposes, but when rouge on the cheeks looks like a real blush, it can be endearing to otherwise threatened men. New recruits to a college fraternity undergo a hazing ritual. They engage in a variety of self-embarrassing behaviors, by way of showing themselves subservient to the older members. No doubt those with more Social Anxiety blush profusely, if they ever even end up accepted by the fraternity.

Then there is the military. The military (as well as many other organizations) utilizes a consciously reinforced version of hierarchy to get things done. Rank is an overt marker for hierarchical status in the military, corporations and academia. This kind of follow-the-leader approach has many advantages for reducing arguments and maintaining effectiveness. On the other hand, there are also disadvantages for the organization, and for society as a whole. Following the leader can be a disadvantage for best decision making. In "The Charge of the Light Brigade," Alfred, Lord Tennyson (English poet, 1809–1892) wrote how "Into the valley of death rode the six hundred!" Brave indeed they were, but they knew they were sacrificing their lives in the service of a blundered command.

In World War II, an unexpected German counterattack caught the Allies by complete surprise, and became known as the Battle of the Bulge. The Allies suffered heavy casualties (as did the Germans). Meanwhile, a U.S. Army Intelligence sergeant was doubly dismayed. His well-documented report predicted the planned attack, was passed up the chain of command, and was then ignored. The data didn't conform to the generals' belief that the Germans were too weak to attack. Although he was later promoted and medaled for this work, the sergeant remained forever shy about both his achievement and his promotion.

How does civilization really level the hierarchy? Alcohol. When used in moderate amounts, it is a "social lubricant" that dissolves biologically evolved hierarchies and lets people talk more easily to each other. In Japan, for example, hierarchies are strictly observed in the workplace. However, the more important social interactions take place every day after work, when teams and their leaders drink together before going home. Under the pharmacologic influence and symbolic protection of alcohol, a subordinate can open up to his boss (women employees aren't usually allowed to accompany them).

At baseline, the Socially Anxious beta-dog humans avoid risk, keep to themselves, and are not adventurous.[53] Now, imagine early man having drinks around an ancestral campfire. So much easier to relax and mingle with the alpha dogs after a bit of home brew.

There is even a study in which volunteer college students were forced (forced!) to drink either alcohol or orange juice, and then shown images of threatening or nonthreatening faces.[55] Surprise—sober subjects paid faster attention to the threat posed by the photographs of angry faces, and faster still if they had diagnosed Social Anxiety. After drinking alcohol, however, the Social Anxiety increased attentiveness effect was not only gone (or should we think temporarily "cured"), but the Socially Anxious actually paid even less attention to threat than the others. So if there are scary looking people in a bar, does it help or hurt to drink more than usual?

Speaking of cultural reflection of instinct, nowhere in music is the Social Anxiety of newfound fame better described than in these verses selected from the Band's "Stage Fright:"

Now deep in the heart of a lonely kid
Who suffered so much for what he did,
They gave this ploughboy his fortune and fame,
Since that day he ain't been the same.

See the man with the stage fright
Just standin' up there to give it all his might.
And he got caught in the spotlight,
But when we get to the end
He wants to start all over again.

I've got fire water right on my breath
And the doctor warned me I might catch a death.
Said, "You can make it in your disguise,
Just never show the fear that's in your eyes."

Now if he says that he's afraid,
Take him at his word.
And for the price that the poor boy has paid,
He gets to sing just like a bird, oh, ooh oohooh.

Your brow is sweatin' and your mouth gets dry,
Fancy people go driftin' by.

The moment of truth is right at hand,
Just one more nightmare you can stand.

INSTINCT AND SYNDROME WORSENED BY CULTURE

Civilization can also make Social Anxiety worse, and not just by letting success-phobic people become successful. All too often, human culture takes Social Anxiety at its biological face value. Shy people are left to themselves or are overwhelmed by their more highly ranked colleagues. The last person chosen for the baseball team may be the shyest player, not necessarily the worst. Leaving someone off the team can even be a way to pick on them deliberately.

There are many reasons that deliberate bullying can happen, but one reason is that bullies are trying to prove or improve their rank. Who to pick on? Seemingly weak, defenseless and low-ranking folks are the easiest targets, and least likely to fight back. After all, why get yourself hurt? Even for those with noble goals, there is a tendency to pick the easier target. As the bumper sticker says, "People are more violently opposed to fur than leather, because it is easier to harass rich women than motorcycle gangs" (Dave Barry, American humorist, 1947–). Unfortunately, there are many out there who insecurely feel that they must raise their social rank, and so their attention is drawn to those with more overtly subordinate instincts. Bullies and victims alike are very attentive to hierarchy.

TURN THE SYNDROME AROUND: ADVANTAGES OF COUNTER-INSTINCTIVE BEHAVIOR

Case study: Counter-Instinctive Behavior

Not so long ago, in a small suburban home in Sydney, there lived a girl in a human family. She was shy as a child, with few friends, and an eagerness to stay home when she could be playing with others. In high school, though, she realized that friends were a good thing. She started to talk to people as often as she could muster up the courage. To ease her anxiety and fears of embarrassment, she was acutely attentive to their reactions. She analyzed carefully even her slightest miscue, and every nuance of their reactions. Although this did not lessen her anxiety, it did steadily improve her ability to make comfortable conversation with classmates, and she knew that was progress. Using the same approach, she started to speak up in class. She didn't feel emotionally close to people, but she did have many more friends. She felt better whenever she put down the unpopular kids, and bragged about how she sometimes poured liquid soap through the vents in their lockers. By her senior year, she even ran for class president, becoming vice president as runner up.

After school, she took a job as a sales associate in a department store. Just as she had trained herself to analyze her "friend" performance, she now focused on her "salesperson" performance for customers. She wore elegant, brand-name clothing, expensive shoes, and often pulled out her Mercedes-Benz key chain. She quickly became a top salesperson; customers loved her, and bosses wondered how she did it. Her anxiety increased of course, and sometimes she felt so "stressed" that she would hide for a while in the employee lounge. At six feet tall, Poppy was indeed a "tall Poppy"— the kind of stand-out success who might be cut down by others (indeed, an Australian politician actually once called for "cutting the heads off the tall poppies"). However, she did like her success and recognition; she hoped to have a real Mercedes soon, and she was especially proud that customers kept asking for her. They were hardly emotional intimates, but they were a constant source of social reassurance.

At a young age, she was promoted to a local sales-training position. Still fearful of self-embarrassment, she used that emotional energy to learn how to teach and reach salespeople, even though she made a point of never thanking subordinates. There was a bit of a crisis when she was asked to keynote a national sales-training conference. Sure, she knew what to say, but this great leap forward in prominence was something she was not yet ready for. She "stressed" for weeks about her presentation, produced a great set of slides, wondered whether she had been set up to fail, and was noticeably tense during her talk. She passed it off as being "under the weather" and decided next time to have a massage and a drink beforehand.

Unfortunately, senior management remembered her tension, and they no longer saw her as a potential national-sales-training leader. This was both a disappointment and a relief for her, but left her recurrently frustrated over the next many years in her local-sales-training job.

Maybe If Things Had Been Different...

One senior manager had been there himself, and still saw her potential. He asked her to have a formal executive-skill assessment, which then suggested a confidential clinical evaluation. "Social Anxiety?" she said, "no one is more out there than me." Still, she learned the difference between how she felt inside and how she acted outside. Propranolol (a beta-blocking hypertension drug) before talks helped reduce her "stress" a bit. Daily sertraline (an SSRI antidepressant) helped much more, and also let her explore her self-embarrassment fears, her hidden fear of authority, and the coping style that led to her sales success. In fact, once she felt better, she rapidly proved herself in her next talk. During some time in therapy, she sorted out her inner workings. The inner Stage Fright was gone. By the time she was moved to the national office, she was comfortable enough with her station that she could clearly make a point of thanking even the lowliest members of her team.

SOCIAL ALARMS PROMPT SELF-IMPROVEMENT

Dale Carnegie could not have known the *DSM-IV* criteria for Social Anxiety, but he had this stuff all figured out long ago. "Instead of worrying about what people say of you, why not spend time trying to accomplish something they will admire," was another piece of his advice. It is advice that many people try to follow deliberately, and sometimes even unwittingly. Afraid of embarrassing themselves, and afraid lest people think they have overstepped their instinctual station, some people try to prove themselves worthy. Their fear becomes a guide to the task at hand: If they fear it, they will do it.

Their exquisite sensitivity to self-embarrassment makes them ever alert to the details of their own performance and to the reactions of others. The beta dogs become ever better at appeasing the alpha dogs, and they prosper as a result. This is especially common in extroverted professionals like actors, salespeople, musicians, models and courtroom lawyers. Many will emphasize that they were shy, awkward and withdrawn until they roared out of their shell. Ingrid Bergman (Swedish actress, 1915–1982) said, "I was the shyest human ever invented, but I had a lion inside me that wouldn't shut up!"

This kind of continual self-improvement helps people get better and better at public speaking, meeting people, and performances of all kinds. Subtle put downs and actual critiques are painful, but they are quite useful when fully digested. From selling products at retail work to selling companies in investment banking, the best salespeople are those who can manage the nuances of the relationship and close the deal. As Dale Carnegie said, "There is only one way...to get anybody to do anything. And that is by making the other person want to do it."

The same underlying uneasiness can also be helpful to those who overcome their fears deliberately rather than unthinkingly. As the *Wall Street Journal* noted of one unusually articulate CEO:

"Ian Cook, the chief of Colgate-Palmolive Co., characterizes himself as introverted. He believes his strong listening skills played a role in his steady advancement since he joined the consumer-goods manufacturer in 1976 as an assistant product manager. "I listen intently," he says. "I am extremely attentive to language and body cues." Still, when the British executive landed his first senior management spot more than a decade ago, he remembers being uncomfortable addressing large groups of staffers. "He was humorous but a little stiff in the process…He wasn't engaging various parts of the audience with his eyes…He tended to look down at the podium." Mr. Cook says coaching from colleagues and advisers improved his presentation delivery. "Unshackling from the podium was a defining moment," he concedes. "I had to learn."[56]

In addition, acting like an alpha dog will sometimes make people think that you really are an alpha dog. If you take someone else's coffee, or put your feet up on the table, people will think you more powerful.[57] Of course, if you act like you own the place, some other people might just see you as rude.

UNINTENDED CONSEQUENCES

Counter-instinctive behavior has other downsides: ongoing fear, lesser enjoyment, less relationship intimacy, and less adaptability to circumstances. Following the fear can be problematic—counter-instinctive behavior is more shaped to the fear than to the actual circumstance. Counter-instinctive bosses who come off as brusque commanders or as insecure deciders are less effective than those who master the air of the quietly confident alpha dog. Most importantly, careers that people instinctively fear aren't necessarily what they are most comfortable with. Maybe that saleswoman would be happier as an accountant, or that actor as a schoolteacher.

If the countershy behavior is not directed to productive purpose, it can emerge as a defiance of an inner bottom-dog instinct, with angry challenging behavior, aggression or reckless social thrill seeking, with counter-productive consequences.[58] Remember those low-ranking gorillas tagging the top gorilla? Imagine if they tagged a little too hard or a little too often.

WHERE DOES THIS COME FROM, ANYWAY?

The Genetic Root of All Instinct

Social Anxiety tends to run in families. It is more common in an identical twin than in a nonidentical twin, and is more common in those with genetically decreased serotonin function. It must have an inherited component, but although the details remain uncertain, there are more genetic explanation possibilities coming down the pike.[59] Likewise, studies of gene-by-environment effects in Social Anxiety are afoot. In all probability, genetic influences are significantly moderated by environmental factors.[60] Not everyone with the genes gets the syndrome, nor do they get it to the same degree or even in the same way.[61] Indeed, the syndrome can emerge even in those with the normal version of the serotonin-activity gene, but their Social Anxiety is less likely to respond to SSRI medications.[62]

Inner Workings

There is an embarrassment center in our brains. Researchers found this center by recording a group of people with brain diseases as they sang along with the Temptations' song, "My Girl." Then they played their own voices back to them without the music.[63] How embarrassing. Neurochemically, human Social Anxiety is influenced by the serotonin neurotransmitter system. Remember that study about social behavior among locusts? Normally loners, they become more social when they gather in swarms, and this is triggered by an increase in serotonin levels. Serotonin makes them less shy, even though locusts probably never worry about embarrassing themselves.

Rhesus macaque monkeys are sensitive to hierarchy issues in the troop. Monkeys with lower genetic levels of serotonin function don't like looking at photographs of monkey faces, and especially not at the eyes.[64] In fact, they have to be bribed with juice even to look at a photo of a high-ranking colleague, whereas their colleagues with higher serotonin levels will give up some of their juice to do the same thing. It takes all kinds. In vervet monkeys, a little serotonin goes a long way. Give them fluoxetine or tryptophan (two ways to increase serotonin activity), and they rise swiftly to the top of a leaderless troop. When the stuff wears off, they go back to where they were.[65] The amount of human blushing in Social Anxiety is associated with the genetic decrease in serotonin function.[66] Patients often feel more socially confident on SSRIs, especially after a bit of therapy. So maybe our biological social rank (there are many nonbiological social-rank factors as well) is related to gradations of serotonin activity, though human research hasn't reached the levels of our monkey cousins yet.

HOW TO FIX IT: EVOLUTIONARY PERSPECTIVE EXPLAINS MODERN TREATMENT
Coping and Self-Improvement

We've already talked about Dale Carnegie's self-improvement approach—overcome fears, and succeed at feared tasks. Garrison Keillor (American host of radio's *Prairie*

Home Companion, 1942–) has another treatment idea. His Powdermilk Biscuits "give shy persons the strength to get up and do what needs to be done." Since the active medication ingredient is not known, it may be that a symbolic biscuit of emotional strength can help a shy person rise to the top. Likewise, the Cowardly Lion in the *Wizard of Oz* needs a medal of courage to feel like the king of the jungle that he wants to be. Biscuits, medals, college degrees, large houses, and other symbols of authority can offer at least a small increase in people's perceived social rank.

Evolved Treatment

Not surprisingly, people with Social Anxiety tend to shy away from treatment. After all, few situations would make them feel more subject to scrutiny than a careful psychiatric history. When they do arrive in the office, it is typically for some other crisis.[67] Modern medication treatment that is most effective includes the SSRI antidepressants. They work by increasing the effects of serotonin (the brain's social director), but it isn't known if they have some more chemically specific effect for Social Anxiety. We talked about how epigenetics can reduce gene functions by attaching methyl groups to DNA, so it is even possible that SSRIs return serotonin function toward normal by undoing epigenetic methylation of certain genes.[68] Somehow, SSRIs do make people look and feel less submissive and subordinate.[69]

If you have Social Anxiety and you are planning a speech or performance, the perception of threat could put you in a high state of physiological arousal ("stress"). Beta-blockers (such as propranolol) taken just beforehand can reduce the symptoms of arousal and also the physical symptoms of Social Anxiety itself. Beta-blockers reduce sweating, racing heart, and some other symptoms. Social Anxiety also causes "regular anxiety," especially before a performance. A benzodiazepine such as clonazepam or diazepam ahead of time can reduce the feeling of anxiety, but does much less for physiological activation, and, in the long run, it is not a great idea. Beta-blockers and benzodiazepines do nothing for underlying concerns about embarrassment and social rank.

Psychotherapy is helpful as well, especially in combination with medication. Conventional relationship psychotherapy[70] helps to understand and correct patterns of shyness; it is not enough to just use medication. When people have a lifetime of experience with Social Anxiety, it becomes ingrained, even if the neurochemistry has been corrected. Psychotherapy helps recognize the hidden expectations and fears that have built over time, and how they influence relationships. Good conventional psychotherapy can benefit even more with an added evolutionary perspective. People need to relearn where they feel comfortable in their personal social network, and where they would like to feel comfortable in the future. While this seems simple enough, the actual psychotherapy is more complex, and takes some time for best results.

Cognitive behavior therapy offers an enhanced version of the self-help approach. The goals there are more on the surface, and they include reducing avoidance of public speaking, of meeting people, and of dealing with hierarchies at work. At the same time, attention is paid to recognizing and correcting unwarranted fears. Practice makes perfect, you might say. However in the end, this kind of approach helps people succeed despite the unwitting notion that their rank is too low. That notion lingers, as can unpleasant emotions. So here, too, therapy works better with medication.

4

A SURE AND TIDY NEST
(CLEAN, ARRANGE, SAVE, AND BEHAVE):
OBSESSIVE-COMPULSIVE DISORDER

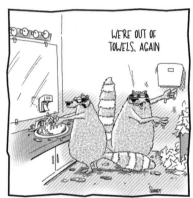

RACCOONS, THE OBSESSIVE COMPULSIVE
HAND WASHERS OF NATURE

"Cleanliness becomes more important when godliness is unlikely."
—P. J. O'Rourke (American writer and humorist; 1947–)

"Organizing is what you do before you do something, so that when you do it, it is not all mixed up."
—A. A. Milne (English Humorist; 1882–1956)

THE SOCIAL INSTINCT

When we live together in a group, there are things that we need to do. We do them for ourselves, we do them for our families and communities, and we do them around the house. Sometimes it is hard to remember them all, and sometimes our ancestors had no clue why they were so important. What is an ancient human to do? It helps to have built-in instinctual behaviors to get things done. Some concerns come automatically to mind, even to obsessional extremes. Some behaviors are so hard wired that we feel compelled to do them. The syndrome known as Obsessive-Compulsive Disorder (OCD) can be broken down into four components: There are prompts to clean, arrange, save, and behave. It is not just us; our less conscious animal friends have the same adaptive instincts. Milder versions of these traits also make it easier for us humans to make the best use of these four inborn OCD component groups when we add in modern cultural, technological and learned improvements. And where are these behaviors most important? Around the nest, of course.

BACK IN THE DAY: THE SYNDROME IN
PRIMEVAL HUMAN SOCIETY

Case Study: How It Might Have Helped Long Ago

Sometime before the dawn of civilization, there was a young woman in a human troop, living in a streamside lean-to house in the African Rift Valley. She was a very methodical woman. Every morning, she checked the wooden poles of the lean-to and the branches and brush that covered the roof. Everything had to be just right. Otherwise, any major rain storm could collapse the house, drenching the family and destroying her carefully saved food hoard inside. She also checked the earthen berm that protected the house from the stream during floods. Mud packing could crack or fall off, so repairs were needed all the time. Even when satisfied, she would still worry all day about the house and the dam, and would often return to recheck it.

Next on her list was breakfast. She would carefully wash stored food in a small spring that entered the stream near the camp. She was especially careful with food that someone had already started to eat. She did this even though she had no idea that germs existed, that they could carry disease, or that they could travel from one person to another.

All of these activities took time and effort, but the house was solid, the camp rarely flooded, and the troop was a healthy bunch in a very well-tended nest. Knowing that she was around, the others could rest easy around the hut, and devote their thoughts to the search for game, and to the constant watch for predators on the savanna.

BASIC PRINCIPLE: THE HERD AT HOME

It is easy to imagine ancient societies (and more primitive species) in which mild OC traits were very helpful in maintaining hygiene, building things, saving supplies for future needs, and reducing risk of disruptive sexual or aggressive acts. These are very important tasks, especially when people live close together in families or tribes. We humans have been doing this for a long time. What serious risks did our ancestors face? Above all, there were infectious diseases, predators (both human and animal), supply shortages (especially food and water), and in-fighting.[1] How nice if they had built-in habits for preventing disease, checking for security, saving for a rainy day, and making nice. An Israeli archeological site from some 750,000 years ago found that our ancient (post-bacterial) ancestors were a tidy bunch (the popular press article was titled "The Origins of Tidiness").[2] Their living spaces had separate areas for different kinds of work and for different kinds of refuse, and they didn't even have vacuum cleaners or computer programs to help or advise them.

AMONG THE ANIMALS

Animals have some behaviors that seem just silly to us, but quite natural to them. So when our Cassidy started digging in his empty water bowl as a young puppy, it was because his ancient wolf ancestors knew instinctively to dig water holes deeper when their primeval water holes ran dry. Even as an adult, he would drag the bowl with a digging motion to signal that he needed more water. We people know how to turn on a faucet for water (Cassidy never figured this out—though he did learn that humans do have indoor water holes where drinking is not allowed), but our emotions and behavior remain more instinctive—more biologically based—than we have known. As if to freshen the bedding, Cassidy would scratch the carpet before lying down to sleep. Comfort? Hygiene? Who knows? Tail chasing is another curious canine behavior. It seems to be particularly common in terriers, and responds to anti-OCD medications.[3] Perhaps an overreaching grooming behavior? After all, terriers are known for their dogged persistence.

Animals have both the usefully mild and clinically problematic versions of OCD. Most of them do not consciously count and hoard resources, few are aware of the germ theory of disease (except maybe some cats as they wash their food), and prob-ably none are inspired by religious or intellectual morality to control their aggres-sive behaviors. Yet all of the OCD behaviors, in milder form, are essential to animal survival, and no doubt prompted by instinctive biological cues. Those instincts help both the individual and the group, and they have a lot to do with keeping house and hanging out with the home crowd.

Obsessive-Compulsive Disorder may even serve some unexpectedly specific social purposes. Remember those socially conscious baboons? It seems that keeping track of so many social rankings requires an obsessively huge amount of calculation, and the social areas of their brains became enlarged as an evolutionary adaptation that allowed this complex task. According to one theory, larger and more complex brains evolved, not for reasoning or memory, but mostly for social skills.[4] Reasoning and memory were more of an afterthought (pun alert).

Dogs lick their paws and cats groom their fur (a kind of cleaning, of course). This attention to hygiene is presumably built in. However, that doesn't mean that animals can't learn new ways to achieve those goals. In a famous study, researchers observed that Japanese monkeys taught successive generations how to wash sweet potatoes. This, they pointed out, suggests the existence and transmission of cultural behaviors in a nonhuman species.[5] Amazing. At the same time, it suggests that monkeys like their potatoes clean, and are predisposed to learning a way to get off the dirt. Not only that, but this behavior has social-hygiene and social-bonding benefits beyond just the individual monkey, and it is learned in a social context. Some animals have clinically diagnosed OCD cleaning rituals, which respond to the same medications as human OCD: Dogs lick their paws to the point of inflammation and pain; parrots pull out their feathers.[6]

Animals are attuned to symmetrical arrangement behavior as well. A bird will carefully arrange sticks into an evenly round nest. Even spiders weave complexly symmetrical webs (a nest for dinner guests, if you will). These are not conscious decisions but instinctual mechanisms that promote the survival of those species.

Hoarding is how animals stock up on food for the winter or for lean times. Chipmunks and birds hoard nuts (and even remember where they stashed them, for the most part). Pack rats collect stuff like, well, pack rats. Then there are pack mice. In one Alaskan study, mice were bred over many generations into two separate strains— one that builds large nests, and one that builds small nests. This turns out to be selection for generalized hoarding behavior, because the large-nest mice also tend to bury more marbles (think seeds or nuts) than the small-nest mice.[7] When the large-nest mice are treated with medication for human OCD, they make smaller nests and bury fewer marbles. Whatever OCD is, mice can be bred to have more of it.

Stepping back and taking in the big picture, this OCD stuff is mostly about family nesting (and a bit of grooming). On the television series *Meerkat Manor*, the cute meerkats take careful care of their nest entrances. They seem to know the four basic tenets of real estate: location, location, location, and street appeal.

How about ants?[8,9] Peter Miller summarizes the behavior of four successive groups of ants leaving a nest in the morning. First the patrollers inspect the terrain, and they are ready to rumble (or not) with patrollers from other competing nests. Then the maintenance workers clean out trash from inside the nest, and dump it outside. The midden workers then neatly arrange that detritus into a localized pile. Finally, the foragers search for food, and bring it back to save in the nest, (perhaps hoarded for future needs). Behave, clean, arrange, and save, just like human OCD. Remember, though, that these aren't conscious decisions by the ants, nor are they following conscious directions. They just do it. Their behavioral roles are determined by an interaction between genetic factors and chemical messages sent by others from the nest.

TIMES HAVE CHANGED

Enough with ants. What about humans today? Do we still need these automatic thoughts and behaviors? Aren't we past that already? Can't we keep house without them? Besides, some people have obsessive thoughts and compulsive behaviors that are way beyond anything that might have been useful to ancient humans or modern apes. In other words, humans with OCD may miss out on the wider world because they obsess about details no longer central to our existence. Don't miss the forest for the trees, as the saying goes. There are a number of book titles with that phrase, several with advice on how to take in the larger view rather than just the details (some others seem to have borrowed the phrase for books about forestry). There is even a book for writers called *The Forest for the Trees* (Betsy Levine) with advice on how to get your writing done. Time to look for that one!

HOW INSTINCT BECOMES SYNDROME
IN MODERN HUMAN SOCIETY

Instinct and Worldview

Depending on which symptoms they have, people with OCD think that they have to clean more, plan more, save more, and control their behaviors (or at least make amends for them). The world seems to them like a vast problem that they absolutely must try to bring under control. Indeed, the world does present these and other problems to people and societies. Cleaning prevents disease, arranging solves practical problems, saving prevents material shortages, and behavioral self-control prevents discord. The problem, of course, is that true clinical OCD goes beyond the realm of actual needs and benefits and into a world of wasted or self-harming thoughts and efforts. With true OCD, even too much is not enough.

Case Study: Instinctive Syndromes in Modern Society

Just this year, a young man in a human family lived near a river in New York. He spent an awful lot of time keeping everything clean. For many hours a day he thought he was fighting the good fight against dirt and germs. Much of that time was spent in the bathroom, and much more in the kitchen. At least, those were places where there were germs that mattered. However, no matter how much he cleaned, he was certain that danger and contamination lurked everywhere. He also cleaned every speck of dust from closets and hallways, washed sheets and towels daily, and never let his children play in the garden. There was dirt out there! He certainly didn't drink the river water or the New York City tap water (reputedly the cleanest in the nation). Only bottled spring water would do. His family kept telling him to cut back on the cleaning, tried to distract him, and ultimately urged him to get help. Their one success was buying plastic plates that could be thrown out rather than cleaned. Stop cleaning he couldn't; he had to make things cleaner and cleaner still. When the children were grown, his wife moved out of the nest.

Nor did his preoccupations stop at the workplace door. In the office he was known for his slow work, and people figured that the paper-towel-lined bathroom stall had something to do with him. He was a loyal and methodical worker, but the boss was at a loss for what to do. No end of coaching, advice, exhortation, and performance evaluation had ever had any effect. When layoffs happened, he was one of those let go.

Maybe If Things Had Been Different…

Before moving out, his wife gave him one final ultimatum: either he gets help or she leaves. Terrified though he was, he could not agree to let up against the germs. However, he did let her take him to the psychiatrist, and he did take the pills (high-dose fluvoxamine, an SSRI antidepressant used for OCD). He inspected each and every pill before taking it with three sips of water before, and another three sips after. Many weeks later, he started talking in therapy, and around that time he stopped washing the sheets every night. Within months, his cleaning routine was down to one hour a day. The couple celebrated with a glass of honest-to-goodness real New York City tap water. Out of the loop on the clinical treatment, the boss was relieved by his new and improved employee, but mystified about why his exhortations had suddenly started to work.

HOW DOES THAT MAKE YOU FEEL?

Obsessive-Compulsive Disorder doesn't always feel so bad, at least if you are careful to follow its impulses.[10] It is the raw primal sensation of your instincts telling you that you had better keep your clan's nest clean and sanitary, your things properly arranged and protected, your needed resources saved for that all-too-certain rainy day, and your disruptive impulses controlled. If you resist the instructions, you may feel like disaster is around the corner. It provokes an overwhelming urge to, well, obsess about these nesting issues and to compulsively attempt solutions. The evolutionary advantage of OCD is that you don't forget some very necessary concerns and tasks. Our ancestors wouldn't want to find themselves living in filth (though since they didn't know about germs, they weren't actually germophobes), unable to find or protect their homes, left without food or tools in an emergency, or stealing each other's food or spouses. The instincts behind OCD help prevent those problems. Point of order, here: Many psychiatrists think that OCD isn't actually an "anxiety" disorder instinct, but rather a disorder of impulses and compulsions that people feel obliged to obey.

Can't abide public restrooms? Don't be absurd, restroom-acquired infections don't happen (pretty darn rarely these days). However, our instincts don't understand reason—they are more responsive to concerns about being near other people, and near their waste products in particular. So, when our human reason lets us use that restroom, we feel an urgent need to clean, clean and clean more. Few people with OCD realize that the highest restroom concentration of bacteria is actually on the handle of the exit door (no worries, still not much of a health risk). It's hard to enjoy a sunny beach resort if the possibility of restroom germs is an overshadowing preoccupation.

WHAT THIS SYNDROME IS

Like our other instincts, OC traits were known in ancient times. Pharaoh asks Joseph to interpret his dream of seven fat cows and seven thin ones (Genesis 41). Joseph prophesizes seven years of bumper crops to be followed by seven years of famine. That being the case, he advises Pharaoh that in the years of plenty, Egypt's grain should be hoarded for the lean years. We also learn that Joseph cleans himself before meeting Pharaoh, arranges the granary distribution system, counts the saved grain, and is known for his wise and proper behavior. All four core OC traits turn up in the same short chapter, thousands of years ago.

Freud noted these very same four factors in *Civilization and Its Discontents*, though not all in one breath. He included them as the components of what he called "anal personality." Little is new under the sun. And here, too, Freud was again especially concerned with wicked sexual and aggressive thoughts and with the notion that they are at the root of OCD and so many other evils.

Overt OCD is much more common than we used to think. In the old days, it wasn't something that could be treated effectively, so there wasn't much point in taking a careful history from patients. With the advent of effective treatments, it turns out to be fairly common. If you can treat something, it is more important to recognize it. The lifetime rate of formally diagnosable OCD is about 2.3% of the population, with many more having milder forms.[11] In milder form, the obsessions and compulsions can be embarrassing, eccentric, time wasting, or judgment impairing. In more severe form, OCD can render some people incapable of functioning in society. They are so preoccupied with thoughts that they can't stop thinking ("obsessions") or behaviors that they can't stop doing ("compulsions") that they don't have time for anything else. (Syndrome details are in the appendix). The toll on time management is considerable. On average, people with OCD spend 5.9 hours each day preoccupied with obsessive thoughts, and 4.6 hours with compulsive behaviors. Most also have at least one other anxiety or depressive disorder to complicate their lives.

Confirmation that OCD is an overlapping set of four different subtypes is relatively recent. Only in recent years have researchers used statistical methods to look carefully at which of the many OCD symptoms cluster together in the same patients ("factor analysis"). Many studies now show the same four Factors: cleaning habits and contamination concerns; ordering, counting and symmetry; hoarding behavior; and aggressive, sexual and religious thoughts with checking rituals. These symptom clusters do overlap, so that someone with OCD can have symptoms from more than just one.[12,13,14] The actual symptoms are a complex collection, duly listed in the Yale-Brown Obsessive-Compulsive Scale (YBOCS),[15] and in the shorter Florida Obsessive-Compulsive Inventory (FOCI, included in the appendix). Some studies suggest there are actually five clusters, but while we wait for that dust to settle, let's take a more detailed look at these four subtypes.

Clean: Cleanliness Is Kind of Like Godliness

This statistically derived Factor includes overriding concerns about cleanliness, and resulting compulsions to keep things clean. For those of us with OCD tendencies today, we have Supernormal Stimuli[16] that are like nothing that evolution ever prepared us for. It is way too easy to overclean. We have washing machines, dishwashers, soaps, cleansers, solvents, antibiotic sprays, scrubbers, sterilizers, and so much more. Sometimes we do everything in the name of cleanliness. This can be a good thing. Some of us like to feel clean; it does keep the germs down, and sterile technique is essential for modern surgery. On the other hand, some hospitals have banned decorative houseplants, even though houseplant-transmitted human disease is essentially unknown. Some suburban parents scrub the house, and don't let the children play in the yard (where the dirt is, not to mention those feared filthy kidnappers). This can take some of the fun out of life. More than that, it may decrease the ability of our immune systems to fight off disease and increase our risk of allergic disorders. The germs notice our fear of them, too; too much exposure to unnecessary antibiotics, and they evolve themselves into medication-resistant strains.

Still, we do think that cleanliness is next to godliness. If experimental subjects are put in a room that seems cleaner (i.e., freshly scented with citrus), they tend to act in more charitable and trustworthy ways.[17] At the same time, when we transgress, we look literally to wash away our sins with soap and water, as so often depicted in movies. About William Shakespeare's (British playwright, 1564–1616) Lady MacBeth we hear of "an accustom'd action with her, to seem thus washing her hands. I have known her continue in this a quarter of an hour." So it is no surprise then, as she muses on the moral stain of her role in the death of King Duncan, that she rubs her hands and proclaims "Out, damn'd spot! Out I say!" Research subjects who are asked to think of past moral transgressions become more able to think of cleanliness-related words, more likely to use antiseptic wipes, and more likely to think of compensatory moral behavior.[18]

Arrange: Getting Your Ducks in a Row

This Factor includes symptoms like repeating and ordering rituals, so that people don't forget to plan ahead. Remember the carpenter's rule? Measure twice, cut once. That kind of checking makes for a better kitchen table (the meeting place of so many human nests). However, when some people check, double check, triple check, and far far more, then they are beyond the bounds of a useful way to ensure the quality of their work. Those kinds of checking rituals can take so much time, emotional effort and energy that OCD can lead to all-consuming compulsions.

Carpenters also need to have the right number of nails. Unless they have a vast supply, they count them to be sure. Kitchen tables shouldn't fall apart. However, some people can't stop counting. They count squares on the sidewalk, letters on a page, books on a shelf, and more. It may feel purposeful to them, but these counting behaviors are also compulsions.

Finally, carpenters also want to make sure that corners are square, and that parts fit just right. Symmetry is very important. However, some patients with OCD can't stop staring at the area rug on a psychiatric office floor. It lies right next to a cabinet, and it is easy to see when the edges are not precisely parallel. It doesn't really matter to anyone else, (especially when the rug moves out of alignment again after every office cleaning), but it bothers them; it distracts them, and they obsess about it. Imagine if a carpenter couldn't stop checking the angles on a table that was already done. He might never put that table to use.

Obsessive-compulsive traits help us to arrange and improve our thoughts, logic and actions. However, clinical OCD can have us indulge in over organizing—paying way too much attention to details and to factors irrelevant in modern life, and drowning in marginally relevant details. In business they talk about "analysis paralysis." This refers to trying so hard to perfect a solution that nothing actually happens. Analysis paralysis can waste time, effort, money and opportunity. Many a college student has spent so much time crafting a paper to perfection that it was late enough to be marked down a grade. Doing much and getting little done is called chasing your tail. This is one way that people and those terriers end up procrastinating. And, yes, analysis paralysis can happen in overly detailed psychoanalytic psychotherapy as well.

We have endless modern tools and whole industries for arranging, organizing, counting and the like: computers and software, household-container systems, the library's Dewey Decimal System, universal resource locators (Internet URL addresses), advanced mathematics, and much more. All these things are exceedingly helpful for us, except, of course, when they are not. Science provides a good example. We are much better at accumulating and analyzing new data on known theories than we are at finding new theories. The real progress in science comes from looking at things differently, not just from using existing explanatory models to organize additional data.[19] Speaking from experience, some of us have spent countless hours trying to fix a balky computer, only to find out that the simple solution was somewhere else. As a patient asked just this week about a balky printer, "Is there any paper in there?" Ockham strikes again.

Saving for a Rainy Day, or He Who Dies with the Most Toys Wins

Hoarding is about, well, the obsession and compulsion to hoard. Some people need to save everything, because they can't bear to throw anything away. Human pack rats we call them, and hoarders even have their own television programs these days. So much detritus accumulates in their homes that some rooms are closed off, while mere pathways allow passage through others. Of course, it doesn't seem to them that they have a problem. What bothers them more is when there are attempts to clean out their house.

There is also oversaving for the rest of us. We have far more ways to save now than did our primeval brethren. We have water reservoirs, oil reserves, grain silos, kegs of beer, wine closets, freezers, savings accounts, gold bullion, stock markets, storage lockers, and this list goes on. If we use all these things right, we are much less likely to run out of anything important. All for the better, of course. However, for those who need to make extra sure, this is a problem waiting to happen.

For some people, too much is not enough. They hoard stuff that has actual value, but way more of it than they will ever need. It isn't just for pleasure, for happiness, for hierarchical prestige, or for drawing people closer. It is large quantities of actually valuable stuff. This has advantages, too. Economists will point out that wealth accumulation has value for individual motivation, for the general economic welfare ("capital formation"), for the growth and survival of a corporation, for corporate economies of scale and for philanthropy. However, these are not the only reasons that people acquire 10 houses, 20 cars, billions of dollars, and heaven knows what else. If your instincts tell you to save, too much can never be enough. Howard Hughes (American aviation pioneer, filmmaker, industrialist and philanthropist, 1905–1976) is perhaps the most famous public figure with OCD. He accumulated accomplishments, careers, girlfriends and vast wealth, but he spent his final years largely isolated and holding on to his holdings. It is sobering to realize that since he died with the most toys, he must have won.

Behave: Warned by Wicked Thoughts

This factor is about automatic moral thinking: except that it looks like a preoccupation with transgressions sexual, aggressive, moral, religious and accidental. Epictetus (Greek philosopher, 55 –135) had this figured out: "If you desire to be good, begin by believing that you are wicked." This brings us to the notion of overbehaving. Some people will drive safely down a street, only to be overcome with the need to turn back and make sure they haven't unwittingly run someone over. Scrupulosity is overbehaving with religious overtones. Some feel compelled to atone for real, contemplated, or imagined offenses. They pray incessantly for their sins, yet they may still be preoccupied with thoughts of violent or sexual transgressions. This is not the same as religious morality, and it goes beyond what even the most orthodox of religions call for.

Worst Case Scenarios

Sometimes things can get really bad. Some are so caught up in their Obsessive-Compulsive world that there is little of it that they can describe or even let other people know about. Their very hidden inner world makes them appear only passive and mildly preoccupied on the outside. At the psychiatric office, they will typically arrive with a concerned spouse, have limited participation in ordinary life activities, and yet have little concern themselves. One man with this presentation was presumptively ("empirically") treated for OCD despite his absence of obvious symptoms. He finally did reveal his long-standing symptoms to a second psychiatrist after his first partial response to medication. The new psychiatrist, unaware of the presumptive diagnosis, heard the newly revealed symptoms and mistakenly concluded that the medication had somehow caused the OCD.

Some spend countless hours cleaning themselves, their homes, and their food. At the end of the day, they still feel that cleanliness has not been achieved. What they do have is hands that are red and raw, and furniture with the finish worn off from so much cleaning. Still others are preoccupied with arranging and rearranging books, spice bottles, DVDs, papers, numbers and more. If anything is out of place, it has to be fixed immediately. Severe hoarding leaves an apartment looking like the underground nest of some burrowing mammal. Periodically, there is a news story about a hoarder who passed away, and whose body was belatedly discovered amid the hoard. Extreme scrupulosity can leave people paralyzed and unable to make decisions. The nest requires the utmost of exacting attention.

SUBTLE AND CLOAKED SYNDROMES

Whatever instincts lead to OCD, a smaller dose also helps many people excel at staying clean, at counting and organizing, at saving for a rainy day, and at checking their antisocial impulses. With OC traits it seems likely that milder versions are actually very helpful for the success of individuals and of society. In fact, all our modern gadgets and tools can be thought of as devices that amplify our ability to carry out the useful dictates of OC traits.

Think of that bird building a sturdy and symmetrical nest. This is a good thing for the bird family, for nature lovers, and even for those who collect bird's nests. It is likely that the bird's nest-building abilities are somehow related to whatever causes human OCD, but there is no way we would want to "treat" the bird for its preoccupation with symmetry. That notion is for the birds, and not so good for the birds.

The difference between OCD and OC traits is roughly analogous to the disease and nondisease forms of sickle cell anemia and thalassemia. Both of these blood diseases cause severe illness and fatality when untreated, yet they are relatively common in West African and Mediterranean populations respectively. How can this happen? It turns out that each disease is controlled by a single genetic variation. We all have two copies of every gene, one from each parent. If you inherit a disease copy of these genes from each of your parents, you have two copies, and you get pretty sick. However, if you inherit just one copy of the gene from just one parent, the milder version protects you against malaria. Full OCD isn't likely to be a single gene syndrome, but whereas full OCD is a serious problem, mild OC traits can be an advantage for people who need to do their work cleanly, perfectly, frugally, or harmlessly.

Then there is the point that OCD is not Obsessive-Compulsive Personality Style, nor Obsessive-Compulsive Personality Disorder. This point calls for a word on personality. Everyone has a personality style (or a combination of styles), and this is not a bad thing; these styles make people more interesting and distinctive and give us something to talk about at cocktail parties. Personality styles are clusters of habits and behaviors that tend to occur together, sort of like the symptoms that make up the syndromes of diagnoses. At some point, though, the style becomes rigid enough and pronounced enough that it is self-defeating or emotionally painful. That's when a personality style becomes a personality disorder.

Back to OC Personality Style. Many people have OC Personality Style. Think of accountants, doctors, and engineers. Jobs that require precision and accuracy may attract this personality style, and they reinforce those behaviors as well. All else being equal, we want financial and medical accuracy, and we don't want poorly designed bridges that will fall down. However, an engineer with full-blown Obsessive-Compulsive Personality Disorder might be so preoccupied with perfecting a design that he might never finish or might overdesign the bridge in an impractical way.

So it is easy to confuse OCD with OC Personality Style and with OC Personality Disorder. Although they are not the same thing, and they don't always overlap, they may represent a spectrum of intensity.[20] On the milder side, there are some harmless and isolated symptoms that sound like fun (in a geeky sort of way). One patient had a lifetime habit of "counting" words, meaning that she would add up her own numerical values of the letters in the word. Those that added up to 123 were special, and she kept a life list. A particular pleasure for this successful woman was when she would find a new word for her list. A skiing accountant had a habit since childhood of counting chairs on the chairlifts. Revisiting a ski area allowed the delight of reconfirming the number of chairs. Last but not least, there are those patients who make sure to organize and neaten the piles of waiting-room magazines. Thank heaven for them.

Increasing interest in OCD has also lead to questions about possible variations and related syndromes. Muscle and vocal tics (often with foul epithets—Tourette's syndrome, if severe), are likely candidates. One group of syndromes bears a striking resemblance to the grooming behaviors of our animal cousins.[21] Remember those parrots pulling out their feathers and those dogs that lick themselves raw? Compulsive hair pulling ("trichotillomania," which includes mouthing the root end of the pulled hair) and skin-picking ("psychogenic excoriation"), are two human examples. Some 42% of patients with psychogenic excoriation also have OCD,[22] and they may improve with OCD treatment.[23] In the context of social nesting behavior, these compulsions bring to mind images of ape families grooming each other and themselves for health, emotional attachment, or for attractiveness to mates.

WHAT THE SYNDROME ISN'T

Even if you allow for a spectrum of OCD severity, it isn't the same as ordinary cleanliness, orderliness, saving and proper behavior. All these are considered virtues in our society, taught to children (with varying degrees of success), and encouraged by school, workplace, government and religious rules. Even people with little of these native instincts will work to stay clean for school, be organized for work, save money in a government-mandated retirement program, and behave themselves for their religion.

THE AGES OF OCD ANGST

OCD-like behaviors start appearing early in normal childhood. Concern for cleanliness, arranging toys exactly, collecting things, and behaving in just the right way peak at about two years of age.[24] It's a cute and normal developmental phase, but clinical OCD can start soon after, with exaggerated obsessions and compulsions that stretch into the realm of problematic behaviors.[25] Clinical OCD can also first develop (or become apparent) at much older ages, sometimes in response to stressful life events.

There is another, more intriguing trigger. Many women develop OCD or worsened OCD late in pregnancy or post-partum, with a particular focus on cleanliness and arranging behaviors, and on controlling harmful thoughts about the newborn.[26,27,28,29] Some men have lesser symptoms after childbirth as well. Nesting anyone? Think of the presumably automatic behaviors of lesser mammals after childbirth. They clean up the newborns and the afterbirth and they keep the nest tidy. No doubt birds and other animals have similar behaviors that increase the odds of newborn survival.

There are some mothers who struggle with thoughts of harming their child. One possibility is that the thoughts serve as a warning to be extra careful with a fragile newborn. A study of parents without OCD states:

> In the immediate postpartum period, more than 80% of mothers and 70% of fathers worried about harm befalling their babies: an illness threatening their health, a developmental hardship, or a defect in their appearance. Many parents reported the persistence of graphic images in which they failed as parents or harm befell their child. Several imagined dropping or throwing the baby, scratching the baby with too-long fingernails, hurting the baby in a car accident, and watching pets injure the baby—even though they would never actually act on these thoughts. Others worried about the possibility of child molestation and Sudden Infant Death Syndrome. Many parents reported that these disturbing images prompted them to make the environment even safer for their infant.[30]

Cleanliness, tidiness, and protective concern increase the likelihood of survival.

However, there is also a darker possibility. At least two observers have reported that impoverished women will sometimes allow death for their newborn infants ("neonaticide") when resources are especially wanting, or when the infant is seen as weak or defective.[31,32] Although profoundly disturbing to our sensibilities, such a mechanism could protect scarce resources for the community, and improve the perceived average productivity ("fitness") of those who survive to adulthood. Infanticide was common in primeval humankind and in societies such as ancient Greece and Rome. Then, too, the purpose was resource-preservation and deliberate selection of the strongest. Modern theologies have prohibited the practice, as in the Quran's injunction (17:31): "You shall not kill your children due to fear of poverty." Tamarind monkey mothers don't listen to theologians. They kill or let their infants die if there is a shortage of resources.[33]

There is also a more protective possibility for these disturbing thoughts. Perhaps the nesting instinct of new mothers includes defending against invaders and predators. In some species, those predators might include siblings, fathers, other adults in the group, and outsiders of all species. Having aggressive thoughts already in mind makes for a quicker defense. Most of us know never to come between a wild animal and its children. We might just want a closer look at those cute bear cubs, but Mama bears would not take any chances when their broods are at risk from human strangers.

There is also yet another intriguing trigger possibility for OCD. Some cases of human OCD begin or worsen after an infection with streptococcus bacteria. The cute acronym PANDAS stands for a more complicated but descriptive syndrome name (Pediatric Autoimmune Neuropsychiatric Disorders Associated with Streptococcal infections). Although PANDAS was first described in patients with new-onset OCD after a strep infection, another study looked at old medical charts and found that strep infections in children predicted later onset of OCD and tics.[34] Once the PANDAS syndrome is established, other infections may also worsen OCD.[24] Indeed, at least one immune-system chemical is increased in people with OCD and Tourette's syndrome.[35] It may not be just strep. People with OCD are also more likely than others to have evidence of past exposure to toxoplasmosis, a common parasite.[36]

Long ago, some primeval ancestor developed automatic mechanisms for dealing with contagious disease. The OCD symptoms serve not only to keep the individual clean, but also to provide a social warning to others to keep their distance from infection. Notably, the OCD related symptoms of PANDAS include motor tics and the offensive epithets of Tourette's syndrome. It is as if we are programmed to announce "infection here—keep your distance."

HOLDING US BACK

Despite the evolutionary and modern advantages of some Obsessive-Compulsive traits, those with the full-fledged syndrome have significant problems in our societies. Mostly this happens when cleaning or arranging behaviors become severe enough that there isn't time enough left for everyday life. People with OCD are significantly more likely to be unmarried, unemployed, and unhappy with their lives.[37]

Romance

Of course, nesting behavior is a kind of mating ritual in many species. Male birds build actual nests to entice females. Courting human males and females try to be on their best behavior. This includes showing cleanliness; carefully arranged grooming, clothing and scheduling; saved resources at their disposal (a nest egg for a house would be nice); and well-controlled impulses (certain ones, anyway). Indeed, both OCD and falling in love are associated with increased function of serotonin, that "social director" of neurotransmitters.[38,39] Clinically problematic OCD adds another layer to the story. Any pro-romantic inclinations are complicated by the adverse effects of obsessions and compulsions on closeness and intimacy.[40] Closeness is tough when your thoughts and behaviors are somewhere else.

Workplace

Work isn't so easy either. Disability is as common in OCD as in other anxiety disorders, and it is highest in those who have the most intensive symptoms. Procrastination is just one problem at work.[41] Despite, and often because of, intense deliberation, work just doesn't get done. Task completion can be so problematic that it can even look like passive aggressive behavior.[42] Work disability is usually accompanied by limited functioning in social relationships, marriage, and life enjoyment generally.[43] Disability is even more common when there are other emotional syndromes present, but work performance does get better as OCD improves with treatment.[44] Too much Obsessive-Compulsive stuff is still too much.

SYNDROME AND SOCIAL STIGMA

When you ask patients about anxiety and depressive symptoms, they are thoughtful and serious. However, when you get to OCD symptoms they often giggle, (unless, of course, they are really depressed or have OCD themselves). Maybe people instinctively see it as a sort of diagnostic curiosity without real angst, so they feel free to laugh. In a similar way, people are often teased for observable mild compulsions, such as carefully arranging the silverware at a restaurant or arranging books on shelves by strict height order. Everyone knows the value of neatness, but sometimes it is just too obvious to everyone. When observable symptoms are more severe, there can be concern bordering on revulsion: hands rubbed raw by washing, exact and obligate placement of objects on a desk, hoarding of useless things, and preoccupation with aggressive or sexual thoughts. When these seem creepy to people, they step away for fear of behavioral contamination. There but for the grace of God go they.

INSTINCT AND SYNDROME TURN UP IN CULTURE

We've already seen how modern technology and culture responds to, mimics and expands our interests and abilities in cleanliness, organization, saving and proper behavior. It is worth looking a little further into the role of religion. Religious rituals are both an outlet for these OC traits, and also an endorsement of them. Most religions pay close attention to all four Factor subtypes (especially if you consider avoidance of wasteful material things to be a form of saving—a penny saved is a penny earned). Cleanliness is next to godliness indeed. There are also English language idioms that reflect this particular interplay of OCD subtypes. You hear a lot about clean living, keeping your hands (and nose) clean, clean-cut, and dirty politics. No doubt there are similar idioms in other languages.

In the film *As Good as It Gets* (1998), actor Jack Nicholson nicely portrays a successful author burdened by OCD. His forays into the outside world are limited, and when he arrives at his favorite restaurant he carefully arranges his sterile napkin and plastic utensils, to the dismay and amusement of those around him. Rituals occupy his time at home, and he has at first little time or need for social interaction. Actually, OCD has become quite the engaging diagnosis. Likewise, the television show "Monk" portrays a detective with OCD. His OCD interferes with his work, but also promotes an obsessive attention to detail that solves crimes.

TURN THE SYNDROME AROUND: ADVANTAGES OF PARA-INSTINCTIVE BEHAVIOR

Case Study: Para-Instinctive Behavior

Just the other day, in a large office building in downtown Osaka, there worked a software engineer. He spent all day, and much of the night, writing a new video-editing program. He deliberated and planned carefully for every single line of code. Each one had to fulfill a precise function in a precise way. Each line, and each program module was checked and rechecked for accuracy and efficiency. Even after triple checking, he would still often wonder if he did it right. His programs were very, very good, but they took him quite a long time to write, and he was never certain that all was well with a finished module. All in all, his compulsive planning, organization and checking was put to good use, and it paid off in those programs that he eventually managed to complete.

While he was at work, he would clean his hands every 7 minutes (because he was born in 1977), and often surreptitiously under his desk. He brought his own soap, towels and hermetically sealed hand wipes from home, and saved a 7-week supply in a locked drawer. Sometimes he'd worry about impulsively tackling the guy at the next desk, or maybe blurting out some obscene comment to the woman behind him, but much though he worried, he was much better behaved than those around him. All in all, he very much liked his life, but was too preoccupied to feel close to anyone there, or to his wife and kids at home. Actually, since he spent little time at home, his OCD didn't interfere much with his brief visits there. To the office, he was just a hardworking, talented, meek, quiet, and private man who wrote great code, very slowly.

Maybe If Things Had Been Different...

Not long after his parents died, and when his wife started talking divorce, he felt a bit at sea, and wondered what his purpose was. Losing weight and feeling listless, he went to see his doctor, who recognized that ordinary grief had been complicated by a serious depression. The psychiatrist, alarmed by a profound Melancholic Depression, chose to start him on twice the usual dose of fluoxetine (an SSRI antidepressant). Three months later, the depression since resolved with medication and therapy, he made his first mention of the long-standing hand washing, and how it was now down to just a short rinse every two hours. His coding was just as good as ever, but now took less time and much less effort. With fewer impulses to control, he felt closer to colleagues, family, and even his wife. Who knew?

Being human, we try to ignore or override our hidden instincts. For our other four social-instinct syndromes, there are people who feel the call of unpleasant feelings, and intuitively respond by trying to overcome them. That may not happen with OCD. There are some people who are so preoccupied with obsessions that they are emotionally paralyzed and can't actually get anything done. They procrastinate, act passively, and leave their homes, finances, or dirty dishes a mess. Full-time analysis: complete paralysis. However, that is not the same thing as feeling the call of an OCD instinct, and then doing exactly the opposite. Cognitive-behavioral-therapy techniques do teach people to do some of that counter-instinctive behavior deliberately, but there don't seem to be many people who unwittingly try to be grimy, disorganized, spendthrift and nasty. Of course, there are quite a few people like that around, but they are not obviously motivated by counter-instinctive OCD. But, you never know, and anything can happen.

More commonly, people divert their OCD energies to more useful para-instinctive purposes ("sublimation" in technical parlance). They put their overnesting tendencies to good use as technical skills, elaborate attention to detail, and unceasing accomplishment (remember all the careers and accomplishments of Howard Hughes). As Thomas Alva Edison (American inventor, 1847–1931) said, "The three great essentials to achieve anything worthwhile are, first, hard work; second, stick-to-itiveness; third, common sense." Even this sublimation can have unintended consequences. The rest of your life falls by the wayside, your work is diminished, and you feel miserable. If you are already a hyper-organized perfectionist, it is counter-productive to do too much planning. New Year's resolutions are derailed when perfectionists are asked to plot out implementation strategies, and get lost in the details.[45] The road to hell is paved with too-perfect intentions.

WHERE DOES THIS COME FROM, ANYWAY
The Genetic Root of All Instinct

Obsessive-Compulsive Disorder runs in families, and it is more common in the identical twin of an affected individual than in a fraternal twin, so the evidence suggests that there is something genetic for this evolutionarily evolved instinct. However, despite intensive effort, we have only limited information beyond this basic finding.[46] Most likely, there will be many genetic contributors. Because serotonin is a central theme of our six instincts, we should point out that OCD does not appear to be related to genetically reduced serotonin activity.[47] Actually, it could be that certain brain areas have increased activity of serotonin,[38] leading to more of a social nesting instinct, which does seem logical.

Gene/Environment Interactions

Controlled studies of environmental factors that contribute to OCD are just beginning. One recent paper found that early traumatic events increased risk for hoarding behavior, though not for other OCD subtypes. In particular, the triggering events included natural disasters and close encounters with death.[48] It makes sense that those sorts of impending death experiences are more likely to prompt hoarding behavior than other traumatic experiences that don't narrowly focus our attention on physical survival.

HOW TO FIX IT: USING EVOLUTIONARY PERSPECTIVE TO EXPLAIN MODERN TREATMENT

Medication, Psychotherapy, Evolution, and Instinct

Modern treatment includes medication (high doses of SSRIs) as well as psychotherapy. Obsessive-Compulsive Disorder needs higher SSRI doses than depression,[49,50,51] perhaps paradoxically because OCD is associated with already higher levels of serotonin activity. Even though SSRI medicines work for both depression and OCD, serotonin plays very different roles. For example, experimental dietary reduction in serotonin levels (the "tryptophan depletion test") can make depression worse, but it does not make OCD worse.[52] It could be that the high SSRI doses actually have the effect of overwhelming the serotonin system, parts of which then go into a kind of shut-down mode. Therefore, instead of merely enhancing serotonin function, high-dose SSRIs effectively decrease certain serotonin activity.[53,54] Indeed, if OCD patients are given a drug that activates one particular serotonin system, their symptoms temporarily worsen.[55] It could also be that OCD is related to glutamate or other brain neurotransmitter activity, and new medications are under investigation.

Once medication has started to work, therapy includes attention to learning new ways of dealing with the world, understanding triggering events that can exaggerate attention to resource preservation, and repairing social relationships. For example, diagnosable OCD can cause significant problems in emotionally close romantic relationships.[40] Also important in therapy is modification of maladaptive, embarrassing or eccentric behaviors. People are very protective of their nest eggs, and hoarding is an especially difficult OCD subtype to treat. In fact, some patients feel as attached to their hoard as others do to people. Hoarding is so difficult to treat that some clinicians joke about using the bulldozer treatment to remove huge piles of accumulated odds and ends.

When CBT is added, patients learn to recognize that OCD symptoms are not part of their rational selves ("metacognition"). That makes it easier for them to learn to ignore obsessions and compulsions, and they even learn to put themselves through a kind of endurance training that helps obsessions and compulsions fade into the background. Perhaps this process can be enhanced if people realize that OCD symptoms have evolutionary purposes.

With diminished OCD symptoms, people become more aware of angry and anxious feelings that are associated with avoidance or prevention of OCD behaviors, as well as their sometimes exaggerated need for self-reliance. When Jack Nicholson's movie character saw the social disadvantages of his OCD, he finally accepted medication, and learned to diminish his eccentricity. Once medication starts to work, evolutionary perspective is useful in helping patients realize that their obsessions and compulsions are overkill for the actual tasks in their lives.

5

GO ALONG TO GET ALONG: ATYPICAL DEPRESSION

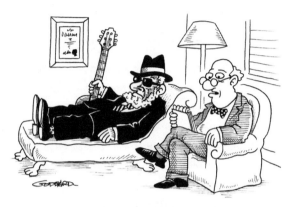

"I see. So what you're saying is that you woke up this morning
and your woman had done left you."

"The deepest principle in human nature is the craving to be appreciated."
—William James (American psychologist; 1842–1910)

"Nature, when she formed man for society, endowed him with an original desire to please,
and an original aversion to offend his brethren. She taught him to feel pleasure in their
favourable, and pain in their unfavourable regard."
—Adam Smith (Scottish economist, 1723–1790)

THE SOCIAL INSTINCT

When everyone sticks together in a society, all sorts of interpersonal frictions
can arise. Even if people know their rank in a hierarchy, there are many other
ways that they can give offense—accidentally, incidentally, or even on purpose.
That can make people angry and uncooperative with them. So what's a society
to do? It helps if there is a social instinct that promotes repentance, thoughtful-
ness and even empathy. Awareness that giving offense can trigger rejection is
heightened by what we today call rejection sensitivity, a core feature of Atypical
Depression.

BACK IN THE DAY: THE SYNDROME IN
PRIMEVAL HUMAN SOCIETY

Case Study: How It Might Have Helped Long Ago

Thousands of years ago, in a forest clearing on the Indian subcontinent, there lived a girl in a human troop. As a child, her attention would often wander as she did her chores, and sometimes one would be left unfinished before she moved on to the next. There was some advantage to the family in this, since it was easier to shift her attention to new chores as they arose, and the girl was someone who liked to do what she was told. As she grew older, there would be times when she did not get the approval she needed from the troop, and sometimes would feel rejected by even the smallest slight. This would make her feel hurt, sad, hungry and tired.

She would retreat from the troop for a while, take long naps and eat as much food as she could find. The naps kept her out of the social whirl, and the food kept her metabolism going in the meantime. Then she would gradually rejoin everyone (faster if she was encouraged to), until the next time she felt rejected, which was often. Without realizing it, she paid particular attention to not offending anyone. Rejection was the last thing she wanted. Not surprisingly, she became known for her inoffensive ways.

Actually, to varying degrees, everyone tried not to offend, and felt hurt by small rejections. This was good news for the troop because it meant that everyone was trying to get along with one another. When it became clear to someone that they had done wrong, their hurt would show their recognition, and their temporary withdrawal and somberness would show a kind of apology. After a period of "repentance," they would reinstate themselves into the troop. People got along pretty well, even with other levels of the hierarchy, although fights with other troops were another matter entirely.

One time, the girl started spending time with a boy in the troop. In the custom of the troop, this suggested a progression to marriage. However, with the boy from a lower-hierarchy rung, her father felt the family risked rejection from the troop (and thus death if they were on their own) and so he scared the boy off. This was a devastating rejection for the girl, and her hurt and sadness knew no bounds. She felt so miserable that all chores were a chore, so hungry that no meal was enough, and so tired that she slept nearly all the time. Even when awake, she would do little more than gaze

passively at the distant Himalayas. This went on for months. She under-
stood the serious consequences if her father failed to maintain proper fam-
ily behavior. But no social time-out or symbolic repentance offered any
hope of relief. Although it was a long time before she risked spending time
with a boy again, she did finally find a mate and a woman's role in the
troop. She was always quick to apologize, and careful not to offend.

BASIC PRINCIPLE: AVOID HURT IN THE HERD

In ancient society, the rejection sensitivity of Atypical Depression made individuals more compliant to the agendas of leaders and group members, and less likely to give offense to anyone. In that way they would avoid feeling rejected. Actual ejection from the group would no doubt have been fatal. When in the tribe, do as the tribe does. It was a wise approach.

Rejection sensitivity has all sorts of advantages for tribal society. It helps people sense and follow cultural norms, learn new skills through imitation of others, and try to avoid confrontation and hostility within the tribe. Those painful little doses of rejection sensitivity make everyone look and act like one big happy family.

AMONG THE ANIMALS

Yankees great Yogi Berra (American baseball player, 1925 –) once said that "you can learn a lot just by watching." Watch a dog sometime. They know when they have broken their humans' rules. They slink into a corner, head and tail down. When you come home from work and see regret written all over them, you know something has happened during the day. Our beta dog Cassidy was especially apologetic once, when after finishing off a pie, he glumly greeted us with his head poking through the plastic window of the pie box top, still stuck around his neck.

When dogs and coyotes play, it is often a playful form of combat—preparation for both hunting and for adult social interactions. As they bite and pounce, they don't mean to hurt each other, but accidents do happen, and animals don't like it when there is a breach in the rules of polite canid society.[1] So, how to keep the peace? When a play-fighting coyote bites too hard, his playmate will let him know, and he will respond with an "apologetic" posture that says he will try to behave himself.[2] He had better, because habitual rule breakers are thrown out of the game. Then they try to look penitent, hoping to be allowed back onto the field of play.

Cassidy knew all this, of course, but the pie was just too good to resist. Just like us, animal regret protects them from social rejection. There is even some evidence that this biological instinct may reside at a regret center in the monkey brain,[3] and more research is yet to come.

TIMES HAVE CHANGED

A little rejection sensitivity now and then is a good thing, because it helps people realize other peoples' feelings and reactions, and it helps them fine-tune behavior to reduce frictions in the group. However, people who are too, too sensitive find themselves easily hurt by minor perceived slights, suffering the slings and arrows of depression, overeating, oversleeping, and more.

Most of us aren't living in small troops of humans anymore. That means that we run into a whole lot of strangers, with a wide variety of personalities, relationships, cultural values, and cultural reactions. It is very nearly impossible to keep track of everyone's particular concerns, and it is all too easy to give offense. Trailed by an attentive sales clerk in a Tokyo department store, a tourist tried politely to wave her off in English and with gestures. Because nothing seemed to inform her, he gently said "no" in halting Japanese, to which she burst into tears and rushed away. The culturally oblivious Ugly American didn't know not to say "no" (better to have said "maybe"). So those with heightened rejection sensitivity find themselves tip-toeing very carefully to protect themselves even from unintended rejections by mortified tourists.

HOW INSTINCT BECOMES SYNDROME IN MODERN SOCIETY
Instinct and Worldview

The core cognitive symptom of Atypical Depression is increased rejection sensitivity: a heightened concern for the possibility of being rejected by others, or by the group as a whole, and a heightened emotional reaction. This is not entirely a bad thing of course, because our comfort and very survival depend on being part of a social group. So, feeling hurt by rejection makes people think hard about how not to be rejected, and how to avoid situations that even raise that possibility.[4] When rejection is felt, people want to pull away and recover. They go into a kind of hibernation, where they eat more, sleep more, avoid pleasurable activities, and contemplate their "misdeeds." Teenagers with more sleepiness and depression are the same ones who crave carbohydrates and chocolates.[5] For some, they sadly end up in this state much of their adult lives. Perhaps this perpetual hibernation protects them from enduring yet more rejection.

Case Study: Instinctive Syndromes in Modern Society

A short time ago, in a human family in an urban Beijing neighborhood, there lived a boy. Quiet as a child, he remained quiet as an adolescent. In high school, he started to realize how unhappy and alone he felt. Having no one to eat lunch with, and afraid of rejection, he tried to sit at a table before anyone else chose to join him there. Even though they did sit down with him, he still ate with apprehension. He ate together with them, perhaps, but always worried about their rejection. He did everything he could to stay in their good graces, though it was actually their bad graces that he most feared.

When he was teased (this was high school, after all), he could never think of a witty response. Instead, he would feel deeply hurt, and often hurry home. There, he would oversleep and feel a sort of dazed lethargy. He'd watch television and laugh at the jokes, but the solace was brief, and the sadness quickly returned. Sometimes he didn't go to school for a couple of days. If this happened during Chinese New Year, his family would have to drag him out for the fireworks and Chinese lion dancing. Even this brought only a brief respite. Eventually, though, he would pull himself back together, and get back to classes.

Although he was careful not to get so close to people as to risk rejection, he did have a small circle of friends—mostly kids as sensitive as him. One day, a good friend saw him pass on the sidewalk, and she did not say hello because she was preoccupied with an upcoming exam. He was devastated—surely, this was a sign of some permanent rejection, so he holed up at home for three whole days.

Over time, he gained weight, overslept, and felt miserable. His caution with people helped him keep a job, but limited his potential. His observable lack of energy and somewhat lower productivity didn't help much either. Not very happy, not a failure, he kept plugging along.

Maybe If Things Had Been Different…

A few years after high school, he read online about Atypical Depression. "That," he realized with only mildly energetic enthusiasm "is me." Some months later, he decided to look into it. On medication (citalopram, an SSRI antidepressant) with a booster (buspirone, marketed for anxiety but used also off-label for this purpose), he felt new energy, new confidence and new optimism. Although his appetite decreased, there was little change in

> *his weight. Some people actually noticed the changes. His work improved; he met some new friends on the job, and he joined a pick-up basketball game down the street. Things were looking up.*

HOW DOES THAT MAKE YOU FEEL?

Atypical Depression is misery. It is the raw primal sensation of our instincts telling us painfully that we must make amends for breaking the code of our tribe. It makes us recognize that we better rethink, repent, and reduce our presence for a while. It is a pervasive urge to hunker down for safety. The evolutionary advantage of this is that it helps us stay friendly with the others in our tribe. Discord and infighting in the tribe would not have been helpful to our ancestors, and besides we could end up on the losing side of a fight. The ongoing rejection sensitivity of Atypical Depression keeps us alert to behaviors that threaten social harmony, and alert to negative cues from others, even when you do behave yourself. Still, when we have ongoing Atypical Depression, we do learn to cope at least somewhat. It does still affect us, but we find ways to keep going even as we feel like hunkering down.

Because we are rational humans, we sometimes try to ignore this instinctual gauge of proper social behavior. Are you afraid to say that you are a liberal (or a conservative)? How silly! We should stand up for our views in a society that values differing opinions (mostly). Still, our instincts don't understand reason; they are more responsive to the fear of putting people off with nonconforming ideas and behaviors. As a result, our human reason can lead us to feel rejected, and then to feel a need to keep that lower profile. Even in a confidential psychiatric office, many people are uneasy talking about such potentially off-putting topics as politics and religion.

WHAT THIS SYNDROME IS

Though the name Atypical Depression is unfamiliar to many, it may be the most common form of depression, despite the "atypical." The name contrasts this chronic depression with the more well-known acute Melancholic Depression, which we'll discuss in chapter 6. Many researchers now joke that Atypical Depression should have been called "typical." One review suggests that the full-fledged diagnosis affects between 1 and 7% of the general population, whereas our own data from corporate employees puts the lifetime diagnosis number at 3.6%.[6] A less strictly defined depression with atypical features may affect 10%.[7] Just think of all the guilty conformists that you know. Atypical Depression varies in severity over time, and has characteristic physical symptoms, which can include frequent episodes of oversleeping, overeating, lethargy, and sadness (but with the ability to cheer up briefly). Importantly, there is always a heightened inner sensitivity to social rejection. (Syndrome details are in the appendix.). Even a co-worker forgetting to say hello can trigger a massive emotional response. Psychiatrists think of this as heightened "rejection sensitivity."

WHO FIGURED OUT THIS SYNDROME?

Atypical Depression is actually a particular type of depression. Psychiatrists were already familiar with Melancholic Depression, which was then thought of as the most representative form. This new type, though, was recognized some 50 years ago as having symptoms that seemed opposite in many ways; for example, appetite increased rather than decreasing, and there were more hours asleep rather than less.[8] Not typical? Must be atypical.

Moreover, Atypical Depression does not respond to the older tricyclic antidepressants, but it does respond quite well to the older still Monoamine Oxidase Inhibitor Antidepressants (MAOIs), as well as to the modern SSRIs (such as fluoxetine, brand named Prozac). This is a good place to point out that the first MAOI was not only the first antidepressant, but it was also originally developed as the first tuberculosis (TB) drug. Somebody made the astute observation that it also treated depression in TB patients. Later MAOI and TB drugs were more effective for their specific purposes, but lost the dual action. Coming full circle, the newish antibiotic linezolid also turns out to be an MAOI, albeit a weak one. How curious is that?

Some 40 years ago, Donald Klein noted the central importance of rejection sensitivity to Atypical Depression, (which was then called hysteroid dysphoria).[9] He and his team also performed a "pharmacological dissection" of Atypical Depression, with their observation that the MAOIs were effective, but tricyclic antidepressants were not. The varied names were sorted out some 30 years ago, and Atypical Depression is now officially recognized as a subtype of depression in *DSM-IV-TR*. In addition, many people with chronic mild depression (dysthymia) have the Atypical Depression subtype on closer inspection. Its proponents would argue, though, that Atypical Depression is actually a separate and distinct illness, rather than a mere subtype, and that atypical is the most common specific form of depression. Because it responds well to SSRIs, it is also the reason that fluoxetine (brand name Prozac) was so rapidly adopted.

PEOPLE DON'T LIKE BEING TREATED LIKE DOGS

Dogs and coyotes sense rejection, and they work to repair the rift if they can. People are like that too, though they can be hostile if they see no way back in. In a Manhattan psychology laboratory, college students with more rejection sensitivity will work harder at ingratiating themselves than others. Of course, rejection-sensitive men and women have different ideas about what kinds of rejection matter to them—men in the study cared more about social-status implications, whereas women were more affected by threats to a close relationship.[10] Truth be told, it is really dogs who don't want to be treated like people. Cesar Millan (television's Dog Whisperer) knows about this. There aren't nearly as many bad dogs as there are human owners who don't know how to treat a dog right.

WORST CASE SCENARIO

What happens when someone has a really bad case of Atypical Depression? They may endure the symptoms for a long time after a minor rejection, and the symptoms can become so ingrained that ongoing rejections aren't even needed. So, they tend to be sad most of the time, sleep as much as they can get away with, feel lethargic anyway, and eat (especially sweets, chocolate and carbohydrates in large quantities). Because of the intensity of their sensitivity, they avoid getting too emotionally close to others (even family) and avoid social pleasures, lest they feel rejected. If people get too close, they'll push them away a bit to protect themselves.

Too much emotional reactivity to rejection can cause another problem. For example, it can be a central feature of some personality disorders. Borderline Personality Disorder, in particular, includes dramatic reactions to perceived or anticipated slights.[11] The seemingly frantic, tragic, hostile and self-harmful behaviors of Borderline Personality are a desperate attempt to control those feelings, but they only make it harder and harder for people to find good solutions in their lives. Reducing their rejection sensitivity is part of their path to a better life.

SUBTLE AND CLOAKED SYNDROMES

There is something called Seasonal Affective Disorder (SAD, as it happens). It is a form of Atypical Depression triggered by short winter days, with their reduced sunlight. SAD is more common in Fairbanks[12] than in Florida of course.[13] The symptoms and treatment are pretty much the same, but SAD is often treated with light therapy. Norman Rosenthal (American psychiatrist, 1950–) figured out most of this in the 1980s.

Then there is Premenstrual Dysphoric Disorder (PMDD; a severe and uncommon form of premenstrual syndrome), which occurs soon after ovulation and ends with menses. Premenstrual Dysphoric Disorder fsymptoms are pretty much like those Atypical Depression symptoms that are provoked by feeling rejected, and that, therefore, predispose patients to less independent behavior. Premenstrual Dysphoric Disorder may also include Panic Anxiety, which also promotes staying close.[14] Controversially, women may be more attractive to men, and themselves attracted to more dominant men, during ovulation than at other times.[15] Other wild mammalian species have sex only when the female is receptive and accepting, at peak fertility. In rats this is related to serotonin again.[16] So, while humans have sex even when procreation is not likely, PMDD could be a vestigial remnant of a more receptive ovulatory phase in primeval women.

Although no one has yet looked carefully, human mothers may have reduced Atypical Depression after childbirth. That is a time when active behavior and a good mood are important for infants (and spouses). (We've already learned that a little Panic can also help mothers stay closer, and post partum depression may actually be too much Panic.) This may be why, in our rat cousins, successful nurturing by the mother requires having enough serotonin around.[17]

WHAT THE SYNDROME ISN'T

Of course, nearly everyone feels a little hurt by rejection or criticism. In small degree, that is not necessarily a problem for them, nor is it evidence of any sort of disorder. If people feel hurt after a really big rejection—abandonment by a spouse, for example—even that seems to be pretty normal. Rejection sensitivity seems to exist on a spectrum of severity. One very rough gauge of diagnosable symptom severity is the answer to this interview question: "If a close friend passes you on the sidewalk, clearly sees you and does not say hello, would you feel hurt?" People with Atypical Depression generally say yes ("How could they do that to me?"), whereas others say no ("Their mind must be in another world"). Actually, there are some people who seem completely insensitive to rejection and criticism. That leaves them with little intuitive emotional input about what other people think and with more freedom for solitary reasoning and behavioral choices, but they have less instinctual collaboration and group membership.

THE AGES OF ATYPICAL DEPRESSION ANGST

When we take a careful psychiatric history, patients typically point back to depressed mood in their early teens, but the rejection sensitivity must go way back further. There are plenty of us who are "sensitive" from an early age. In Iowa, an experiment with 2-year-old children led them to think they had broken the experimenter's favorite toy. That made them feel and show varying degrees of guilt by hiding their faces and averting their eyes, trying not to be rejected for their transgression. Those who showed more guilt had fewer behavioral problems over the next five years. This socially useful kind of rejection sensitivity starts way back then. Hopefully, the children felt better when they were given a kind of ritual absolution after the experiment was over.[18] However, since it takes a while for people to realize the difference between depressive feelings and their connection to perceived rejection, one epidemiologic study put the average age at onset for the less rigorously defined atypical features of depression at 27.[7]

HOLDING US BACK

In modern society, rejection sensitivity can also lead to an unpleasantly conformist and placid role (although some other people are content that way). What you won't find in the *DSM-IV-TR* is how rejection sensitivity makes some people go overboard in trying to avoid rejections. Acceptance can be so desperately needed that they go to awkward and counter-productive lengths to find it.

Afraid of social rejection in high school (and who isn't)? Well, try to be the first to sit at a lunch table. That way you are "accepted" by anyone who sits down with you. Don't want to be called out for your appearance? Just be a slave to fashion (and remember how the "nonconformists" of the 1970s developed a strict uniform of blue jeans, informal shirts and long hair). "Sensitive" people try especially hard to comply with behaviors of the larger group, or at least of some particular sub-group. They want to fulfill the requirements of membership. Go go along to get along. Or perhaps they do unto others as they would have others do unto them.

Less-often remembered is the additional presence of "acceptance sensitivity." People with Atypical Depression have a notably heightened response to positive regard, including such things as party invitations, merit badges, "employee of the month" awards, and to sincere, if minor, compliments. So, they find roles, behaviors and occupations where they are less exposed to the possibility of rejection and more likely to find approval from the group. Rejection sensitivity makes people want to behave, and acceptance sensitivity makes people feel glad that they did. All in all, these sorts of reactions can help people feel more a part of the group. Edgy, perhaps, but bonded.

However, all this can lead to too much conformity for everyone's good. Groupthink can cause lemming-like behavior that leads everyone to the same dismal fate (lemmings are Arctic rodents thought to have the habit of following each other off cliffs). Tulip manias, stock-market bubbles and pet-gerbil hysterias eventually collapse, and everyone wonders why they hadn't seen it coming. (Tempted to breed valuable gerbils as a child, with vivid recollection of the price hysteria back then, there is no mention of it on the internet). Investors (and their computer programs) herd themselves mostly into the same pastures as other investors.[19] What economists call "momentum investing" is all-too-often followed by stock market bubbles and crashes.

Our rejection sensitivity leads us to value (and overvalue) the valuation opinions of others for as long as possible. Laboratory research that shows that a brain center for social valuation of music choices is strongly influenced by the opinions of others, at least in the case of college students deciding what music they like. Each to his own taste? Not exactly. Oh, and about those lemming stories? They may get lost on mass migrations, but they don't actually commit mass suicide or jump off cliffs together. This age-old Arctic myth was popularized in a 1958 movie that used a turntable to launch the poor things off a cliff.[20] Real lemmings don't act like lemmings, even if some people do.

Garrison Keillor (American humorist and radio host, 1942–) points this out nicely: "Experiments with laboratory rats have shown that, if one psychologist in the room laughs at something a rat does, all of the other psychologists in the room will laugh equally. Nobody wants to be left holding the joke." All kidding aside, groupthink is not good for scientific research, other creative pursuits or any kind of problem solving (almost everything needs creativity now and again). Conformist groupthink is not the same as the Socially Anxious "yes men" who use follow-the-leader thinking. Both can interfere with the wisdom of crowds, which relies on combining independent perceptions and ideas.

So, Atypical Depression can lead people to conformism in order to feel more secure. Well, how comforted are they? Not enough, it turns out. In a study of adults at a depression clinic (not just college student volunteers this time), those with Atypical Depression were less likely to feel secure in their relations, and more likely to have "anxious/ambivalent" relationships. Secure? Maybe. Fearful of rejection? Still.[21]

On the other hand, sensitive people are also more sensitive toward others. They are predisposed to increased recognition of the thoughts and feelings of others ("Theory of Mind"). Research shows that this enhanced Theory of Mind is associated with a maternal history of depression in both depressed and nondepressed adult women.[22] This makes them more empathic, or at least more sympathetic. While we are at it, empathy is the ability to recognize the feelings and motivations of others; sympathy is awareness of the expressed concerns or outward displays of others. Empathy leads to compassion, whereas sympathy leads to commiseration or pity. Which would you prefer?

In *The Wisdom of Crowds*[23] James Surowiecki (American journalist, 1967 –) points out that for groups and societies to make the best decisions, harmony is needed, but conformity must not crowd out the combined wisdom of multiple opinions, diverse perspectives, varied information sources and independent judgments. Therefore, maybe what we need is just the right amount of rejection sensitivity, but not so much that it turns into something so painful that it needs help.

THE INSTINCT IS WITH US STILL

We don't want a society full of people who are immune to the rejection and disapproval of others. Think of someone you know who cares not a whit for the feelings and opinions of friends and family, and imagine if everyone was like that. Rejection sensitivity gives us at least a baseline level of concern for the opinions and welfare of other people, and maybe it actually works. In another study of college students (Aussies, this time), sticking their hands into painfully cold water made them feel less guilty about past misdeeds. The guiltier ones kept their hands in even longer.[24] With that in mind, the pain of rejection sensitivity could be an instinctively self-applied punishment for breaking with society, and real physical pain can serve the same purpose. This kind of repentance through pain is complemented by a Massachusetts study showing that imagining social losses prompts an increased desire for social contact.[25]

That's not all we know about students down under. It turns out that people who are made to feel sadder (by experimentally contrived criticism or by sad movies) are also fairer in a psychology-lab test of sharing. Sadness makes them more likely to share their raffle tickets—no doubt to assuage sadness experienced as guilt.[26]

Romance

How do you solve a problem like rejection? It is hard enough to meet a potential romantic partner, so imagine if you were unduly sensitive to rejection. It's enough to make you hold so far back that they can't even see you, or to keep up such an emotional wall that you never actually connect. That can actually be more comfortable for some people, though disappointing nonetheless. Emotional closeness can also develop gradually over time, as long as nothing bad happens. Some sensitive souls find each other and connect on that very level. However, the risk for many is an emotional roller coaster of a relationship.

Rejection-sensitive folks pay more attention to nuances, interpret them more negatively, and react in ways that compromise romance.[27] This can include hostility, or quiet self-silencing.[28] Suffering in silence may have at least one advantage. It reduces the release of the stress hormone cortisol. For the most rejection-sensitive, this silence may be protective against their highly exaggerated cortisol response to rejection.[29] This makes sense, since they do find rejection so stressful.[30] The more often you feel rejected, the more you will find yet other psychological ways to protect your emotions and your biology.

Looking for Love in All the Wrong Places

One solution that people use is preemptive rejection, or as they said in the Westerns, "heading them off at the pass." If a potential partner is getting emotionally closer, then pushing them away (sometimes with hostility they record in their own diaries) is a protection against rejection, except that the partners sense the emotional distance, and then they respond with even more actual rejection[31]—a vicious cycle indeed. Even without hostility, folks with more rejection sensitivity somehow can end up with more rejecting partners. People are attracted to the familiar, and that includes the very rejection that they are accustomed to dealing with. As Rita Rudner (American comedienne, 1953–) said, "I love being married. It's so great to find that one special person you want to annoy for the rest of your life." Sounds real good, but this sort of thing tends not to last for the long term.

Another unwitting technique is to find seemingly unobtainable partners, such as people who are already married, clearly disinterested, or living far away. Any rejection is then buffered by the thought that it was inevitable. "Of course we broke up," one might think, "we never had a chance. There is nothing for me to feel hurt about."

Then there are some who push away the hurt with the thought that it is not about them, it is about their looks. People who are more rejection sensitive (especially as far as their appearance is concerned) are more likely to want plastic surgery. This even remains true after statistics takes out the effects of depressed mood, weight, and self-appraised appearance.[32,33] The hope, of course, is that improving their physical appearance will make them less likely to be rejected. Actually, plastic-surgery patients are generally satisfied with the cosmetic results, but it doesn't do so much for state of mind.

Maybe some chocolate can help. Chocolates are romantic, and chocolate cravings are a very common in part of Atypical Depression. Coincidence? Maybe. (Roses are also romantic, perhaps for their appealing smell, but there is no science yet about rose cravings). People with mild depression do eat more chocolate,[34] and chocolate can increase serotonin activity in the brain.[35]

Something called phenylethylamine (PEA) may be the active ingredient in chocolate. It actually works as an antidepressant for mice.[36] Phenylethylamine may also be a tiger pheromone[37] that lures prey with a scent of romance or affection. Indeed, since PEA reduces fear in mice,[38] mice should be careful about the scented lure of tigers.

When rejection sensitivity does lead to feelings of guilt and eagerness to please, people are much more likely to say "I'm sorry" to their partner, but only if they overcome the hurdle of recognizing that there is actual potential in this approach. Studies show that those two words go a long way to helping relationships, even experimentally in college students.[39] A comedian was once asked how he stayed married for 50 years. "Easy," he said, "every night I whisper the same three words into my wife's ear: I *am* sorry."

Workplace

People with ordinary Atypical Depression do often run into problems at work. They feel lethargic, so they may be seen as lazy or underachieving by others, even when they are trying their hardest. Because of their chronic depression, they may seem cold, serious, or distant to co-workers. That distance can increase because of the need to protect against rejection. That same sort of anxious/ambivalent relationship in romances can be a problem with colleagues too. Then again, Atypical Depression can lead some people to try hard to rejection-proof their behavior and performance. Some even try extra hard, as we will see. However, all this can suddenly be undone by loud carping about perceived mistreatment, triggered by some minor rejection or criticism.

What happens to them in the workplace? Well, to start with, they are less likely to be there. Adults with Dysthymic Disorder (a different and more general syndrome of chronic mild depression, but useful as a rough proxy for a group with Atypical Depression)[40] are less likely to be working (only 36.2%) than never-depressed adults (52.0%) in one study, and more likely to be on Social Security Disability (13.9% versus 2.9%). Needless to say, it is also true that not working can be demoralizing. However, people with Dysthymia are also much more likely to say that their emotions interfere with their social lives and with their accomplishment generally.[41] Even when they try their darndest, they may need a Herculean effort to overcome their symptoms and get their work done. It's not easy being tired, sad, sensitive, and self-protective.

INSTINCT AND SOCIAL STIGMA

As befits a syndrome that evolved for instinctively social purposes, other people do notice Atypical Depression. The resulting "stigma" is partly a subtle reaction to sensing the rejection sensitivity of others, and it increases if onlookers witness a particularly obvious reaction. People react by keeping a certain emotional distance from people who are "too sensitive" if they don't want those people to feel hurt, or else they try the reassurance route. Either way, the relationship that results is colored by anxious uncertainty ("how will this turn out?") and ambivalent attachment ("should

I stay or should I go?"). It can be like walking on eggshells, with careful attention to proper behavior all around.

People also react to other symptoms. Low-energy people are seen sometimes as lazy; people who eat too much are seen as unable to control their diet; people who sleep too much are considered unmotivated. Not too far off the mark for an instinct that is designed for hunkering down and keeping a low profile.

Speaking about stigma, it is even tempting here to wonder about a connection to the seven deadly sins (or at least to four of them). Keep in mind that to the early Christians and the traditionalist Catholic Church these seven sins are cardinal sins, because they were thought to predispose people to even more serious vices. The mnemonic "SALIGIA" is derived from the first Latin letters of the seven deadly sins: *superbia, avaritia, luxuria, invidia, gula, ira, acedia* (if you will: pride/hubris, avarice/greed, lust/excessive attention to others, envy, gluttony, anger/wrath, sloth/despair). Lust for others (and not just the carnal kind) sounds like the loneliness of rejection sensitivity. Gluttony resembles the increased appetite for food, wrath the snappish reaction to rejection, sloth the lethargy of depression, and despair the depression itself.

However, for the three deadly sins that remain, let's get some help from Greek mythology. There was the envious Daedelus (who killed his nephew for first inventing the saw); his son, the hubristic Icarus (who flew so high that his wings were melted by the sun); and avaricious King Midas (who gained the golden touch, but turned his food and daughter to the precious metal). These are three ways to pump up your ego and feel less rejected by society, but all at the risk of incurring the wrath of the Gods. Envy, hubris, and greed make us think of Narcissistic Personality. The more pronounced version called Pathological Narcissism brings us back to that concern for the greater vices. The Narcissism portrayed in Greek mythology is all over the news even today. Indeed, people with Narcissistic Personality are especially sensitive to social rejection, which they perceive as loss of social desirability ("narcissistic injury" in the trade), and they are more likely to retaliate with anger and aggression, or even to direct their hostility at bystanders.[42]

Carrying this cheeky notion a few thousand miles further, how bad are the seven deadly sins in Sin City? Some folks from Kansas State University actually looked into this. Using publically available population statistics as proxies for the sins (a few choices to quibble with there), they surmised that Clark County (Las Vegas) had the rest of Nevada pretty much beat, though not necessarily the whole rest of the country ("rigorous mapping of ridiculous data" reported the *Las Vegas Sun*).[43] Additionally, one not-so-far away modern Hungarian has thoughtfully pondered if the seven deadly sins (just like Atypical Depression) are each related to serotonin in the brain.[44]

INSTINCT AND SYNDROME TURN UP IN CULTURE

So how does society handle a problem like rejection sensitivity? We have all sorts of rules and customs to help us get along. "Do unto others as you would have others do unto you" is a mantra for this goal. Secret ballots in a democracy let people vote their consciences without fearing rejection. The military requires soldiers passing on a sidewalk to acknowledge each other with a salute (Nancy Petersmeyer; American military psychiatrist, 1954–). Some grade schools prohibit parties that don't invite every child in the class. Every society has a way of reducing direct criticism and rejection (even those that do encourage direct confrontation at times). Nobody likes to be dissed.

There are some times, though, when overt rejection is necessary. Colleges send rejection letters that emphasize the size and talent of their applicant pool, as well as the impersonality of their selection process. In Japan, the college rejection is less personal because it is mostly based on one standardized national examination score. The art of "Dear John" letters (and conversations) is in their attempt to redefine rejection as good fortune: "It's not you, it's me"; "You can find someone better than me," or, these days, "I'm just not ready to commit." Society also helps people cope after the fact. There are legal, cultural, social, and religious mechanisms for repentance, encouragement of conformity, forgiveness, consolation (and consolation prizes), apologies, and, of course, lawsuits.

Society utilizes rejection sensitivity as well. Do bad things as a child? Get sent to your room or to a corner for a "time-out." Do bad things as an adult? Get sent to prison. Do really bad things? Get put into solitary confinement. Then, there is military basic training. Criticism and implied social rejection are direct, intense, and absent any evidence of sugarcoating. There is no attempt to avoid rejection sensitivities, because the whole idea is to make soldiers "toughen up," so that ultimately they can rely on each other despite touchy situations that might arise from time to time.

The musical style and lyrical themes of American blues music include a never-endingly creative reflection on the sadness and rejection sensitivity of Atypical Depression. It is hard to miss all those songs about losing lovers and leaving town. However, the simple lyrics of this one verse from Robert Johnson's (American bluesman, 1911–1938) classic song "Crossroads" capture the essence:

I went down to the crossroads,
Tried to flag a ride.
I went down to the crossroads,
Tried to flag a ride.
Nobody seemed to know me,

Everybody passed me by.

Heartbreaking. And reassuringly soulful to the sensitive spirit.

The forward-thinking last verse of Elmore James' (American bluesman, 1918–1963) classic song "Done Somebody Wrong" even anticipates the value of treatment:

The bell has tolled, my baby done caught that train and gone.
The bell has tolled, my baby done caught that train and gone.
It was all my fault, I must have done somebody wrong.
Everything that happens, you know I am to blame.
Everything that happens, you know I am to blame.
Gonna find myself a doctor, perhaps my luck will change.

To look at this social instinct from another perspective, Hank Williams, Sr. (American bluesman with country trimmings, 1923–1953) vividly describes the kind of anxious and ambivalent attachment of a woman with Atypical Depression in these selected verses from "Cold, Cold Heart":

I've tried so hard, my dear, to show,
that you're my every dream.
Yet you're afraid each thing I do,
is just some evil scheme.

Another love before my time,
made your heart sad an' blue.
And so my heart is paying now,
for things I didn't do.

In anger unkind words are said,
that make the teardrops start.
Why can't I free your doubtful mind,
and melt your cold cold heart.

You can almost feel her self-protection against even the possibility of rejection.

TURN THE SYNDROME AROUND: ADVANTAGES OF COUNTER-INSTINCTIVE BEHAVIOR

Case Study: Counter-Instinctive Behavior

Not very long ago at all, in a mansion-dwelling human family in Chicago, there lived a boy. A sad and "serious" child, he sat quietly in school, and watched videos at home. It wasn't that he didn't like people, but they didn't understand his seriousness, and he couldn't respond to their lighthearted banter. So he pushed himself though life. The slightest slight would send him into a tailspin, with an urge to sleep, eat and withdraw. He needed a solution, and he found one—just fight it off! When he felt tired he would exercise. When he wanted to oversleep he would set an extra alarm. When he felt extra hungry, he would diet. And when he felt hurt, he would respond with tolerance or even kindness, even though his irritation would often still show.

As a result, he became a driven soul. Every waking hour was filled with constructive effort. He achieved more than average, but he couldn't slow down. He won prizes, but couldn't pause to enjoy them. He couldn't even lie passively on the Lake Michigan beach for more than five minutes. He would have to get himself up to do something, anything constructive. He had a wide social circle, but no close friends.

Not surprisingly, his driven dedication made him a successful lawyer, who pulled all-nighters, expected others to do the same, and quickly moved up the ranks at his firm. They were glad to have him; he made partner at a young age, and he was the rising legal star of the Windy City. He was still on that treadmill when he started to feel empty. Sure, he was a big success, and had a larger mansion than his father, but wasn't there something more? After a vacation to Hawaii (not a moment left unscheduled, of course), he decided to quit the law. Newly ensconced in a yet larger mansion on Maui, he set to work. Complex home improvements were followed by a real-estate-development company, and he even took on a few legal clients. It was a second stage of success, but the emptiness had not changed. A third divorce left him barely solvent and more careful about his money. He hardly spoke to his three children. Why wasn't there anything more?

Maybe If Things Had Been Different...

When the managing partner learned that he planned to quit the firm for Hawaii, he called him in. "I've known you for a long time," he said, "and it won't be any different for you there. Wherever you go, there you are. I love Hawaii myself, but I go there to get away from work and schedules. Nothing but swimming and golf is all I do there. Your real problem is inside you." The now-grown boy thought about this, and before taking a giant leap across the Pacific Ocean, he decided to investigate. There were many consultations, many books, many time-consuming hobbies, and many failed efforts to do nothing for a full hour at the beach. Finally, one *psychiatrist asked if he felt sad or alone. A terrifying thought, but it hit home. Fluoxetine (an SSRI antidepressant) relieved some of the sadness. Psychotherapy helped him understand how sadness and rejection sensitivity had shaped his life and personality. Drivenness became mere hard work. Now he could stop and celebrate a legal victory, and even lie on the beach. That one took a bit more practice—it took some time for the fear of overwhelming aloneness to die down. Best of all, and to his utter surprise, he felt emotionally closer to his family and friends. No longer a Cold Cold Heart.*

SOCIAL ALARMS PROMPT SELF-IMPROVEMENT

They say that firemen are different from everyone else because they run toward the flames, instead of in the other direction. It doesn't seem natural to risk a burn, until you realize that flames to them are an opportunity to serve society, and to prove their mastery. Situations that threaten rejection are like that for some people with Atypical Depression. They seek it out to prove and improve themselves. It hurts, but they grin and bear it; they gradually learn how to reduce the rejection, and they gain mastery over the situation. "I take rejection as someone blowing a bugle in my ear to wake me up and get going, rather than retreat."—Sylvester Stallone (American actor, 1946 –).

What does this look like? It looks like grim driven Type A workaholics who can't stop even to breathe. Unlike merely hardworking people, these folks can't let themselves savor a victory and smell the roses, because they have to keep pushing to fend off depression and fear of rejection. As one patient put it, whenever he felt tired he went to the gym, when sad to work, and when hungry to a diet. He spent his time surrounded by people, but that didn't mean he felt warm and fuzzy with them. He mastered much more than just the rejection sensitivity, but he realized at some point that he felt socially detached and unfulfilled.

Grim determination and endless hard work is not all bad. It helps individual success, and it contributes to society as well. As Barbara Corcoran (American real estate entrepreneur, 1949 -) says, "Ask yourself the question of how good are you with rejection. When you get slammed on the head personally, professionally—when you're handed insult—when people don't believe—when your parents didn't love you good enough—when your brother says you'll never be anything—how good are you at standing back up? If you can bounce back faster than the next guy...that's a natural entrepreneur wired for success in business."[45] However, there is more than one way to work hard. Workaholism is not just hard work; it is not the most efficient work, and it is not merely some kind of voluntary addiction. It is a coping strategy for mild depression, and a stressful one at that.

UNINTENDED CONSEQUENCES

So there is another price to pay. "All work and no play makes Jack a dull boy" says the proverb (and "makes Jill a rich widow," added the wit Evan Esar). The problem is that Jack is a depressed boy to begin with, and all work is how he copes with no play. (More in chapter 10 about how Jack's depression-fueled work habits might make Jill a rich widow.) Not only that, but he feels alone and struggles with irritability. Indeed, British civil servants who work extra-long hours are more likely to suffer from episodic depressions as well.[46]

WHERE DOES THIS COME FROM, ANYWAY?

The Genetic Root of All Instinct

While we wait for good genetic findings on this under explored syndrome, clinical observation suggests that it runs strongly in families. If it is anything like other common psychiatric diagnoses, then it is most likely genetic but significantly influenced by environmental factors.

Gene/Environment Interactions

How might environmental effects work? Harry Harlow (American psychologist, 1905–1981) was famous for his controversial work with maternally deprived monkeys. Raised without their mothers, they had a hard time growing up and had serious emotional problems as adults. They were helped quite a bit if they had a warm, cloth-covered monkey dolls to hold in infancy, but it wasn't the same. Now imagine if you were raised in an orphanage without parents, if one or both of your parents passed away in your childhood, or if they were so emotionally detached that there was little emotional or physical warmth in your early life. You probably would be pretty unhappy then, and there would be lasting effects as well. Rat research helps us find what happens inside. When rats are separated from their mothers and reared alone, their brain serotonin just isn't what it might have been.[47] This could be because of the lack of a close relationship or because the lack of social interaction practice prevents proper childhood brain development. That kind of maternal deprivation experience might bring out underlying genetic tendencies for anxiety and depression (epigenetic factors at work, perhaps). Although this may not be specific to Atypical

Depression alone, it is easy to imagine that those rats and Harlow's monkeys felt pretty rejected.

The Primeval Origin of Instinct

First of all, rejection can be a real pain. Somewhere way far back, rejection sensitivity may have the same roots as physical pain. In fact, it may have a lot in common with physical pain. In Michigan, researchers showed rejection-sensitive people photographs of the exes who had recently broken up with them. This caused increased brain activity in the same region as physical pain induced by heat.[48] One brain center for two kinds of pain; as we saw earlier, rejection hurts.

In Kentucky, on the other hand, researchers ease the pain. It turns out that acetaminophen (brand name Tylenol) reduces the amount of reported everyday social pain, and even reduces brain activation to experimental social rejection in a laboratory computer-screen ball-toss game. (Actually, it was the computer that pretended to be a rejecting companion.)[49] Who knew? And no, acetaminophen and other pain killers have not been shown to be good treatments for Atypical Depression. More powerful narcotics may help social sadness temporarily, but the risks of addicting pain killers far, far outweigh their benefits.

Rejection sensitivity is one part of the puzzle, and the consequent depressive symptoms are another. What kind of primeval physiologic mechanism did evolution shape into the other Atypical Depression symptoms? It is hard to miss the comparison of Atypical Depression symptoms to winter hibernation (itself a form of withdrawal from group activity). Hibernating animals eat as much as they can, then slow down their metabolism to conserve energy and survive the winter. Although we don't actually hibernate much, some of us do have Seasonal Affective Disorder (SAD), the daylight-sensitive form of Atypical Depression that is more common in Fairbanks than Florida. If Atypical Depression developed from primeval hibernation, then SAD could just be a vestige of that heritage (more on that later). Then again, maybe it was adaptive for our hunter-gatherer ancestors in the northern climes to semihibernate when there is less food, colder temperatures, and the tensions of closer quarters. Indeed, chronically depressed mood is genetically linked to a gene that regulates our sleep-wake cycle ("circadian rhythm").[50]

Studies of chipmunks suggest that the serotonin system plays a central role in inducing their hibernation phase and greatly reducing their body temperature, and that a serotonin blocker can both induce hibernation of waking animals in the laboratory, or even wake them from hibernation.[51] So maybe an SSRI would increase serotonin activity, and keep them awake through the winter. That is nice for people with SAD, but it would be disturbing for a chipmunk in the wild. Their well-laid plans for a comfortable nest, a store of body fat, and a long winter snooze would fall by the wayside, in favor of a cold, dark, foodless, and rejecting winter world.

Inner Workings

What else do we know about people with Atypical Depression? Well, we know that they pay more attention to how other people feel, as we might expect. For example, one research method involves showing subjects photographs of faces that are manipulated so that a smile could appear only on the left side of the face, or only on the right side (one example of "chimerical faces"). Research subjects with Atypical Depression are much more reactive to the emotional cues in the manipulated faces, (which tend to be handled by the right side of the brain) than are other people with depressions.[52]

Not surprisingly, rejection sensitivity predicts exaggerated brain activity in response to photographs of people with faces showing disapproval, and in one particular part of the brain.[53] Along those lines, when adolescents played a computer ball game with two other "kids" (just the computer actually), those with more rejection sensitivity described more hurt when excluded, and their brains also showed greater activation.[54] Perhaps the scientists were inspired by those of us picked last for childhood baseball teams.

All that attention to other people's feelings can make you empathic. There are even certain brain locations that are activated by empathy.[55] When observing someone else's social exclusion, the more empathic adolescents went further to console them in some emails they were then asked to write. They also showed more activation of their own brain center for rejection pain. They know what it feels like, and they feel it in the same part of their brain. Empathy (in proper proportion) is a very good thing for any society.[56,57]

Neurotransmitter studies are just beginning, but in a study that compared Atypical Depression to Melancholic Depression, people with SAD were much more likely to have genetically reduced serotonin activity.[58] Along similar lines, serotonin activity enhancement with SSRIs works very well for Atypical Depression symptoms. (Though SSRIs are not necessarily sufficient for the seven deadly sins.)

HOW TO FIX IT: USING EVOLUTIONARY PERSPECTIVE TO EXPLAIN MODERN TREATMENT

Coping and Self-Improvement

There are coping skills for Atypical Depression. If you are aware of your rejection sensitivity, then you can try to remind yourself when you are making mountains out of molehills. The hardest part, of course, is that when you think you see mountains, it is very hard to realize that they are only molehills. For the oversleeping, overeating and lethargy, you can train yourself to override these symptoms. However, these things are not easy to do; they do little for the underlying biology, and they can have unexpected consequences.

Evolved Treatment

The right treatment for Atypical Depression is already pretty good. So how does modern treatment deal with symptoms that were once evolutionary adaptations, and now remain biologically ingrained? The most effective treatment includes SSRI antidepressants and psychotherapy. The SSRIs diminish the heightened rejection sensitivity, though it doesn't disappear completely. They also reduce the physical depressive symptoms. People do not say they feel "high" or "always happy." They often do say that they feel more "normal" or more confident. The SSRI benefit probably has something to do with the association of serotonin enhancement with a generally greater feeling of social closeness. Indeed, it may even be that Atypical Depression is closest to the core of our five social instincts. Adding a second medicine that increases serotonin levels by another route is one way to further improve medication treatment of Atypical Depression. To be sure, some psychiatrists think that the 1950's era Monoamine Oxidase Inhibitor ("MAOI") antidepressants are more effective still.

Medication alone isn't usually enough. There are underlying emotional issues that are linked with Atypical Depression, and there are also relationship patterns and emotional expectations that have developed as a result of long experience with the syndrome. If one has been so sensitive to rejection for a long time, they unwittingly developed ways of protecting their feelings, even at the risk of limiting their relationships or career. Psychotherapy involves overcoming excessive fears of rejection, recognizing patterns of "self-defeating" behavior (actually, it is "self-protective" for the rejection sensitivity), improving relationships (remember that Hank Williams song about ambivalence and anxiety?), and learning more flexible social roles. A large part of this is understanding the conflicts between rational wishes and instinctually derived emotions. From the evolutionary perspective, psychotherapy can help people learn new ways of dealing with and avoiding social rejections and their consequences, and developing more emotional intimacy.

The combination of medication and new awareness of cognitive mind-sets ("metacognition") makes it far easier to see molehills for molehills. Another way to build on this improvement is through CBT. Even so, the end result might be that you have better coping skills, but that some symptoms and behavior patterns remain. This kind of approach may help you become more counter-instinctive, and is typically more appealing to people who already lean that way. Later on we'll talk more about the downsides of counter-instinctive behavior.

Maybe we don't have to be so preoccupied with conformity, obsequiousness, and avoiding rejection. However, we probably do need enough to keep our world (and our society) a friendly and harmonious place.

6

FEELING SO USELESS YOU COULD DIE: MELANCHOLIC DEPRESSION

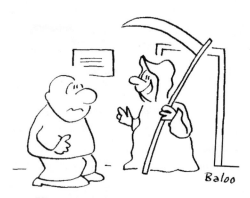

"Don't worry, I'm not death —
I'm just a bad head cold."

"Would I were dead, if God's good will were so, For what is in this world but grief and woe?"

—William Shakespeare, Henry VI Part 3 (English playwright; 1564–1616)

"How do geese know when to fly to the sun? Who tells them the seasons? How do we, humans know when it is time to move on? As with the migrant birds, so surely with us, there is a voice within if only we would listen to it, that tells us certainly when to go forth into the unknown."

—Elisabeth Kubler-Ross (Swiss psychiatrist; 1926–2004)

THE SOCIAL INSTINCT

Primeval social groups depended on everyone doing their part for the greater good. Otherwise, they could be short on resources and long on complaints. So, most of the time, everyone must have pitched in. Time came, though, when some felt that their job was done, their purpose gone, their contribution too small. Maybe an inborn instinct would help the group—an instinct that would prompt a graceful demise, and offer the group one less drain on scarce resources of many kinds. The severe depression we today call Melancholia may be just that instinct.

BACK IN THE DAY: THE SYNDROME IN PRIMEVAL HUMAN SOCIETY

Case Study: How It Might Have Helped Long Ago

Ages ago, in a human troop on the Central Asian Steppes, there lived an older woman. She had lived a good life, raised many now-grown children, starved and feasted, and recovered from physical illnesses and injuries. One day, her youngest child died after a fall out of a tree. The woman grieved her lost child, but soon felt somehow guilty, and became hopeless about the future. She cried, slept poorly, stopped eating and avoided the others. Compassionately (and at some short-term cost of their resources and time), the others did not leave her by herself. They took turns sitting by her side, plying her with food, and grooming her hair. Eventually, she recovered, accepted the painful loss of her child, and re-entered the life of the troop almost as if nothing had happened.

Some years later, and a bit the worse for wear, the woman found it difficult to keep up with the other women. Try as she might, she would fall behind on their travels, and could not finish her share of the chores. She had long since stopped helping to tend their sheep. She began to think that she was a permanent burden on the troop. Once again, she fell to hopelessness, guilt, crying, insomnia and weight loss. She felt especially sad in the mornings. Although the other women once again tried to care for her, she was not consolable, and thought herself not even worthy of consolation. As the woman became increasingly weak, thin and tired, she came to think that her body was withering away. She had vague thoughts that her body might be rotting inside like spoiled meat she had once seen. One day she started to cough up a bacteria-laden green sputum, and just a week later, she passed away in her sleep. The troop mourned her loss, and then went on with the activities of their lives.

BASIC PRINCIPLE: TAKING ONE FOR THE HERD

In ancient societies Melancholia may have been a biological method of culling nonessential members from the tribe, thus allowing scarce resources to be shared by a group now smaller by one member. What kinds of resources were scarce? No doubt it varied by time, place, climate and custom, but food, water, shelter, clothing, mates, caregivers' time, and defenses against predators are just a few possibilities.

It seems pretty doubtful that our primeval ancestors actually wanted their elderly and infirm to die. Clearly, other species mourn the death of a group member (no matter what its cause). Most poignant are accounts of apes, chimps, dolphins and elephants. Just like us, they seem to know the permanency of death, and they grieve the loss of friends, relatives and leaders. Remember those apocryphal stories about elderly Inuit (once known as Eskimos) set adrift on ice floes to die? Melancholia is kind of like a self-induced ice floe instinct, except that those Eskimo tales may not actually have happened. Another Arctic myth debunked.

But is there another benefit as well? Left alone, Melancholia will often get better eventually, so shorter-term Melancholia could also have had an adaptive role in rehabilitating still productive troop members. Faced with a hopeless or desperate situation, Melancholia could have served as an instinctive defeat mechanism. If and when recovery set in, adverse circumstances could diminish, adversarial people could move on, and painful losses could recede from memory. Deposed troop leaders, for example, could productively re-enter the group at a lesser rank after a period of outward passivity.

AMONG THE ANIMALS

In other species, Melancholia analogues may be seen in hopeless situations, such as monkeys who can see their mate cohabiting with another in a different cage, infants separated from their mothers, and pets that lose their masters. Also, troop leaders who are dethroned will sometimes fall into a torpid state. To human observers, all of these become withdrawn, disinterested, and lose their appetites.

TIMES HAVE CHANGED

We don't know if Melancholia is more common today than in the past. Although there is some research that finds that Major Depression in America may be more common now than it used to be, we have to remember that Major Depression includes many diagnoses, of which Melancholia is only one. At first glance, an increase in Melancholia would be hard to figure. After all, we live in the most technologically advanced society the world has ever known; we can travel long distances in short hours, and our health care is better than ever at treating physical illness, relieving distress, and prolonging life.

However, some consequences of this are that we have more people than ever who are retired, living apart from loved ones, socially isolated, chronically ill, and feeling themselves a "burden" on others. It is most often the ill, elderly, and alone who suffer

Melancholia. Along similar lines, the highest rate of completed suicides is among men in their late 60's—men who have lost a work-focused life, and now feel apart and useless in the world around them. As Plutarch (Greek historian, 46–120) noted, a sense of uselessness can befall even successful people who think they have reached the point where there is no higher mountain to climb: "When Alexander [the Great] saw the breadth of his domain he wept, for there were no more worlds to conquer."

Elderly people with little perceived purpose in life are nearly twice as likely to die as their peers who do see an important role for themselves.[1] Undoubtedly, people of all ages are most concerned about their social usefulness. In one study, a large group of elderly people were ranked by how useful to others they thought themselves. Those who felt least socially useful had about a threefold increase in physical disability and death over the next seven years.[2]

To be old is for some people to feel unwanted. Jerry Garcia (American blues and bluegrass musician, 1942–1995) sang about being "Old and in the Way":

Old and in the way, that's what I heard them say.
They used to heed the words he said, but that was yesterday.
Gold will turn to gray and youth will fade away.
They'll never care about you, call you old and in the way.

People are more naturally attracted to youthful cuteness that reminds them of adorable infants than they are to elderly frailness. Even standards of adult beauty include child-like large eyes, small noses and trim physique. One older woman patient, alone and lonely despite her servants, hoped desperately that dressing like a 20-year old would win her new entrée to the social whirl. She was so focused on her age that she dismissed the possibility that her awkward social behaviors could possibly play any role at all.

HOW INSTINCT BECOMES SYNDROME
IN MODERN HUMAN SOCIETY

Instinct and Worldview

Not surprisingly, the core cognitions of Melancholia include guilt (think "burden"), loss of pleasure ("anhedonia"), and hopelessness. These thoughts are biologically amplified by Melancholia, and set the stage for a mindset that it is time to make your exit. This mindset is even more striking when Melancholia progresses. Symptoms then reflect the notion of no longer belonging among the living: delusional guilt (i.e., preoccupation with exaggerations of past misdeeds), delusional poverty (i.e., irrationally fearing financial bankruptcy, even when finances are actually quite good), and delusional illness (including the notion that one's living body is quite literally rotting away).

Case Study: Causing Problems in Modern Society

Just last year, in a human family in Vancouver, a man retired at age 72. He had lived a long and fulfilling life. Troubled by Panic Anxiety from an early age, he never gave in to apprehensions about feeling trapped in enclosed spaces. Blessed with a successful, if all-consuming, interior-re-modeling career, a healthy family, and some money in the bank, he looked forward to watching sports, playing golf, and spending time with family. Then things started to happen. His only nearby child moved to another province; his wife passed suddenly from a heart attack, and he found himself lonely for the old social contacts of his office.

With few people to talk to, and nothing pressing on his agenda, the man did not know what to do with himself. Rather than enjoying a well-earned retirement, he felt useless, and old Panic Anxiety returned. Football games were less fun if there was no one to discuss them with; his finances needed no real attention, and food shopping was a chore. He wasn't the kind of person to make new friends, much less to try dating after all these years. As his Panic and anxiety were supplanted by overwhelming sadness and fatigue, he gradually withdrew to his bed, often with an ignored game on television. He slept poorly, woke up at 5 A.M., didn't enjoy food, and kind of wasted away. Family would call now and again, and he would always put on a good show. When they would ask him to visit their house in the mountains, he treated the invitation as mere family obligation. He never mentioned his cough, nor the green sputum. Eventually, he passed away in front of the television.

Maybe If Things Had Been Different...

During one phone call, the man's son noticed a sadness, and even thought that he heard stifled moans and coughs. After much insistence, the man finally listened to his son, and went to his internist. On bupro-prion (an antidepressant), and an antibiotic for his pneumonia, the man gained strength and found renewed purpose. He started weekly trips to the mountains, took pottery classes on Grenville Island, flew out to visit his son, started to mentor a young woman with a home-repair business, and even joked about finding a date online. He barely had time to catch his breath.

HOW DOES THIS MAKE YOU FEEL?

Melancholic Depression is an all-consuming sickness unto death. It is the raw primal sensation of our instincts telling us painfully that it is our time to shuffle off this mortal coil. Our instincts say that our time is done; our contribution is no longer sufficient. It is a pervasive urge to pass from this world. No longer do we feel any need to eat, produce, laugh and socially bond with others, or even to sleep (one purpose of which is to review social memories in dreams, in order to improve social skills). There is no evolutionary advantage for the Melancholic themselves. The evolutionary advantage resides in the help to their tribe in maximizing the use of food, space and other resources. Even so, Melancholia is often an instinct too easily triggered. Although it may lift even on its own, a first episode suggests a growing sense of pointlessness, and greatly increases the risk of another.

Because we are still rational humans, we try to ignore this instinctual prompt to remove ourselves (as well we should). Don't want to give up this world? Of course not—there is much left to enjoy, and there are new ways to contribute. However, even at this penultimate moment, our instincts don't understand reason: they are responsive more to a sense of pointlessness. So, our human reason can lead us to push on despite despair, and more so when we know that Melancholia can get better with care. We may yet spend more time at some sunny beach resort, helping the community, remembering old friends and meeting new ones.

WHAT THE SYNDROME IS

Melancholia must have been known for millennia, and it clearly appears in the Old Testament (Psalm 38):

O LORD, rebuke me not in thy wrath: neither chasten me in thy hot displeasure.

For thine arrows stick fast in me, and thy hand presseth me sore.

There is no soundness in my flesh because of thine anger; neither is there any rest in my bones because of my sin.

For mine iniquities are gone over mine head: as a heavy burden they are too heavy for me.

My wounds stink and are corrupt because of my foolishness.

I am troubled; I am bowed down greatly; I go mourning all the day long.

For my loins are filled with a loathsome disease: and there is no soundness in my flesh.

I am feeble and sore broken: I have roared by reason of the disquietness of my heart.

Even though this syndrome was described in biblical times, Melancholia is a word you have to be careful with. It has had so many meanings now and over time[3] that it is worth the pointing out that we are only talking now about one particular and officially recognized meaning. We are not talking about mere sadness, sweet sadness, or mournful contemplation. Melancholia is that long-recognized form of severe depression in which people can't eat or sleep or smile. The sadness and hopelessness can be overwhelming. The inability to experience pleasure ("anhedonia") is dramatic. Unlike the other four other social-instinct syndromes we have discussed, Melancholia is an acute condition, though often recurrent. (Syndrome details are in appendix.) It is sometimes thought of as a distinct and pathologically exaggerated variant of normal mourning and grief.

In the essay "Mourning and Melancholia," Freud waxes eloquent about this distinction:

In mourning it is the world which has become poor and empty; [while] in melancholia...the patient represents his ego to us as worthless...and—what is psychologically very remarkable—by an overcoming of the instinct which compels every living thing to cling to life.

Unlike ordinary mourning and grief,

The distinguishing mental features of melancholia are a profoundly painful dejection, cessation of interest in the outside world, loss of the capacity to love, inhibition of all activity, and a lowering of the self-regarding feelings to a degree that finds utterance in self-reproaches and self-revilings, and culminates in a delusional expectation of punishment.

In more modern times, Donald Klein coined the phrase "endogenomorphic depression" to reflect the clearly biological origins of Melancholia. This syndrome is a specific type of depression, and it is hard to miss if you are looking. However, there is a big problem. Ever since the *DSM-III* and *DSM-IV* introduced the more global Major Depression, clinicians and researchers have paid less attention to the Melancholia type. As we learned before, Melancholia is lately a renewed focus of attention.[4,5] It is hard to know how many people have full Melancholia in their lifetimes, since little research has addressed that question. Although Melancholia is a specific form of illness, it can look different in different people. How a symptom looks is shaped by interaction with personality, culture and circumstances. If a homeless man in a hospital bed with cancer bemoaned his poverty, there would be little reason to presume the emotional impoverishment of Melancholia, but if the billionaire with the same cancer in the next room said the same thing, suspicions would more likely be aroused.

Melancholia is more common in people who have one of the chronic disorders such as Social Anxiety, Panic Anxiety, or Atypical Depression. In fact, the path to Melancholia often begins with worsening of one of those other diagnoses—Panic in particular. As James Ballenger (American psychiatrist) put it, "If you're facing terror every day, it's gonna bring Hannibal to his knees." It is also more common in people who suffer serious physical illness or overwhelming losses, and most common still in people with illness or loss on top of a chronic emotional syndrome.

Melancholia may follow the death of a spouse or child, real financial destitution, serious physical illness and other major or symbolic losses. Importantly, it tends to follow events that cause a significant loss of perceived societal or personal purpose. One elderly woman fell into Melancholia after she read the obituary of a boyfriend from some 40 years before. Although she had not seen him since then, she had followed his career and increasing fame in the papers, and her thoughts of their romance had been her constant companion. Although diagnosed Melancholia is more common in women, it is especially common in recently retired men, as is suicide. Some people say they just want to curl up in a ball and die.

That brings us to Freud's "Death Instinct." He postulated an underlying and ongoing drive to return from life to the inanimate earth. His "Death Instinct" appears during life as self-destructive behaviors, or more importantly, as outwardly directed aggression and violence. Among other things, this concept was his attempt to explain the aggression he saw as pervasive in the human condition, and in the horrors of the World War I.[6] However, our social instinct for death is not always lying in wait. Melancholia appears suddenly in response to great loss. It is an instinctive biological response to the perception that other people would be better off without you.

WORST CASE SCENARIO

Severe Melancholia is a striking illness. People eat virtually no food, do not smile, sleep very poorly, and have no interest in people or pleasure. Nothing can cheer them up. The extreme sadness rubs off, so that those who visit them walk away feeling pretty gloomy themselves. As time goes on, they can become emaciated from weight loss, withdrawn into a private world, subject to infection and physical illness, and prone to suicidal thoughts. Actually, the risk for actual suicide attempts may briefly be higher still should they start to recover. That is when they have renewed physical energy to act, but before their hopeless and suicidal thoughts have had time to diminish.

In the Cotard syndrome (Jules Cotard, French Neurologist; 1840–1889), people think they are already dead. Although this can happen as a result of brain injury, it is usually part of a Melancholic or Psychotic Depression. Psychotic Depression (see Chapter 7) is a form of Melancholia in which people have fixed false beliefs ("delusions") that their bodies are rotting, that they bear the guilty responsibility for unimaginable calamities, or that they have become dead.

WHAT THE SYNDROME ISN'T

Everyone gets sad sometimes, and many people have bleak periods now and again. Grief brings great sadness, but it does not cause profound hopelessness or guilt. Melancholia is not mere sadness, bleakness, grief, or even hopelessness. It is a distinct and pervasive depression that is very different from ordinary everyday emotions. In older usage, it sometimes referred more generally to sadness or depression. "He is of a very melancholy disposition" wrote William Shakespeare, perhaps suggestive of modern Atypical Depression. Severe Atypical Depression is not Melancholia, but can be mistaken for it, and can even trigger it (sometimes called a "double depression"). Our Melancholia is also very different from the romantic notion of melancholy. "Melancholy is the pleasure of being sad," said Victor Hugo (French author, 1802–1885).

It is worth noting that Melancholia and serious physical illness often occur together and also that they are easily confused with each other. A non-Melancholic cancer patient may have little appetite or energy. A Melancholic patient with severe weight loss may have endless tests for cancer before psychiatric causes are ever considered, and sometimes not even then. A new patient with weight loss, sadness and little energy might have serious physical illness, Melancholia, or both.

THE AGES OF MELANCHOLIC ANGST

The last four chapters were about chronic syndromes that all begin in childhood or adolescence. Melancholia is an acute illness that is uncommon in children, more possible in adolescence, but most common as we get much older. The kinds of severe losses and illnesses that trigger Melancholia are more common at later ages, and most common among the elderly.

HOLDING US BACK

The main social role limitation of Melancholia is, well, an inability to be social. In modern society, Melancholia makes it difficult or impossible to continue in usual social and occupational roles. People are too sad, tired, weak, and detached to keep up relationships or do their jobs. Sleep loss and weight loss put people at greater risk for starvation, physical illness, and death. Some surgeons have long said that they won't operate on someone with a serious depression, because experience tells them that the odds of survival are reduced.[7] Could it be that depression is a purely or partly rational helplessness in the face of physical illness and old age? Of course. However, if you re-examine depression by leaving out any physical symptoms directly attributable to physical illness, you end up with a depression diagnosis that is an even better predictor of death in the hospital than a standard diagnosis of depression.[8] Indeed, the risk is about seven times higher in one Brazilian study, even after adjusting for other factors. In addition, a 30% increased risk of mortality continues outside the hospital for years after diagnosis of depression in elderly Californians.[9]

At least one study suggests that the increased mortality in the depressed elderly is mostly infectious disease and cancer.[10] Those with the more severe Psychotic Depression are the most preoccupied with the anticipation of death, and the most likely to die.[11] So if Melancholia is not recognized and treated, it may carry through on its primeval instinctual purpose. Even so, many people, even with unrecognized and untreated Melancholia, will be cared for by family or other caretakers. Special foods, sleeping pills, conversation—all these may help, and sometimes may even lead to recovery.

THE INSTINCT IS WITH US STILL

Not too long ago, many elderly died from pneumonia—so many that it used to be known as "the old man's friend" (William Osler, Canadian physician and "founder of modern medicine," 1849–1919). Melancholia accelerated the demise of the dying. Infections like pneumonia happen more easily with Melancholia, especially if untreated, because the depressive symptoms are overlooked or rationalized away. Depression predicts mortality in people with cancer, even when it doesn't predict progression of the cancer itself.[12,13] What do cancer patients most often die from? Infections, caused by poor nutritional status, immune suppression, damaged tissue—and no doubt Melancholia.[10] Alexander the Great, who wept when he ran out of lands to conquer, died young at age 32 from infectious typhoid fever,[14] not long after further despairing over the death of his lover Hephaestion.

From the viewpoint of primeval-society resource allocation, these deaths are "adaptive." Does this instinct still have value in modern society? Well, from a civilized and humane point of view, the answer is a very clear no. But for that tiny minority who have a very narrow focus on societal resources, it would help reduce health-care costs in the seriously ill elderly, and those costs spiral far higher than the costs of their food and shelter. Fortunately, few would argue outright that instinctual Melancholia should be a deciding factor in health-care utilization. Unfortunately, Melancholia takes its toll too often nonetheless.

Romance

True Melancholia is not the romantic melancholy of yore, to be relieved by true love. On the contrary, Melancholia leaves little interest in romance, in sex, or even in companionship. Melancholia can certainly be triggered by loss of a romantic partner through death, divorce or departure. Then again, unexpected romance can offer a cure and a new sense of purpose.

Workplace

Work holds little interest, and Melancholic employees will often stay home or quit. Some employees do follow their routine and do their best. What results is typically rote work effort, depressive presentation, poor communication, impaired social skills, lateness, absenteeism, and little initiative or creativity. Work can be an island of purpose in their lives. However, Melancholia can jeopardize their jobs when their performance or interpersonal skills drop, or when it increases workplace physical risks. Some employees should be encouraged to take a brief medical leave while they recover, with the expectation that they will be better than ever on their return.

SYNDROME AND SOCIAL STIGMA

The compassionate reaction of most people today to someone with Melancholia is to protect and care for them, and nurse them back to health. Even then, there is often an instinctive reluctance to rationally acknowledge Melancholia in others. People may sense the pervasive sadness, and they may "understand" the most obvious cause of the Melancholia, such as loss of a spouse, financial ruin, or a diagnosis of cancer. However, even with their protective instincts aroused, they may seek to "protect" the victim of seemingly inevitable Melancholia from seemingly pointless interventions. On the level of their own social instincts, they want to respect the "natural" social mechanism of Melancholia in others.

In one case, when two observing psychiatrists happened to recognize Melancholia in a medical inpatient with cancer, they left a note in the chart about the necessity of treatment. The internal medicine staff was so concerned for the patient that they immediately and prematurely discharged her, in order to prevent unnecessary psychiatric "intrusion." Their rational knowledge that Melancholia is easy to treat was overridden by their instinctive need to protect the emotional status quo of a patient whose cancer wouldn't go away.

Melancholia is not to be ignored, no matter how obvious its cause may seem. There is a telling tale they discuss in medical schools. The psychiatrist tells the oncologist "your patient is depressed," to which the oncologist responds "well of course he's depressed, he has cancer." "Well," says the psychiatrist, "if I had cancer, I'd hardly want a depression to go with it." This joke reflects a very real problem that continues unabated despite decades of research and countless different approaches at engaging oncologists and other physicians in better psychiatric diagnosis and treatment.[15,16]

INSTINCT AND SYNDROME TURN UP IN CULTURE

If you are going to have Melancholia, now is probably the best time in the history of man. It is easily treated, if and when it is diagnosed. Modern society tries to provide the elderly, infirm and Melancholic with the same resources and humanity as everyone else. Indeed, there is even a renewed emphasis on seeking and respecting the contributions and wisdom of all. Modern society has new methods of treating the health and companionship losses that lead to the syndrome. Companionship and purpose are offered by social programs for the elderly, by volunteer opportunities to help the blind, and by opportunities for retired executives to share their business expertise.

Even so, there are dark clouds on the horizon. Increasing numbers of elderly citizens strain societal resources. Rising health-care costs raise questions of health-care rationing ("death panels"), which would disproportionately affect those who are Melancholically resigned to their fate.

Despite our good intentions, if not because of them, modern society can increase the risk of Melancholia. Men and women who find purpose in work often are faced with voluntary and sometimes mandatory retirement, and then with decades of "golden years." Those who find purpose in social relationships are faced with rising divorce rates, children moving far from a now-empty nest, and separation from their family in retirement communities and nursing homes. Modern medicine keeps people alive with serious physical illness, but often with ongoing symptoms and physical limitations. In the tradition of Niko Tinbergen (Dutch ethologist 1907–1988), these social and physical ills are Supernormal Stimuli to our instincts. We endure illness and age far more pronounced than anything evolution anticipated.

Compared to our four chronic instinctive syndromes, there are fewer songs about acute Melancholia. Although there are many songs about death, dying, and grief, Melancholia is not an instinct that prompts people to write songs about the experience. John Lennon (English musician, member of the Beatles, 1940–1980) singing "Yer Blues" is a strikingly specific exception, even noting thoughts of bodily decay, suicide, and distaste for the joy and purpose of music in these selected verses:

I'm lonely
Want to die
If I ain't dead already
Ohhh girl you know the reason why.

The eagle picks my eye
The worm he licks my bone
I feel so suicidal
Just like Dylan's Mr. Jones

Black cloud crossed my mind
Blue mist round my soul
Feel so suicidal
Even hate my rock and roll

TURN THE SYNDROME AROUND: ADVANTAGES OF COUNTER-INSTINCTIVE BEHAVIOR

Case Study: Counter-Instinctive Behavior

Quite recently, a powerful man in a human family succeeded beyond his wildest American dreams. It wasn't just that he had finally taken charge of his Texas company, but his long-term strategy was finally paying off, in a way that no one had expected, but that everyone couldn't help but notice now. As a result of his efforts, his company's main competitor was struggling and slipping. In fact, they even sent a back-channel message that they would consider being bought out rather than go bankrupt. What a victory! At last everyone could see the wisdom of his persistent efforts.

At first he basked in the glow. Quietly on the outside, of course, for that is the kind of man he is, but bask he did nonetheless. Soon, though, he began to flounder. He was outwardly quiet about that, too. With victory accomplished, what was left for him? Sure, his family was intact, but that was not how he defined himself. After years of pursuing his business strategy to this dramatic point, he was at a loss for what to do next.

He became inwardly even more quiet, ruminated pointlessly and avoided making decisions. He slept poorly, though strong sleeping pills helped. Food was tasteless, but he ate exactly the same food as before, prepared for him in exactly the same way. He even kept up his exercise routine, though it wasn't any fun and the weights felt so much heavier. He didn't think of himself as sad, though he sometimes thought that work wasn't so much fun anymore. He kept his social calendar the same, and was deliberately attentive to his social graces. Even so, close friends noticed that he was just going through the motions. Sometimes, to himself alone, he thought that there wasn't really any purpose anymore. Throughout this three-year travail, no ophthalmologist could stop the water from coming out of his eyes.

Although nobody knew it (not even the man himself), this wasn't the first time. Over the years, as he fought for his strategy against long odds and against the opposition of his peers, he had had just this kind of funk before. By not realizing it was there, he did not succumb, and he was able to keep pushing through. He had passing thoughts of the concrete and channelized Trinity River that ran through Dallas. Unwittingly, it reminded him of himself. Alone, charmless, and unnatural, it did manage to carry water, but to what end? Since he suffered so quietly, others left him alone.

Other people at work noticed only that the old spark was gone. When time came for his review by the board, they rewarded him for his success with a handsome retirement package, and decided to look for a younger and more charismatic boss.

Maybe If Things Had Been Different . . .

Maybe yet one more ophthalmologist could help solve that eye water problem. This one decided not to repeat the usual tests yet again. Instead, she pointed out that the tears were part of Melancholic Depression. In psychotherapy and with an antidepressant, the man felt dramatically better three weeks later. His appetite was back, his sleep was good, he laughed at jokes, and he started thinking of new purposes for his life. The Trinity River reclamation project was first on his list.

Relieved of this long and powerful effort to overcome his instinct for a final exit, he confided in another board member. "Yer Blues? Been through this myself," the other man said. "After I closed the big deal it seemed like I could never top it, and so what was the point of it all? Melancholia. Me! Got that better fast, and been riding that deal ever since. At 65 the wife and I even started to ski with the grandkids. What a life!"

SOCIAL ALARMS PROMPT SELF-IMPROVEMENT

Other than a display of passivity or subdued behavior after a major change, it isn't that counter-instinctive Melancholia is often helpful to an individual. However, it is a way that we can use conscious thought and decisions to survive despite our difficult circumstances and biological hopelessness. By fighting the Melancholia and surviving, we can live to fight another day. When Demosthenes (Greek orator, 384–322 BCE) said "he who fights and runs away will live to fight another day," he was guiltily trying to explain away his premature flight from a battlefield. The battle in Melancholia is against perceived purposelessness, and the instinctively initiated Melancholia is hardly cowardice. It is, eventually, a message to find new meaning and a new day.

One way that fighting against Melancholia can be helpful is when others unwittingly sense it. In the midst of an economic downturn, a laid-off and grouchy executive had trouble finding a new position. Given his credentials, it was easy to get interviews, but then it would be hard to hide his bitter perspective. Eventually, the job hunt seemed hopeless, and he was gloomily aware that his unhappiness had moved on to something different, pervasive and severe. Perseverant as he was, he decided to go ahead with yet another pointless interview despite his lack of energy. This time, he was quieter, and the interviewer felt an unwitting compassion for him. To his surprise, he made the short list and was scheduled for further interviews. "Who knew?" he later thought.

WHERE DOES THIS COME FROM, ANYWAY?

The Genetic Root of All Instinct

There is little specific research on the genetics of Melancholia, and there is less still on early gene-by-environment interactions that could increase the later risk of the syndrome. Some studies say that genetically low levels of serotonin activity may double the risk for Melancholia,[17,18] but other studies say that genetic factors do not increase the risk.[19] If there is a relationship, it could occur through some kind of indirect effect, because low-serotonin function predisposes people to three of our other four instinctive syndromes, and those in turn predispose to Melancholia. Even so, it is still possible that genetically low serotonin function directly increases Melancholia risk, especially since we know that those genes reduce the effectiveness of medication treatment in Melancholia.[19]

The Primeval Origins of Instinct

A death instinct can be useful for a species. There is one kind of death instinct that operates at the DNA level (that is, if DNA could have social "instincts"). The Hayflick limit (Leonard Hayflick, American anatomist and microbiologist; 1928 –) is the maximum number of times that a given cell type can divide, replicate, and replace itself. Each replication shortens one particular part of the DNA ("telomeres," that are otherwise genetically meaningless), leading ultimately to DNA that is too short for more replication. The evolutionary advantage of this process might be through prevention of DNA copy errors, or limits on rapidly dividing cancer cells in animals. Either way, it may cause some of the problems of human aging as cells can no longer replace themselves, and it may limit us to a theoretical maximum life span of 140 years. Our modern bacterial relatives have no Hayflick limit, and our own cancer cells have managed to escape the limit by reactivating an inactive ("dormant") gene that produces those DNA telomeres. Turning that gene back to "off" may come in handy someday to treat cancer, and turning it on carefully might slow the aging process.

There is a second kind of death instinct that operates at the cellular level (*apoptosis*—from the Greek for "falling off," and, no, cells don't have social instincts either). Why would cells do themselves in? The adaptive purposes may include anatomical development, tissue regeneration and renewal, and defense against infection or malignancy.

With these other death instincts in mind, there is another remarkable bit of biology to ponder in our context of Melancholic Depression. Whole organisms can also have programmed death (*phenoptosis,* from the Greek for "programmed death"). There is an Australian marsupial mouse that dies soon after mating (that would be the male, of course).[20] Similarly, when salmon swim upstream to spawn, they die soon after completing their task. Their lives' purpose is done, and it turns out that death in both species is brought on by a dramatic increase in glucocorticoid levels (i.e., cortisol from the adrenal gland). If you take out their adrenal glands, then they stay alive.[21] Although it could be that this same mechanism evolved twice in quite unrelated species ("parallel evolution"), it could also have evolved just once in some distant common ancestor, no doubt sometime later than those ancestral bacteria.

Maybe we humans are yet a third example of this process.[22] In Melancholic Depression, there is also a substantial increase in levels of cortisol (the "stress" hormone). There is even an experimental diagnostic test that shows that cortisol levels cannot be artificially normalized in untreated human Melancholia. Fortunately for human males, there is still more to life after mating (and mating rarely turns men Melancholic). However, there does come that time when some men and women think their life tasks are done, when Melancholia ensues, and when their cortisol system changes in a way that invites death.

Indeed, serious physical illness and serious emotional stress are each often accompanied by increased cortisol. Is that merely bodily reaction to stress, with increased cortisol thereafter causing Melancholia? Or, could it be the other way around, that

Melancholia maintains the increased cortisol activity? Regardless of whether the chicken or the egg came first, once the heightened cortisol state exists, it can do real damage. To understand this, there is a medical illness of increased cortisol levels (Cushing's Syndrome). Not surprisingly, depression is common in Cushing's (score one point for the chicken).[23] Also, the skin becomes thin, wounds take longer to heal, the immune system is impaired, and blood sugar levels increase.[24] This is just like a picnic for bacteria, fungi, parasites, and other disease-causing bad guys, and lethal infections can result. If Melancholia is a death instinct, then cortisol leads us to our demise.

Did this death instinct evolve from something else? Maybe Melancholia didn't pop up out of nowhere. Not long ago, someone noticed that physical illness can provoke an immune response that leads to a depression-like "sickness behavior," namely fatigue, impaired concentration, and feeling socially detached.[25] This got people thinking. If you give healthy people a chemical ("endotoxin") that only looks like living bacteria to their immune systems, they stay healthy, but they show the same sickness behaviors. Likewise, if you give them a typhoid vaccine (no live typhoid is included), subjects feel tired, confused, can't concentrate, and change how they process the social information in peoples' faces. Quite literally, they see people differently, and feel more apart from them.[26,27] Some people, despite their best efforts, can't tell the difference between mild physical illness and mild depression. They survey their bodily sensations for signs of fever, cough, or other symptoms that might help them answer the question.

How would sickness behavior help? It would preserve bodily energy for the arduous task of fighting infection and repairing physical injury. Meanwhile, it would promote social withdrawal to reduce the odds of spreading infectious disease within the group. Sometime later, sickness behavior evolved into Melancholia. Protecting the group against infection grew to encompass protecting the group against the infected member. So, perhaps primeval sickness behavior that prevents epidemics evolved into a physically or emotionally induced Melancholic death instinct that stops use of group resources. The effects of perceived "unwantedness" and social rejection may act through the very same pathways as physical illness.[28]

Actually, this cortisol finding has given us a laboratory test for Melancholia. The story begins in 1960, when Willam Bunney (American psychiatrist) and others noted that patients at the start of a severe depression tended to have increased levels of the stress hormone cortisol. In 1968, Barney Carroll (Australian psychiatrist, 1940 –) and others down under reported that patients with ongoing Melancholia had cortisol levels near normal, but that those levels did not decrease when they were supposed to (cortisol levels normally go down when you give them the synthetic hormone dexamethasone). So an abnormal "dexamethasone suppression test" (DST) is a marker for Melancholia. Intensive research followed, largely by Barney Carroll and Edward Sachar (American psychiatrist, 1933–1984) documenting this remarkable DST finding.

Pretty soon, in 1980, *DSM-III* came along. Melancholia, instead of being a distinct syndrome, became an infrequently used subtype of Major Depression. Alas, when other researchers relied on this less specifically defined group of Major Depression, the DST findings disappeared, and the level of interest plummeted. There was much controversy at the time, with psychiatrists trying to tell each other what to think.[29] Even so, the DST has not disappeared from research, and it remains a laboratory test with promise for Melancholia diagnosis, insufficient-treatment response, and suicide risk. Indeed, among patients with Major Depression, the DST predicts Melancholia and psychosis.[30,31] The DST also returns to normal when there is a full clinical recovery.[32] Remarkably, one study showed that when patients are hospitalized after surviving a suicide attempt, an abnormal DST from that time predicts a seven-fold or more increase in completed suicide in later years.[33]

By the way, the male marsupial mouse, on the path to meet his maker after mating, also develops an abnormal DST. So, even the mouse might be Melancholic.[21] There is something about Melancholia. When there is too much cortisol activity, something wicked this way glum.

HOW TO FIX IT: USING EVOLUTIONARY PERSPECTIVE TO EXPLAIN MODERN TREATMENT
Coping and Self-Improvement

Although people do get by without treatment, coping and self-improvement are problematic with Melancholia. Even those few who do muster up the rational desire to stay active and get well are nonetheless at risk for further illness, perceived social isolation, and even suicide. Better to get good help.

Evolved Treatment

Melancholia treatment should not be left to self-help for the helpless. Modern methods make it easy to treat with one of the antidepressant medications, combined with psychotherapy. As usual, SSRIs may help by increasing the level of serotonin activity and thus increasing social functioning. So, how do the other antidepressants work here? All antidepressants may have the effect of reducing the effects of increased cortisol.[34] Recently, there has been interest in the use of specifically anticortisol drugs (that are not otherwise known as antidepressants) as a more direct treatment for psychotic Melancholia [35] and for Melancholia with high cortisol levels.[36] Therefore, some antidepressants may work because they blunt the cortisol mechanism of the death instinct.

Although either medication or formal psychotherapy alone can often be successful, the combination of the two is more reliable, faster and safer. Psychotherapy for the Melancholic death instinct at first resembles the approach to those who are truly dying, with extra attention to risks for suicide. People fear losing their social network, fear social isolation, and fear being forgotten. Blind Lemon Jefferson (American bluesman, 1893–1929) captured this essence in song when a dying man says, "There's one last favor I'll ask of you, see that my grave is kept clean."

In those who will go on living there is hope for overcoming loss and anger, and for refocusing relationships. Psychotherapy for Melancholia also includes regaining purpose, role and hopefulness, instead of thinking of oneself as socially nonproductive, and feeling the guilt of "being a burden." Our modern society allows for more role and relationship change than that of our primeval ancestors. Developed countries are not so resource strained that they must let some members die off from Melancholia in order that others might have enough food to survive. Once the Melancholia itself has resolved, other important issues remain for psychotherapeutic attention. Even though Melancholia is easy to treat, the triggering physical illness or social losses continue to present pressing problems and painful memories to those rescued from a premature demise.

7

CONSCIOUSNESS LOST AND
INSTINCT RUN AMOK:
SCHIZOPHRENIA AND PSYCHOSIS

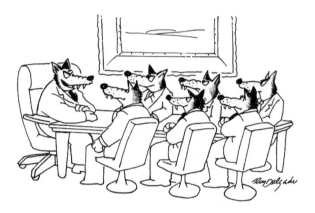

"Then it's agreed. We'll go with our animal instincts."

"Wisdom begins in wonder."
—Socrates (Ancient Greek Philosopher; 470 BC–399 BC)

"The very essence of instinct is that it's followed independently of reason."
—Charles Darwin (English naturalist: 1809–1882)

THE SOCIAL INSTINCT

In the beginning, there was instinct, and it was good. Bacteria responded to the sensation of food by consuming it, and if a simple multicellular creature sensed a physically hostile environment, it would instinctively back off. However, as species evolved, there came a need for greater perception of the outside world. Touch, smell (including taste), vision and hearing allowed earlier detection of food, danger, topography, resources and social community. These signals were first processed and assessed by instinctive mechanisms. Scent trails help an ant to find food, and then to return to the nest. A lizard finds a warm rock, and then heats itself by resting in the sun. A mouse recognized family by smell, but doesn't think to itself "oh, that's my cousin Mickey." Indeed, a mouse is unable to realize that it has a thinking brain, much less realize that another mouse also has a thinking brain. Baboons recognized fellow troop members, and know their relative rank in the hierarchy, but although there is some sort of higher mental processing, they don't literally say to themselves "her number 4 outranks my number 37, so better for me to be deferential."

Humans, more than any other species that we know of, are aware that they think, are aware of what they sense, are able to rationally examine their thoughts and senses, and are able to realize that other humans do the same (dolphins are the foremost example of similar abilities in other species). Consciousness has enormous evolutionary advantages. We humans can rationally assess our circumstances and our plans (not that we always do, of course). By knowing how much food we have, and how best to get more, we can reduce the odds of starvation, and we can feed a larger community. We can also develop new methods of agriculture, new food crops, cooking with fire to enhance the caloric value and taste of food,[1] and such delightful new recipes as ratatouille niçoise, bananas Foster, and the Philadelphia cheese steak. Conscious reasoning has vast adaptive value for human survival in agriculture, risk avoidance, tool use, manufacturing, science, art, learning, and in social behavior. There is value still for those species with smaller levels of Consciousness.

This ability to think about thinking has been the subject of philosophical contemplation for millennia. It even prompts us to wonder whether we exist at all, and yet suggests to us that we do. To quote Descartes again: "I think, therefore I am." Consciousness happens. It isn't something that we choose to do. So as an innate pattern of human behavior, Consciousness meets the definition of an instinct. Our sense of free will—that we can make rational decisions about what we do—stems from this instinctive Consciousness. Oftentimes, though, we have a hard time differentiating between our rational thoughts and our Consciousness on the one hand, and our other unwitting instincts on the other. More often than not, as we have seen, our free will contains the hidden influences of instinct. This admixture of rational thought and instinct is especially true for the social biology that we are considering. Furthermore, when it comes to understanding unchangeable false beliefs or perceptions ("psychosis"), the problem is not the presence of the Consciousness instinct, but rather its weakening or absence. Absent that conscious moderation, we experience the heightened arousal of our social instincts as raw and often frightful perception. Our animal cousins, our ancestors, and our selves have hidden biological engrams that warn us of the primeval consequences that could befall those who fail to obey their social instincts.

CONSCIOUS REASON BALANCES UNCONSCIOUS INSTINCT

The reasons for our social decisions are complex. When we are among strangers at a business party, some of us will feel a sudden Panicky need to flee for home. Our sense of hierarchy may influence whom we talk to and whom we feel threatened by. Our nesting instincts may lead us to straighten out the food table, or to avoid shaking hands with all those people who might carry germs. Our fear of rejection will guide us on how comfortable to be at approaching potential new friends. If that was all the guidance we had, we would each fall into some stereotyped social role defined by our varying biologies. Fortunately, all of those social instincts are moderated by our Consciousness instinct. Our reason allows us to talk to the alpha males and females, without fear of some sure and certain punishment for our insolence in approaching them. Reason even reminds us of the need for caution and respect with them.

THE MIND/BODY PROBLEM

John Locke (English philosopher, 1632–1704) suggested that Consciousness is "the perception of what passes in a man's own mind." So Consciousness (and its progeny, rational thought) is a social self-awareness that acts as a supervisor of our hidden social instincts. It allows us to override our biological social instincts, and thus permits us more rational social behavior, cooperation, communication and language. One small part of this is the ability to argue with each other, rather than meekly obeying instinctive cues.[2] Similarly, language may have a central function as a moderator of social perception. In one experiment, when subjects were told bad things about someone, they stared longer at photographs of that person. Gossip tells us whom we need to keep an eye on.[3] Consciousness may well have started as a largely social instinct.[4]

As a secondary benefit, we also have greater conscious awareness of environmental resources, and we have developed technology that allows us to better utilize those resources for our communities. Finally, on an individual level, people who can most easily and rationally describe their inner selves also report a more meaningful experience of life.[5] Locke would not be surprised. Only a few other species are even capable of physical self-awareness. For example, some apes, crows and dolphins can recognize themselves in a mirror. Basically, if you put a colored tag on them, they can see that tag in the mirror, and then look for it on themselves.

Once you realize that you have your own mind, the next step is to realize that other people also have their own minds. In psychology and philosophy, this is called Theory of Mind (ToM). Theory of Mind is essential for rational consideration of social interactions. It is not just the ability to overcome your inner social instincts—you also need to realize that other people have rational and instinctive thoughts and feelings as well. It is mostly a people thing, though some other species may have some limited ToM as well. It seems unscientifically clear that our alpha dog Bonnie often knows what people are thinking. Although she can't think in words (does she have an inner bark?), she has some awareness of when to deliberately offer a ball to play or when to suddenly reverse direction when playing chase in the yard.

PROBLEMS ENSUE WHEN CONSCIOUSNESS IS OVERCOME BY INSTINCT

Our Consciousness has been hugely adaptive for our species, but there are times when it is no longer able to balance and moderate our core social instincts. Those are problematic times, when raw unmodified instinct rises to the fore. When this effect is powerful enough, what we see is an unchanging loss of contact with conscious reality, and a particular loss of normal social functioning. The unmoderated social instincts are now appearing as what we call "psychosis," or as the particular group of psychoses called Schizophrenia.

In 1887, Emil Kraepelin (German psychiatrist, 1857–1926) introduced the term *dementia praecox* (from the Greek for "precocious dementia") to encompass his pioneering syndromal descriptions of Schizophrenia. He realized that the many psychotic symptoms of madness were part of one group of biological syndromes. In 1908, Eugen Bleuler (Swiss psychiatrist; 1857–1939) coined the term *Schizophrenia* (from the Greek for "split brain"). By that he meant that Schizophrenia is a group of illnesses where the brain splits apart the real-world conscious mind from the inner unconscious, and where that inner unconscious can thus come to dominate.[6] If you assume that this unconscious included social instinct, Bleuler was way ahead of his time. By the way, Schizophrenia has absolutely nothing to do with either multiple personalities, or with the idea of consciously obsessing about two opposing ideas or strategies.

Jonathan Burns (South African psychiatrist) suggests that Schizophrenia happens when social adaptations clash with real-world genetic and environmental events.[7] Randolph Nesse (American psychiatrist, 1948 –) chimes in about the "cliff-edged" advance of social-fitness functions.[8] Increasingly strong social instincts are adaptive only up to a point. When they become too powerful, they take us over the edge of a psychotic cliff. As have other research papers, a general population study in New Zealand found that there is a wide severity spectrum of psychotic symptoms, extending well into the "normal" population. What they also found is that people who had commonplace anxiety and depressive disorders were more likely to have isolated psychotic symptoms, and much more likely to go over the edge into catastrophic psychotic illness.[9]

LEARNING BY TREATING

Before we go into a more detailed theory, let's ground the theory with a little more of what we know about Schizophrenia and psychosis. To begin with, for the past 60 years we have had medications that are effective in reducing psychotic symptoms. The antipsychotic effects of phenothiazine medications were discovered as an accidental by-product of research on antihistamines (used for allergies). Chlorpromazine (aka "Thorazine") became widely used in the early 1950s, and works by blocking the effect of a particular brain neurotransmitter ("dopamine"). Indeed, if you compare clinically effective doses of the different antipsychotics, those doses correlate almost exactly with the various drugs' ability to block dopamine activity in laboratory studies. In other words, it is the dopamine-blocking ability of a given drug that predicts how effective it is as an antipsychotic; dopamine is key. Later generations of antipsychotics work the same way, and although no more effective, they do have significantly lower side effects. Reserpine is a naturally-occurring drug that also blocks dopamine and has long been used as a folk medicine for psychosis, but not without considerable risks. So this bit of pharmacologic dissection suggests that the many forms of psychosis all seem to involve a relative increase in dopamine sensitivity.[10] Thus sprang forth the Dopamine Theory of Schizophrenia.

HOW DOPAMINE HELPS

Having introduced dopamine to this evolutionary discussion, the next question is: What does dopamine normally do for us? Dopamine is part of the reward system in the brain, and helps us form and recall emotional memories of things we like. When we find something we want (e.g. food, sex, etc.), some pleasurable dopamine is released in our brain. From then on, when we catch a hint of good things around us, dopamine release tells us to go out looking for them.[11,12] Dopamine plays the same kind of role in other animals, even in quite primitive species.[13,14] Indeed, by increasing our focus on satisfaction of our appetitive instincts, dopamine effectively decreases the role of our rational conscious thought. So, whereas serotonin is the "social director" of neurotransmitters, dopamine is the "appetitive director."

That is why dopamine can be fun for people. When people listen to music, the resulting dopamine release makes people want to move in more than one way—they dance, but also seek out pleasure, novelty and inspiration.[15] Blame it on the dopamine, you might say. Music also helps babies to fall asleep, and it helps people feel better about their woes. Singing the blues isn't wallowing in misery, or mere entertainment—it is a form of self-medication and relief from conscious distress.

As William Congreve (English playwright, 1670–1729) said: "Music hath charms to soothe the savage breast, to soften rocks, or bend a knotted oak." Of course, music is also a stimulus for romance and seduction. "If music be the food of love, play on" as William Shakespeare says in *Twelfth Night*. And he didn't even know about dopamine.

From the lowered dopamine side, Parkinson's disease (a neurological movement and tremor disorder) is associated with reduced dopamine activity and thus with reduced pleasure and novelty seeking.[16] A drug that treats Parkinson's through dopamine enhancement ("L-DOPA") also enhances anticipation of pleasure.[17] Parkinson's treatment can also go overboard. Pramipexole (brand name Mirapex: a synthetic dopamine enhancer that is used for Parkinson's) can so dramatically amplify pleasure- and novelty-seeking that it sends patients off on gambling, shopping, binge-eating and sexual adventure sprees—and can also trigger psychosis.[18,19,20] This just goes to show what kind of appetitive instincts can lie beneath our civilized veneer.

Dopamine also plays a central role in the memory of frightening situations. Traffic police who stand bravely amid oncoming cars all day have increased dopamine levels.[21] Perhaps this may explain their supposed appetitive affection for doughnuts, but it also gives new meaning to the idea that traffic can drive you crazy. Dopamine helps us remember and recall frightening ("aversive") situations.[22] It may have helped us to avoid lions back on the African plain, (not to mention toxic plants),[23] but more important is that it helps us recognize angry and scary people. People who have genetically increased dopamine activity are more sensitive to laboratory procedures that trigger a fear response.[24] With their low dopamine activity, untreated Parkinson's disease patients have reduced ability to recognize anger, but not necessarily reduced ability to recognize the other emotions.[25] In addition, when you study brain activity, Parkinson patients show a reduced brain reaction to fearful situations.[26] Dogs who are afraid of thunder respond well to dopamine-blocking medication, but not so well to medications for Panic or for anxiety[27] Our beta dog Cassidy handled thunder much better after a canine dopamine blocker. Likewise, one patient with neither psychosis nor anxiety disorder—but in a legitimately frightening ongoing situation of personal risk—felt much better on a dopamine-blocking antipsychotic than on medications for Panic and anxiety.

We already know that dopamine activity can enhance the pleasure of our appetites, and also increase our fear of anger. Both of these dopamine actions point our thoughts more toward our biologically instinctive reactions, and away from Conscious rational thought. The role of dopamine in psychosis may prove to be crucial but indirect, and it is not the only neurotransmitter story for psychosis. Recent work has expanded the focus to other neurotransmitters, including to glutamate and to anxiety-related gamma amino butyric acid ("GABA").

THE MISSING THINK—LOSING YOUR THEORY OF MIND

So if the psychotic Schizophrenias have something to do with social instincts, then is there something distinctive about social functioning in psychosis? Indeed there is. Patients with Schizophrenia have decreased ability to think things through consciously. To look at this thinking problem, let's start with Theory of Mind (ToM—that ability to recognize that other people also think and feel). The diminished Consciousness in Schizophrenia reduces the ability to recognize other people's Consciousness in a laboratory test,[28,29] especially in those with paranoid delusions.[30] Having Schizophrenia means not having much social interaction with other people, and reduced ToM is the best predictor of this.[31] In one brain-imaging study, patients and normal controls were asked to look at visual images of geometrical triangles that moved randomly, or else that moved with seeming intent. Those with Schizophrenia had a harder time seeing the intent, and they had decreased brain activity in important brain areas. Even so, those who also had greater activity in their frontal cortex did a little better at prediction, perhaps because they could still use their rational thought to compensate for their ToM limitations. In Schizophrenia, we are less aware of other people, we are less able to assess them and their social intent, and we have less ability to talk with them. In Schizophrenia, our social life becomes more of an internal process and less of a real life interaction with other people.

In the laboratory, those basically normal students who do occasionally hear voices (which isn't always Schizophrenia, but which is a related symptom) are less able to use their frontal cortex to deliberately block their recognition of pictures they have already seen, as compared to students who never hear voices.[32] Likewise, there is also a decreased capacity for abstract thought in Schizophrenia. Give someone with Schizophrenia a proverb like "people in glass houses shouldn't throw stones," and they are likely to tell you only that broken glass is a bad idea. These kinds of thinking problems happen in pretty much any kind of psychosis.[33]

But wait a second. Clearly, someone with active Schizophrenia can be overwhelmed by unchangeable false beliefs ("delusions"), by voices ("auditory hallucinations") and by a somehow dysfunctional brain ("cognitive impairment"). For example, people who hear voices also have poor insight into their illness.[34] So are the thinking problems a cause of psychosis, or do they result from psychotic confusion? One way to answer that question is to look at nonpsychotic young people who are at "high risk" for Schizophrenia, many of whom later do develop Schizophrenia. They do seem to have the same kinds of thinking problems as those with the established illness. They are not very good at conscious processing of social and emotional information[35,36] or of facial expressions,[37] and they tend to be less socially interactive.[38] They do better at social tasks if they have some extra time to think,[39] and when they focus on ToM tests, brain scans show that they need to make intensified mental effort to answer them.[40] So, diminished Consciousness must already be there before psychosis even begins.

One intriguing possibility is that ability to understand others' minds in psychosis is impaired by an inability to simulate what others are thinking.[41] Studies suggest that imitation and simulation are important parts of how we understand other people. Perhaps we could say of other people that "they are what we do." There are even "mirror neurons" in the brain that work at that very task, and simulation ability is important for all of us. Recent studies looked at presumably healthy people who had cosmetic Botox (botulinum toxin brand name) treatment of facial muscles.[42,43] Because Botox reduces wrinkles by paralyzing facial muscles, it is more difficult to display our own facial emotions. So if we can't make facial expressions, then it is hard to recognize the expressions of others through mimicry. As a result, having Botox makes it harder to understand other people's facial emotions. This could make for some confusing cocktail parties. Our wrinkles look better, but we can't tell if people like it. In one companion study, a thick gel on the face (something like heavy pancake makeup) forced the facial muscles to work extra hard, which actually made it easier for subjects to recognize others' emotions.[44] Botox may make us look younger, but it gives us a poker face, and makes other people more inscrutable to us.

CONSCIOUSNESS AND SOCIAL INSTINCT UNBALANCED

Although limited Consciousness of social cues is a social problem (and also a problem for real poker players, who need to assess their opponents' emotions), it is not by itself a psychotic illness. Psychosis happens when inborn social instincts overwhelm conscious social processing—through some combination of decreased Consciousness and increased social instinct. Let's start with decreased Consciousness, and look at situations where the Consciousness functions of the front part of the brain (in the surface layer of the "frontal cortex") are reduced, impeded, or distracted.

One possibility is that some people have less brain to think with—not the whole brain, but the frontal cortex parts where we think consciously, and where we process social cues and instincts, that is, our social minds. There is a long research literature on reduced function of the frontal lobe in Schizophrenia,[45] and it turns out that there is a thinning of the frontal cortex in both Schizophrenia and in true Bipolar I Disorder.[46] This thinning seems to be there from the beginning: in people at high risk for Schizophrenia[47] and also at first onset of psychosis,[48] and it doesn't worsen with the severity or duration of illness. So thinning of the frontal cortex probably isn't caused by psychosis or by antipsychotic medication. Not only that, but a thinner cortex is associated with less awareness of being ill,[49] and with reduced attention span.[50] Thus sprang forth the "Hypofrontality theory" of Schizophrenia.[45]

THE GENETIC ROOT OF ALL INSTINCT

Clearly, Schizophrenia runs in families, and much effort over many decades has gone into looking for evidence of specific genetic factors, but as Randolph Nesse points out: "The evolutionary question about Schizophrenia is why selection has not eliminated the genes for this highly heritable disease that so dramatically decreases fitness."[51] The search for susceptibility genes has had only modest success. As we will see, there are at least two genetic variants that may overarchingly predispose us to the Schizophrenias and to psychoses of all types. One of these genetic variants increases the amount of dopamine activity, and the other one reduces the effectiveness of the conscious thinking part of our brains in the frontal cortex (i.e., The Dopamine Theory and the Hypofrontality Theory).

Under our evolutionary theory, one reason for the failure to find genes highly specific for Schizophrenia generally is that the various Schizophrenias derive from several different, if overlapping, social-instinct subtypes. Each subtype must have its own separate pattern of inheritance, and each one of those is far more complex than the intricate genetics of a sneeze, a yawn, or a smile.

One line of genetic research has looked at the function of our dopamine appetitive director. The dopamine receptor D2 gene ("DRD2") controls the level of certain dopamine receptors, and a particular variant can increase the level of dopamine activity. That would increase dopamine's appetitive effects, and thus would increase the activity of some social and other instincts. So what do we know about DRD2? For one thing, the variant form is more common in Schizophrenia than it is in normal controls in Bulgaria, Spain, Australia, and probably everywhere else.[52,53,54] Most people don't always think straight. But with dopamine increasing all that instinctive pressure, it is even harder for these people to think straight.[55,56] So, they tend to think less and are more likely to follow their instincts in laboratory studies, even if there is some kind of penalty as a result.[57] Because they are more preoccupied by instinctive reactions, it is similarly harder for them to notice a second visual image that is presented very quickly after a first.[58] Basically, when instinctive fears are aroused, the fears persist in a way that crowds out other thoughts.[24] So when we're considering our social instincts, increased DRD2 dopamine activity can make those instincts and their underlying fears rise to the fore.

A second line of genetic research has looked at the frontal cortex—the thinking part of our brains. We already know that there is a thinner frontal cortex in Schizophrenia. There is a genetically determined protein ("Neuregulin 1" or NRG1) that plays a major role in forming nerve cells and their connections, and there are quite a number of different versions of this protein. Variations of NRG 1 are associated with a frontal cortex that is smaller or has fewer nerve cells[59,60] and that has a failure to communicate well with some other parts of the brain.[61] Neuregulin 1 variants also make some people have to work their frontal lobes harder at laboratory mental challenges, even at ages 10 to 12, long before any psychotic illness would start.[62] So it is not surprising that NRG 1 is associated with Schizophrenia in Icelandic, Scottish, Swedish, and other studies.[63] It is also possible that epigenetics (where activity of some genes is reduced during life by attached methyl groups) plays a companion role in determining the types and levels of frontal lobe activity.[64] Epigenetic mechanisms could be how developmental and environmental factors take effect, and they could be a clue to new treatments.[65]

HOW COULD THESE GENES POSSIBLY BE HELPFUL?

A best guess is that Schizophrenia itself is not evolutionarily adaptive for people who have it—they tend toward great unhappiness and have few children—and neither is it adaptive for their immediate families through altruistic or other benefits to the gene pool of the extended family.[66] However, if humans still have genes floating around that increase dopamine activity or that limit the abilities of our conscious social mind, then there must be a reason. If some of us don't think the same as others, therefore they must be better at something.

In some measure, increased dopamine activity leads to novelty-seeking and creativity. That has helped the human race, and in these times that try men's goals, a little more creativity would come in handy. An "impaired" frontal cortex reduces conscious oversight and thus gives us more access to biological social instinct. Scientists, doing as scientists do, managed to put the human enhanced dopamine gene (DRD2) into unsuspecting mice. The mice then became hyperactive when put into novel situations.[67] No word, though, on whether they became handier with tiny little paint brushes. Neuregulin 1, despite reduced frontal cortex brain function, is associated with greater creativity.[60] In the right dose, this too would allow more novelty seeking, creativity, and social instinct to poke through. Instinctual gut feelings, when you can conceptualize them, are an invaluable source of information for inspiration and decision making.

This makes you wonder if there could be yet other kinds of creativity not directly or indirectly linked to social instinct. This recalls the observation of Thomas Kuhn (American philosopher of science; 1922–1996) that true scientific advances come from unwittingly-realized new conceptual models ("paradigm shifts" that are most often realized in the shower) rather than merely from rational scientific investigation.

As a society, we need a balance of the factors that differentiate creative and not-so-creative people. An unfortunate by-product of that balance is that some people have so much of those biological creative factors that they fall off of Randolph Nesse's "cliff edge," into the realm of psychosis.

CONSCIOUSNESS LOST

Things go terribly wrong when we develop an imbalance because of reduced conscious control or because of increased instinctive drive. On the Consciousness side of the equation, too little ability to modify or enhance social instincts leaves us with little but instinct to guide us. There are a number of ways that Consciousness can be impaired. Most important for Schizophrenia and psychosis is the kind of biologically reduced social consciousness and social mind that is associated with a thin frontal cortex, with NRG 1, and with unknown other factors. However, there are other known mechanisms, and the risk of psychosis is especially high when there is more than one.

Psychosis is common in Alzheimer's dementia, where there is a progressive reduction in frontal-lobe consciousness, memory and rational thought.[68] Since this is presumably a function of the dementia itself, it is not related to NRG 1 genetics.[69] Psychotic symptoms are more common in those with the most impaired thinking.[70] Altogether, some 41% of patients with dementia develop either delusions (36%) or hallucinations (18%) or both over time.[71] That presents a treatment problem, because antipsychotic medications have higher risks of death and medical complications in elderly demented patients.

Psychosis can also happen with medical illnesses that affect the frontal cortex. In late-stage syphilis that affects the brain ("neurosyphilis," once known as "general paresis of the insane"), the infected frontal cortex becomes smaller and presumably less effective.[72] Because the resulting psychosis looks very much like Schizophrenia, the role of syphilitic infection is all too easy to miss.

Sleep is another kind of Consciousness lost. Consciousness begins to fade as we enter "twilight sleep." That's when many nonpsychotic people will hear a voice calling out their name. These "hypnogogic hallucinations" are more common in people who are also more sensitive to environmental sounds generally.[73] Along similar lines, if you tell college students in an experiment to not think about something ("whatever you do, do not think about white bears"), then they will actually think more about that something (i.e., white bears) when they are in twilight sleep.[74] The thought that they had tried to push aside comes back when their conscious control fades. Fortunately, these experiments do not summon forth real live bears.

During actual sleep there is even less Consciousness. As Immanuel Kant (German philosopher, 1724–1804) said, "the lunatic is a dreamer in the waking state." Dreams, then, are a nearly pure reflection of inborn social instincts as modified over time by social learning. That's why they are useful when psychotherapy is focused on understanding ourselves. As Freud pointed out, dreams are the "royal road to the unconscious." Most likely, dreams are that social-learning and instinctual-modification process in action, as we sort through recent events to adapt our social understanding. It is worth noting that nonpsychotic people have nonpsychotic dreams. Although dreams can be magical, psychotic events don't happen in ordinary dreams.[75] The dreams of psychotic people contain the same kinds of fixed false beliefs as when they are awake.

Serious sleep deprivation can produce psychotic symptoms that are not good for us.[76] For example, at 56 hours without sleep, people have reduced frontal-lobe activity, increased anxiety and moodiness, and paranoid thoughts.[77] Last, but not least, severe anxiety, depression or fear can overwhelm our minds, and crowd out our ability to reason.

INSTINCT RUN AMOK

The second side of the mind/brain equation is the instinct side: that is, we can also become unbalanced by exaggerated instincts that overwhelm our mind's ability to regulate them. Let's start with how dopamine leads us into temptation. We see a hint of a tasty experience, and the flowing dopamine prompts us to seek out fulfillment for our appetites. So far, so good. However, we have social instincts that view our appetitive behavior in the context of social groups. If we go for a forbidden cigar (or ostentatious luxury car), it may trigger Panicky thoughts of catastrophic group expulsion for misbehavior, increased fears of embarrassingly high status in front of hierarchical superiors, of cigar-ash contamination, or of social guilt for offending others. Cigars and luxury cars are metaphors, of course, but sometimes a cigar is more than just a cigar. If you see it as an appetitive extravagance, it may be an intensifier of your lurking social instincts, at the expense of your conscious control.

Dopamine also plays a role in frighteningly aversive situations. Those who have a greater dopamine response to an oncoming Rolls Royce will merely have a greater amount of fear. So far, so good. However, if social fears trigger dopamine release, there is a yet further increase in fear, further exaggeration of social instincts, and thus further reduction in rational conscious control. Owning Rolls Royces does not make most people psychotic, but when there are enough propsychotic factors and heightened social instincts at play, then owning a high-profile possession can help trigger psychosis.

Amphetamines ("speed") and cocaine can cause a time-limited psychosis quite similar to Schizophrenia, presumably by inducing greater dopamine release in susceptible people, and without even requiring NRG 1 or other contributors to decreased frontal lobe function.[78]

Social stimuli can also be toxic to the predisposed. There is an old and largely abandoned theory that Schizophrenia is related to a high level of "expressed emotion" among family members. Even so, one recent study suggests that emotionally overinvolved relatives (that's just one type of "expressed emotion") are associated with more psychotic symptoms.[79] Is this because the family overinvolvement and psychosis have a common underlying cause? Is it because more psychotic symptoms make the family get more involved? Or is it because overinvolvement triggers more of those bothersome social instincts? Perhaps we should go with the last of these, because NRG 1 and reduced frontal-cortex function are also associated with increased sensitivity to family conflict in Schizophrenia.[80] If you are already at risk, then overinvolved family can really get to you.

Anticipation of social conflict can make even mundane events worsen psychosis. One homeless patient with Schizophrenia appeared in the emergency room requesting hospitalization for increased voices. He had saved his money for some very fancy sneakers (the vehicular equivalent, for him, of a Rolls Royce), and was now terrified about returning to his homeless shelter. Homeless shelters have no shortage of expulsion risk, dominance displays, crime, and people quick to take offense. Once he realized that new sneakers had increased his fears of the social world at his shelter, he was much less fearful, and he devised a practical plan for the real possibility of theft. So if frightening social stimuli can worsen psychosis, then maybe the cosmetic Botox we talked about could help a little by reducing awareness of threatening facial emotions. Plastic surgeons would love this. Thick pancake makeup, on the other hand, might make social stimuli extra frightening.

When sufficiently aroused, our five core social-instinct diagnoses can be quite stressful indeed. Through interaction with reduced frontal-cortex function and increased dopamine activity, they are major contributors to psychotic disorders. The usual suspects for anxiety and depressive disorders are also the usual suspects for psychotic disorders. Rational decisions, ironically, don't always help. When we deliberately overrule the prompts of our social instincts, they not only continue to prompt us, but they may actually prompt much more insistently. That has consequences for psychosis and other illnesses.

Likewise, civilization can have unexpected effects. By encouraging counter-instinctive behavior, civilization can also amplify the intensity of social instincts. Imagine someone with Panic Anxiety as they endure dramatically severe levels of Panic if they must travel far away in a claustrophobia-inducing airplane. Indeed, first psychotic episodes are often triggered by travel.[81] And it's not just the direct biological effects of these intensified instincts; too much emotional noise from instincts can drown out our conscious mind. What emerges, then, is that raw and dramatic presentation of exaggerated social instincts as psychosis.

CAN THE USUAL SUSPECTS TAKE US OVER THE EDGE?

Just as Major Depressive Disorder (MDD) is a catch-all for depressive disorders, and Generalized Anxiety Disorder (GAD) for anxiety disorders, Schizophrenia can be viewed as a catch-all for psychotic disorders, as well as a paradigmatic example of psychosis. As it happens, the same five social instincts that lead to specific anxiety and depressive disorders may also help define specific subtypes of Schizophrenia. However, whereas we already have the diagnostic tools to fine-tune depressive and anxiety disorders, we are only now starting to do the same with psychosis and Schizophrenia.[82]

Although the mixed-illness nature ("heterogeneity") of Schizophrenia has long been known, progress has been slow in peeling away distinct kinds of psychosis. One major step was the discovery that some Schizophrenia is actually that late and serious form of syphilis in the brain ("neurosyphilis"). This recognition led to syphilis screening in psychotic patients and effective treatment with penicillin and other antibiotics. Although Mania (now part of what is known as Bipolar I Disorder) has long been recognized as a distinct illness, more recent work recognized the occurrence of a more psychotic form of Mania that has often been confused with Schizophrenia. Other diagnoses pulled out of the Schizophrenia category include Psychotic Depression (a form of Melancholia), and Paranoid Delusional Disorder, not to mention various psychoses caused by medication, substance abuse, and physical illness.

Still, the nature and relationship of these psychoses is not well understood, and more research is needed. For example, research suggests that a "harm avoidance" personality style (which has four subtypes that seem to correspond nicely to four of our social instincts), is higher in schizophrenic patients, and also in their relatives.[83] Although most Schizophrenia research focuses similarly on the overall diagnostic category as a whole, some researchers continue to look for valid subtypes of the "Schizophrenias." One way of looking at Schizophrenia subtypes is by looking at other syndromes that occur together with it (co-morbidity).[84] Not that long ago, those other syndromes were supposed to be ignored in Schizophrenia, on the basis of the theory that Schizophrenia is so overwhelming that the multiplicity of symptoms merely reflects a multifaceted disease.

More recently, scattered researchers have started to note that anxiety disorders are common even in correctly diagnosed Schizophrenia. Even voices in "normal" people happen more often in those with anxiety or depressive disorders.[85] Most recently, researchers have started to identify co-morbid anxiety disorders in a systematic way, with specialized diagnostic interviews and techniques.[86,87,88] One study of early-stage Schizophrenia spectrum patients suggested that 9.3% had Panic Anxiety, 48.1% had Social Anxiety, 14.3% had OCD, and at least 84.9% had at one or more anxiety disorders that preceded psychosis onset. In another study, of people with established Schizophrenia, 24% had Panic Anxiety, 17.7% had Social Anxiety, and 24% had OCD.[89] Those might even be underestimates.[90] We will try to follow in these promising footsteps, as we present our usual suspects in the same order that we introduced them.

Panic Psychosis Case Study: Alone Against the Predators

Not very long ago, an Indiana college student felt very nervous. As she headed toward her first visit to a psychiatrist, she resisted a sudden urge to get off the bus. But as she stayed rooted in her seat, the desire to flee returned abruptly, along with a voice telling her that she must escape from the dangerous intentions of the other passengers. The voice continued for some 20 minutes after she reached her stop. It turned out that her recent anxiety began with the onset of Panic Disorder some two years before, but that this was the first day that she had heard a voice or felt such intense fear. That she had no other prior syndromes besides Panic was uncommon.

In the hospital, medical evaluation was normal, and antipsychotic medications stopped the voice some weeks later. Even so, she remained withdrawn and frightened, with frequent, if subdued, Panic Attacks. After hospital discharge, clonazepam was added to her medications every 12 hours. With that, she felt back to normal, but soon felt a need to stop all medications. With reassurance and family support, she persisted and was later able to talk about deeper concerns in psychotherapy. She completed college, went on about a successful social and professional life, and many years later was doing well with clonazepam as her only medication.

Panic Disorder is very common in Schizophrenia.[84,88] Even today, most clinicians view this as an unpleasant, if unremarkable, symptom of Schizophrenia. Besides, if you were psychotic, wouldn't that make you Panicky too? In our social-instinct theory, though, some Schizophrenia has Panic Anxiety as a core feature of a "Panic psychosis."[91] For one thing, most people start having Panic Attacks well before they ever have psychotic symptoms, and Panics continue even if the psychosis is controlled with antipsychotic medication.[88,92] Panic Attacks are most difficult to diagnose while people are acutely psychotic. Somehow the Panic social instinct takes over from conscious thought and produces a psychotic state.

Nonpsychotic Panic patients have increased brain activity in response to experimental noise.[93] This might have helped listen for predators and to inner cautions when they were away from home way back when. So it is not surprising, then, that patients with Schizophrenia and high anxiety levels (i.e., most likely Panic) have more voices and delusions (aka "positive symptoms") as well as more social withdrawal and lack of pleasure (also known as "negative symptoms").[94] Voices are pretty common in Schizophrenia, and they may be especially common in what we are calling "Panic psychosis." Panic can make the mind go yonder.

If you look very closely at the voices, they tend to come on in a flash. And if you look carefully at that flash moment, patients also tend to have Panic Anxiety symptoms. The association of voices with Panic Anxiety poses another chicken-and-egg problem, but it seems likely that the voice is an additional symptom of a Panic Attack. For one thing, adding fixed doses of certain antipanic medicines, such as clonazepam or alprazolam, will treat both voices and Panic, though it is worth noting that other antipanic medications do not seem to work for this.

Remember how carbon dioxide can trigger Panic in patients with Panic Anxiety? In one study, carbon dioxide triggered Panic in all of eight patients with Schizophrenia and voices.[88] This study also used a new interview method that focused on the flash moment of voice onset, which found that their voices were always associated with Panic symptoms (since Panic Anxiety mixes with voices, an ordinary interview doesn't get enough information when you merely ask about Panic by itself). In some patients who are not on low-dose antipanic medications or on high-dose antipsychotics, the carbon dioxide-induced Panic also brings on voices. This is useful, if very preliminary information, because it may help figure out how to better help some patients.

Julian Jaynes (American psychologist; 1920–1997) asserts that voices are basically messages from the mind,[95] and he might be right. Because Panic Anxiety is an ancient instinctive fear of separation from the group, one valid concern is of facing predators on your own. Indeed, the voices and paranoid fears of Panic psychosis patients are about facing a world of potential predators, pretty much on your own. Jaynes speculated that internal voices were predominant in humans in the past. It is easy to imagine similar instinctive internal fear communications in animals of all kinds (especially infants), and we can only guess how and if they "hear" those warnings. However, our human language allows us to give verbal warnings to ourselves.

Samuel Siris (American psychiatrist,1944 –) has also written about Panic and sudden-onset paranoid thoughts.[96] There, too, it seems likely that Panic onset is associated with suddenly exaggerated fears. For example, a nonpsychotic Panic patient might Panic if he felt closed in on a bus, and then he might make an exit. But when one patient with Schizophrenia got on a bus, he had the Panicky conviction that the other passengers were out to get him, and he got off as soon as possible. Studies have factor analyzed the various kinds of delusions and hallucinations that can be present in Schizophrenia, and there may be at least four subtype Factors of this "psychosis factor analysis," which we will get to in turn. One distinct delusion Factor group is persecutory delusions—the mistaken idea that people are out to get you.[97] Those may also be associated with Panic.

So how is the mind/brain balance unbalanced in Panic psychosis? Although we know that frontal lobe consciousness is diminished in Schizophrenia generally, there have been no studies yet that focus on a Panic psychosis subgroup. We do know that the frontal lobe is at least somewhat less active in nonpsychotic Panic patients[98] but that it improves with Panic treatment. Panic Anxiety may also be associated with more dopamine activity, leading to more social-instinct expression.[99] Exaggerated together, these mechanisms might lead us to hear in human words the raw warnings of our primeval Panic instinct.

There is bad news in that diagnosis of anxiety disorders in Schizophrenia is difficult, but good news in the possibility that we may be able to significantly improve treatment.[91,100,101] Quite preliminary work suggests that some Panic psychosis patients may show significant improvement in all their symptoms with clonazepam and an antipsychotic, and that some, in time, become essentially symptom free.

SOCIAL ANXIETY: MAKE YOURSELF FEEL UNWORTHY OR SHUNNED

We know that Schizophrenia can be associated with Social Anxiety,[102] at least 25% in one study of first episode Schizophrenia, and 39% in a study of outpatients in treatment.[103] Because Social Anxiety mixes with paranoid delusions during psychosis, it is hard to see it clearly during a psychotic episode. Social Anxiety is easier to diagnose when the psychosis has been at least partly treated.[104] However, Social Anxiety precedes the onset of psychosis, and those early symptoms are similar to those of nonpsychotic Social Anxiety patients, so one can also focus diagnostically on the years before psychosis began. Even nonpsychotic people with Social Anxiety are more likely to have some level of paranoia and altered perceptions.[105] Patients with both Schizophrenia and Social Anxiety are less social, less functional, and more likely to commit suicide than those with Schizophrenia alone.

Social Anxiety means being afraid of the powers that be (or "the Man," as "they" are sometimes called). Patients feel that the safe approach is to lay as low to the ground as possible, and to believe that that is where their social rank actually dwells. The psychotic form of Social Anxiety is associated with a fixed delusion of inferior status in the eyes of others, and with concerns about mistreatment and persecution as a consequence.[106] Depending on the culture, that might include delusional notions of having fewer social permissions (including for romance, cuisine and companionship—shades of that baboon hierarchy) or of smelling offensively bad to others (olfactory reference syndrome).[107] Voices may tell you that you are worthless. Along those lines, the most important correlate of Social Anxiety in Schizophrenia is low self-esteem.[108] Indeed, assessed Social Anxiety in Schizophrenia is dramatically associated with perceived unlikeability and incompetence.[109] Do whatever it takes to submissively placate "the Man," or retaliate if it seems necessary. A recent television commercial showed a senior executive signing a document, and he gleefully says, "That'll stick it to the Man." The surprised junior executive at his side responds, "but sir, you are the Man," though he doesn't actually diagnose Social Anxiety in his boss.

And when Schizophrenia is associated with both low self-esteem and high suspiciousness, people are significantly more likely to overread anger in emotionally neutral photographs in the laboratory.[110] The Man can lurk anywhere. In pure form, psychotic Social Anxiety often looks like what is already called delusional disorder, especially the persecutory (paranoid) subtype. The lower the self-esteem, the greater the suspicious paranoia[111]—because "you can't be too careful." The delusions typically reflect concerns about malevolent observation by powerful authority figures, and the details derive from cultural influences.[112] Religious themes, such as fears of Satan, have been around for a long time. Hostile aliens, more common decades ago, are now largely replaced by the CIA and FBI, but with terrorists creeping steadily into the mix.

Psychotic Social Anxiety is associated with both increased paranoia, yet also with a still highly functional Theory of Mind.[113] This combination can present another kind of problematic symptom. If you are acutely aware of other peoples' minds, and highly fearful of other people, you may conclude that other people can read your mind, that people on television are talking directly to you, or that other people can move thoughts in and out of your mind.[111] Voices commenting on your thoughts correspond to the notion that others can read your mind. These are among the Schneiderian symptoms (Kurt Schneider, German psychiatrist, 1887–1967) that are characteristic of Schizophrenia, but whose significance has long been hard to understand. So from an evolutionary perspective, these symptoms are a psychotic ToM. That psychosis factor analysis we mentioned also found one Factor group composed of these very same Schneiderian symptoms.[96] It is worth a bet that this subtype, (and maybe also persecutory delusions) are associated with Social Anxiety. Psychotic patients with a pronounced earlier history of Social Anxiety seem nearly always to have thoughts of mind reading or thought control. Their instinct and their ToM tell them to pay close attention to the minds of the alpha dogs, which, in the patients' minds, are no doubt paying close attention to them.

Since the limited Consciousness in psychosis reduces their ability to test these concerns against real social data, they end up with concerns that come more from their inside world than from the outside world. Parkinson's disease has a high co-morbidity with Social Anxiety.[114] So when patients are given pramipexole (or similar drugs that treat Parkinson's by enhancing dopamine), the psychosis that can occur often looks like the Paranoid Delusional Disorder that would correspond to psychotic Social Anxiety.[115] This psychosis is more likely to happen in those Parkinson's patients who also have a dementia that reduces their conscious moderation of instinct.[116] Social Anxiety gets better with SSRIs that improve social comfort, and so does psychotic Social Anxiety when SSRIs are added to antipsychotics.[108]

OCD: HONING YOUR NESTING, GROOMING, AND SENSES

The occurrence of OCD symptoms in Schizophrenia has been known since the days of Eugen Bleuler but here too there has been little research attention until recently. One review article concluded that more than a third of patients with Schizophrenia had OCD or at least OCD symptoms.[117] A Japanese study of hospitalized Schizophrenia patients found that 14% had full OCD, and another 51% had OCD symptoms.[118] Not only are these big numbers, but the presence of co-morbid OCD predicted more severe psychotic symptoms, and worse outcomes. An Israeli study examined the pattern of OCD symptoms in patients with Schizophrenia. With a little variation, their results are similar to the clean, arrange, save, and behave subtype model that we have been using in our theory.[119] If you look at people with nonpsychotic OCD, some 23% of high-risk patients may go on to Schizophrenia.[120,121] As a result of this recent work, there is now much speculation about the possibility of a schizo-obsessive subtype.[122]

If there is a schizo-obsessive subtype, then what kind of symptoms do we see? First of all, standard OCD symptoms can be present in psychosis, and sometimes in a further exaggerated form. A patient with a compulsion to tap a door three times before entering may develop a fixed belief that the world will come to an end if he does not. Patients with compulsive behaviors may come to experience the compulsions as voices that instruct them what to do (command hallucinations).[123]

There is also a curious interaction between OCD and our five senses: hearing, vision, touch, taste, and smell. A Brazilian research team has reported sample cases of Schizo-Obsessive Disorder and sensory hallucinations: one patient with voices about Satan as her king, (requiring decontamination and religious acts, perhaps to allow her return to society); another with visualization of black dots on the skin (requiring ritual cleaning for perceived feces contamination); one with tactile sensation of urine on the upper legs (requiring avoidance of contaminating others with the offensive self-contamination); and one with fetid personal odor (requiring relentless bathing for the self-perceived offensive smell).[124] In the presence of psychosis, OCD takes potential sensory concerns and turns them into problematic and exaggerated delusions. Not surprisingly, another of the delusion factor-analysis results is a cluster of perceptual symptoms including sight, smell, and tactile hallucinations.[103]

Obsessive-Compulsive Disorders can have similar sensory effects in otherwise nonpsychotic people. Oliver Sacks (American neurologist, 1933–) has written eloquently about musical hallucinations in *Musicophilia*. Musical hallucinations occur in Schizo-Obsessive Disorder,[125] but they also occur in people with hearing loss.[126] Two recent patients were both elderly women with long histories of untreated OCD, significant recent hearing loss, and new onset musical hallucinations. In quiet settings, both of them heard pleasant favorite songs from their younger days, and one of them also heard hallway noises that sounded like voices. They both improved with an SSRI for the OCD, and the musical interludes reached their finales.

In Charles Bonnet syndrome (Swiss naturalist, 1720–1793), new onset blindness can lead to visual hallucinations. Indeed, even prolonged blindfolding of normal volunteers can produce this effect.[127] There is no word yet on whether those visions are more common or more complex in those with OCD as we might expect. There are also patients who turn up in dermatology offices with the absolute conviction that they have parasites in their skin ("delusional parasitosis," also called Morgellon's syndrome) Despite skin biopsies and patient-provided "parasite" samples, very rarely is there any evidence of actual parasites,[128] yet nothing will reassure these patients. Just as nonpsychotic self-scratching ("psychogenic excoriation") is often linked to OCD,[129] so too is delusional parasitosis.[130] Indeed, since these patients do have some sort of reduced cognitive abilities [131] their ancient instinctual concerns more easily become very real sensory perception.

In the absence of enough conscious control, (due either to psychosis or else to a relative sensory deprivation such as hearing or vision loss), OCD somehow allows vague sensations to be instinctually interpreted as primeval causes for concern. If your senses exist to help you to be a fit member of the societal nest, then this limitation of sensory-information processing means you have to be extra careful about parasites and other things. Vague sensations remind you of those OCD obligations to clean, arrange, save and behave in order to be a suitable nestmate.

Treatment for Schizo-Obsessive Disorders is uncertain. Antipsychotics clearly help, but adding SSRIs for the presumably underlying OCD is problematic. On the one hand, the OCD improves, but on the other hand, SSRIs can make psychosis worse, especially in the higher doses needed for OCD. There may be a way out of this conundrum. One patient with Schizo-Obsessive Disorder did very well when his psychosis was treated with an antipsychotic and his OCD with a high-dose SSRI, while worsened psychosis was prevented with clonazepam.

ATYPICAL DEPRESSION: ALL WE NEED IS SOCIAL HARMONY

If we imagine an extreme and unrealistic version of sensitivity to social rejection, we end up with something that sounds a bit like paranoia. For example, a psychotic version might start with: "Because people are undoubtedly rejecting me, I must have done something to annoy them." This leads to a heightened focus on keeping a low profile so as not to offend. Eventually, though, the concern turns from maintaining proper behavior to the sense of rejection—and then on to the notion of anger directed at a world of rejecting people. In other words, their own unmodulated rejection sensitivity leads them to believe that they are the undeniable focus of other peoples' malevolent intent. This is not too different from Freud's idea that some paranoid thoughts come from the conscience ("superego").

There is also a companion possibility. People with Bipolar I Disorder (classically called manic-depressive disorder) have both manic and depressive episodes. Although the depressive episodes can include Melancholia (as well as the ill-defined Major Depressive Disorder), they are most commonly Atypical Depression. Research offers strong support for this clinical impression.[132,133,134] So if other anxiety and depressive disorders have corresponding psychotic forms, perhaps mania is one psychotic form of Atypical Depression. This linkage would correspond to their clinical association, and offers a reassuring symmetry. Expert clinicians know that deliberate interview techniques can sometimes make acutely manic patients briefly seem depressed, though they quickly revert to mania. We should also point out that there seems to be more than one genetically distinct form of Bipolar I Disorder, and maybe even of different forms of mania itself.

THE SWITCH

Somehow, bipolar patients suddenly "switch" into mania. We don't really understand this. Suggested triggers include sleep deprivation, medical steroid use, and maybe some antidepressants.[135] Both positive and negative life events may also play a stressful role.[136] For example, one patient came to the emergency room in a fully manic state after a finally achieved financial goal made him fear the envy and hostility of others. Other patients may suffer rejections such as unexpected divorce, parental death, job loss, or severe criticism, triggering a manic episode.[137]

This makes sense. If episodes of Atypical Depression are triggered by sensitivity to others' emotions and perceived social rejection, then extreme perceived rejection might trigger mania in susceptible patients. There is a common saying that concerned people should "Think globally, act locally" in order to do good in the world. That's what people with Atypical Depression do. When they think they have been rejected for giving offense, they try to mend their ways. Mania can be thought of as something more like "Think locally, act globally." True mania often involves thoughts of a profound ability to simplistically bring about social harmony through universal love and compassion, world peace, and an end to hunger—a kind of psychotic social consciousness. More modestly along those lines, one airline flight attendant decided to follow company instructions to keep customers happy. In her manic state, she thought the best way to do this was to laughingly run down the aisle spraying whipped cream on passengers to either side. Mania often includes paranoia, but with a twist. Instead of thinking that they are followed by FBI agents trying to hurt them, manic people might think the FBI is there to help protect them and support their mission.

Mania often takes on religious overtones, with thoughts of being Jesus or some other Savior, or of taking orders from some higher power. Manic people do sometimes have good ideas, tend to be quite charismatic, and can sometimes do some good. It is quite possible that some secular and religious leaders derive inspiration from episodes of mania. Not only that, but mania can encourage creative, if rather bold, approaches. Joan of Arc (French military leader, 1412–1431) followed visions from God at age 16 to seek peace for France through defeat of the English army. And as the Blues Brothers said in their movie: "We're on a mission from God!" Indeed, in the "Jerusalem syndrome," well known to psychiatrists there, manic patients fly to Israel in the throes of their manic missionary zeal. That psychosis factor-analysis we've been discussing produces a Factor group of symptoms matching mania, with grandiose plans, religious content, thoughts about guilt and sin, and exaggerated self-importance.[97]

What might make the perceived rejection stronger or the response so different in Mania? Looking at mania through the lens of balancing instinct and Consciousness, there are a number of possibilities. Acute mania includes impulsive behavior, which could be due to increased instinctive drives. As in other psychoses, genetically increased dopamine activity could be one factor.[138] For example, mania is associated with reckless gambling, sexual adventures, spending, and substance abuse (sounds a bit like those side effects of the dopamine-enhancing medicine pramipexole). More than that, people make riskier choices on a laboratory gambling task during acute mania.[139] Actually, they make riskier gambling moves in all phases of bipolar illness: manic, depressed, and normal baseline.[140]

The other side of the equation is conscious control. It looks like Bipolar I Disorder is also associated with a variant NRG 1 gene, though perhaps different from the variants in Schizophrenia.[141] Neuregulin 1 variants, of course, can impair Conscious thinking in the frontal cortex, and, the frontal cortex is also less active[142] and has a thinner surface cortex in bipolar patients.[143] A smaller frontal cortex also predicts more frequent episodes of mania, but not of nonpsychotic Depressive episodes.[144] Just what we might expect.

Other than as risk for acute mania, how does this decreased conscious control look? For one thing, patients with a prior history of mania are not so good at laboratory ToM tasks—it is hard for them to figure out what other people might be thinking.[145] Similarly, their frontal cortex plays a more modest role in modulating instinctual emotions.[146] This is also reflected in a tendency during a normal state to rely more on rumination, catastrophizing, and self-blame, and less on rational contemplation in the face of stressful events.[147] As a result, even in a nonmanic state, they may not sense subtle emotional cues in others. If we pay close attention, we can sometimes sense a mild air of social detachment about them.

WHAT ABOUT THAT SEROTONIN SOCIAL DIRECTOR?

If there is some relation between Atypical Depression and mania, then serotonin should play a role in their underlying social instincts. What we find depends on whether we study people during acute mania, or at other times when they may be in a depressed or normal baseline state. There is evidence of increased epigenetic deactivation of some serotonin genes in bipolar disorder at baseline (and in Schizophrenia), perhaps reducing serotonin function.[148] Their family members, even though without clinical bipolar disorder, still have some impaired frontal-cortex functioning that appears when given the tryptophan-depletion test that further reduces serotonin function.[149] So the predisposing serotonin system differences run in families. Questions have been raised about whether use of SSRI antidepressants (and other serotonin enhancing drugs) can trigger a manic episode. Indeed, patients with mania history may have greater risk of SSRI-induced mania if they also have genetically decreased baseline serotonin function.[150]

The risk of SSRI-induced mania goes higher still if the SSRI is enhanced by other medicines that increase serotonin activity to a toxic level ("serotonin syndrome").[151] Indeed, there are even some clinical similarities between serotonin syndrome and mania. During acute mania, there are fewer serotonin receptors in the brain (perhaps because increased serotonin activity reduces receptor numbers through the mechanism of "downregulation").[152] So an intriguing question arises: Could the manic "switch" be a sudden shift from low serotonin activity to very high serotonin activity?

A dramatic increase in the serotonin social director could help explain a shift from quietly acting "locally" for interpersonal social harmony, to dramatically acting "globally" for world social harmony.

The relationship between Atypical Depression and mania raises another intriguing possibility. Just as we speculated that Atypical Depression developed as a further evolution of primeval hibernation, so perhaps mania evolved from the switch from hibernation back to a full and eager waking state. Wilhelm Griesinger (German psychiatrist, 1817–1868) long ago suggested, "in winter—a profound Melancholia has supervened which in spring passes into Mania." (as with Aristotle, his use of the word *melancholia* may differ from the meaning in this theory)[153] More recently, a cartoon shows a polar bear in a psychiatrist's office. Says the psychiatrist: "So then, you're a bipolar bear." Indeed, mania does have a seasonal pattern, and is more common in the spring and summer.[132,154,155] Maybe mania is the ultimate wake-up call. The seasonal patterns of Atypical Depression and mania correspond to changes in our serotonin system.[156] Likewise, there are complex changes in the serotonin system associated with hibernation in squirrels.[157,158]

TREATMENT

These days, there are several medications that are effective for acute mania. Lithium, valproic acid, and carbamazepine all take several days to work, but newer antipsychotics such as olanzapine have an antimanic effect that sometimes start working within a day or two. The older antipsychotics can be helpfully sedating (and antipsychotic, of course), but they don't seem to have a specific antimanic effect. Lithium may increase serotonin activity, but it may also increase conscious control over time by increasing frontal-lobe size and function.[159] The newer antipsychotics block not only dopamine, but also have serotonin effects, which may explain their more specific antimanic benefits.[160] Most curious of all, that tryptophan-depletion test, which reduces serotonin activity (and thus makes Atypical Depression worse), may have an experimental antimanic effect.[161] Mania sometimes includes voices, though this seems to happen mostly in people who also have Panic Anxiety (common in Bipolar I Disorder).

MELANCHOLIA—THE END IS HERE

Psychotic Depression, long ago considered part of the Schizophrenias, is a form of Melancholia. It is the raw unfiltered expression of the Melancholia death instinct. People have extraordinary delusions that they are worthless to society, guilty of horrific crimes, undeserving of life, that their body is physically rotting away, and even that they are already dead (Cotard's syndrome). Nothing, of course, can convince them otherwise. An unusual journal article from 1950 is essentially several pages of uncommonly doleful quotes from patients with Psychotic Depression, organized by theme and strung together into a dramatic representation of this curious thought process.[162] Although this syndrome is more likely in people with a history of anxiety disorders, those historical diagnoses are more common in the younger patients, and less prevalent in those older patients with Psychotic Depression.[163] There is no clearly corresponding psychosis factor-analysis item yet for Psychotic Depression. This could be because Psychotic Depression is less likely to occur amongst those diagnosed with Schizophrenia, less likely to overlap with other psychotic subtypes, less likely to be a persistent illness, or maybe just because the right symptom questions were not asked.

As with ordinary Melancholia, there is an increase in the activity of the cortisol system in Psychotic Depression,[164] and normal means of suppressing cortisol don't work (the abnormal dexamethasone suppression test).[165] One study suggests that the dexamethasone suppression test may be more of a marker for psychosis (or psychosis risk) than for just severity of depression.[166] There is even some preliminary research that cortisol blockers can treat this syndrome. Mifiprestone (the Plan B abortion pill, among other uses) seems to return the patient with Psychotic Depression back to life.[167,168] Conventional treatment, usually a combination of an antidepressant and antipsychotic, is quite effective. The death instinct is triggered by changes in the cortisol system, and voiced out loud through the words of Psychotic Depression.

HOW CAN THIS HELP TREAT PSYCHOSIS?

So if psychosis is instinct run amok, then how do you treat it? The first problem is finding the diagnostic subtypes we've just talked about. Accurate diagnosis is difficult in much of medicine, more difficult in psychiatry, and tougher still when patients are psychotic, confused, and often uncooperative. However, that's no reason not to try. Fortunately, there is a steadily growing body of literature on what to look for, on special interview approaches, and on biological diagnostic tests. With those, and perhaps with some of the newfangled imaging scans, it may become easier to make the right diagnoses. And multiple diagnoses are common. Just as nonpsychotic angst is usually caused by more than one of our usual suspects, so too does psychosis usually have more than one underlying anxiety or depressive disorder.

With any of these diagnoses, the first step is to start an antipsychotic medication. The next step is to use other medications to target the underlying instincts that fuel the psychosis. "Take away the power source," says Dolores Malaspina (American psychiatrist; 1952–).[169] Oftentimes, other medications are needed to manage side effects, and sometimes, antipsychotic doses can eventually be reduced. That leaves us at psychotherapy. Once people are nonpsychotic, they can eventually benefit from more than just supportive approaches, and often even the same kind of conventional psychotherapies we talked about in earlier chapters. One crucial point, though, is that high-quality weekly (or more) psychotherapy visits are absolutely essential during the acute recovery phase, even if there is little to talk about for the 45 minutes. Otherwise, when people feel their improvement, they take it as a sign that things can only get worse, and they stop their medications, or else they run off to some other continent with medications in hand (really).

CAN A FOX BE CRAZY?

Although we don't have much evidence that animals get psychotic, we also don't know how a delusional fox would act, how voices would present in a species without language, and how diminished Consciousness and lessened ToM would appear in creatures that don't have them to begin with. This is a practical problem for medical treatment research. How would you know if you had found a meaningful animal model for psychosis? At the very least, you have to rely more on the biology, and far less on outward behavior or subjective symptoms. It is possible that animals always operate far more on instinct and far less on Consciousness than we do. That would suggest that they have a sort of mind/brain "imbalance" that is normal for them, but that would be highly problematic for us humans. Even so, when mice are experimentally manipulated to "knock out" their NRG 1 gene, there is a change in their social interactions. Instead of moderating their social instincts with some modest mousy Consciousness, they follow new mice friends too a bit too closely, and even walk on top of them.[170]

Dogs also give us pause for thought. They have co-evolved with us for many thousands of years, and have developed some human-like social capacities as a result. Most notably, if we point at something, our dog will look where we are pointing. Only people and dogs can do this instinctively—apes can't even learn this for tasty morsels of food. Dogs (and other animals) can go into stages of what appear to be sustained anger, fear, or pacing (especially in small cages). Dogs are capable of extreme separation anxiety (i.e., Panic) at times, and although we do wonder what they are thinking, they recover quickly when they see us. Some dogs appear to chase small invisible animals.[27] Is this some sort of psychotic OCD mousing instinct to clean up the nest, or are they just playing? Having talked about our social instincts from the individual perspectives of people and some animals, let's step back and think about how these herd instincts play out in groups and civilizations.

PART TWO

Civilization

The Rise of Reason and

the Ascent of Angst

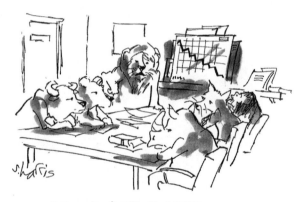

"I BELIEVE IT'S TIME WE STOPPED
RELYING SO HEAVILY ON INSTINCT."

"It is impossible to overlook the extent to which civilization is built upon a renunciation
of instinct."

—Sigmund Freud (Austrian psychiatrist; 1856–1939)

8

HAPPY IN THE HERD:
INSTINCTIVE HERDS AND
PRIMEVAL IGNORANCE

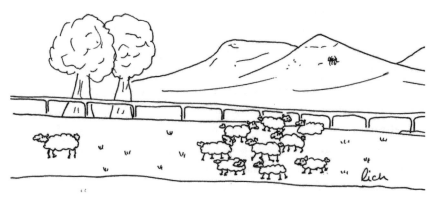

"I do wish she wouldn't be such a human."

"The security of Society lies in custom and unconscious instinct, and the basis of the stability of Society, as a healthy organism, is the complete absence of any intelligence amongst its members."
—Oscar Wilde (Irish playwright; 1854–1900)

"Collective fear stimulates herd instinct, and tends to produce ferocity toward those who are not regarded as members of the herd."
—Bertrand Russell (English philosopher; 1872–1970)

So far, we've been looking at our instincts and diagnoses as they appear in individuals. Now it's time to take a top-down look at how they appear in large groups of people and other creatures. There are families, troops, tribes, villages, cities, nations, societies, and civilizations of people, but for now, let's think of all of these as herds. Herds stay together, act together, and have common needs and goals. Social instincts are the glue that binds members together, and allows them to fulfill their common goals. A herd (or civilization) can be thought of as any group of similar organisms that hang out together in a collaborative way.

From the herd perspective, the social instincts appear as personality traits. This is true in herds of humans, dogs, apes, birds, fish, and even cows. Everyone has many instinctive flavors in their personality, and the clinical personality disorders in us humans are intensified, elaborated, and sometimes complex versions of the basic traits. Here, we'll stick mostly to the underlying core traits. As we shall see from several perspectives, our six social instincts play a central role in the mental state of humans and other relatives.

HISTORY OF THE HERD (OR, RETURN OF THE SLIME MOLD)

Herds have evolved from a very rudimentary beginning. Life started with bacteria-like single-celled organisms. Primitive bacteria lived near each other, but were not very social. Slime molds are a small step up. Although each one is a separate simple organism, there are times when a chemical signal will prompt them to cluster together. Another type of slime mold can meld multiple cell nuclei into a one single containing membrane. In each case, the various cells and nuclei of each herd member do pretty much the same things as each other.

Our ancestors gradually evolved into increasingly sophisticated multicellular organisms, with specialized cells that served different functions for the organism as a whole. A muscle cell is not a nerve cell, and a blood cell is not a skin cell. These complex multicellular organisms in turn started to congregate with each other. Herds of identical creatures have certain advantages. As a group, they can collectively find food, mates, safety and new worlds to inhabit. Remember the locust loners? When crowding triggers serotonin release, they flock together to find greener pastures for the herd. In numbers, there is also safety from predators. This protects not only individuals but also the herd's gene pool as a whole.

Herd behavior seems uniform on the surface, but it requires social instincts for everyone to get along. We humans have long depended on those six social instincts that contribute to our modern angst. Instincts in modest amount, and largely obeyed, produce little angst. Because not everyone in our human herd has the same blend or intensity of these instincts, we all have different personalities. The more carefully you look, and the higher up the evolutionary scale you go, the more personality you find.

EVERYONE HAS A SPECIAL PURPOSE

By way of introduction, herd effectiveness is enhanced when there are varieties of member skills to match with the various available roles. On one level, this can lead to different roles in the herd. Plato (ancient Greek philosopher, 429–347 BC) suggested that his idealized Republic required "a farmer, a builder, and a weaver, and also, I think, a shoemaker and one or two others to provide for our bodily needs." Adam Smith (Scottish economist, 1723–1790) noted in his *Theory of Moral Sentiments* that human behavior is largely guided by social concern for the opinions and feelings of others. In his *Wealth of Nations,* he emphasizes that enhanced economic productivity relies on the division of labor.

As put by Matt Ridley (English author and scientist, 1958–):

> ...we human beings are surely as utterly dependent on each other as any ants or honey bees. As I write this, I am using software I did not invent on a computer I could not have made that depends on electricity I could not have discovered, and I am not worrying about where my next meal will come from because I know I can go and buy food from a shop. In a phrase, therefore, the advantage of society to men is the division of labour. It is specialization that makes human society greater than the sum of its parts.[1]

THE BIRDS AND THE BEES

When Cole Porter (American composer, 1891–1964) said that "Birds do it, bees do it," he may have been thinking about how to best structure a society, or he may have been thinking about something else entirely. William Shakespeare (English playwright, 1564–1616), did dryly note the analogy of human society to bees' in "Henry V:"

> Therefore doth heaven divide
> The state of man in divers functions,
> Setting endeavour in continual motion;
> To which is fixed, as an aim or butt,
> Obedience: for so work the honey-bees,
> Creatures that by a rule in nature teach
> The act of order to a peopled kingdom.
> They have a king and officers of sorts

The role of any given bee is determined by genetic instincts, by developmental and epigenetic changes (through methylation to deactivate some genes),[2] by behavioral and environmental cues, and by visual messages, but not much by rational thought.[3] Biology is destiny for any individual bee, but this makes bee societies very successful at keeping their gene pool going. Indeed, they make up for their lack of rational thought through a sort of collective crowd wisdom[4]—or you can dismiss it as herd mentality. For example, when bees go out looking for food, they'll return to the nest and offer a dance that tells other bees where they were. Any given bee may not give the correct location for food, but when enough bees give the same message, most of the bees know the right place to find lunch. Along similar lines, we humans now have restaurant rating guides that use a similar technique to guide our individual culinary decisions.

Ants have been helpful for package delivery.[4] When they go out looking for food, they leave a scent trail for others to follow. Because ants have a bit of an independent streak, they will sometimes venture off a trail to find something new. Those ants that chance upon the shortest route will make faster round trips, and thus their scent trail will appear sooner and become stronger. When other ants follow the strongest scent, they find the shortest route (unless they stumble onto a still shorter path, or a new food source entirely). Efficient scheduling of package delivery (known as the "traveling-salesman" problem) as well as related issues turns out to be a very complicated and difficult task for a delivery company. Even computer programs are slow and inefficient if they plan delivery routes by evaluating every possible sequence. Ants to the rescue. More modern computer programs that emulate ant behavior produce plans faster and find more efficient delivery routes. This wisdom of crowds improves further if it draws on members with different skill sets, each offering an independent opinion that utilizes their special expertise. So unlike ants, modern scheduling programs also know to include rational human concerns about timing (delivery necessary tomorrow, or maybe anytime this week will do), quantity (a full truckload, or just one envelope), and fuel consumption (the most efficient route also considers fuel costs), and such esoteric knowledge such as the greater speed of right turns than left (unless you are in Britain, of course).

Likewise, different people with different training and practical skill sets add different perspectives to communal herd decisions. Thinking back to our workplace perspective, how do people sort themselves into these different roles? Part of it is appetitive (brewmasters usually like beer), cultural (not many women drive trucks in some places), physical (men nearing seven feet tall are invariably asked to try basketball), opportunistic (be in the right place at the right time), or familial (shoemakers, lawyers, and ministers encourage their children to follow suit).

Part of it also derives from personality. People's personalities guide their interest and career choices. The Strong Vocational Interest Survey (now the Strong-Campbell Interest Inventory) was first developed in 1927 to use personality to direct career choice. The idea was to match your personality to others in the same field. Corporations also use personality tests to match employees with job functions. Our role in the herd derives in part from our personality and particular pattern of social instincts. Jokes about doctors, lawyers, ministers and other professions are funniest when they have a kernel of truth. There is even a joke about the personalities of different medical specialties: Four doctors on a duck-hunting trip decide to take turns. The internist goes first, and on seeing a distant bird asks, "Is it a goose? Is it a sparrow? Is it an eagle?" and by then her bird is gone. The psychiatrist is next, and on spotting a bird asks, "Where does it want to go? What is its motivation? How does it feel?" and by then his bird is gone. The surgeon is next, and on seeing a speck she wheels to the right and drops it with a single shot. Turning to the pathologist, she says, "Hey, you, see if that's a duck."

Just because we fit the personality profile of a given profession, or just because our personality seems to fit the job requirements doesn't mean our fates are sealed. Those kinds of fit don't necessarily predict job happiness, preference, success or talent. Unlike bees and ants, we do make our own choices, although even those choices are still influenced by our social instincts, culture, resources and community.

NOT JUST FOR THE BIRDS

Some birds are pretty smart. Some parrots can use words deliberately, and crows can be highly intelligent. Other birds, though, are not the sharpest beaks in the zoo. Even so, they have mastered the art of flying together in a flock (a bird herd, if you will). Elite jet pilots such as the U.S. Navy's aerobatic Blue Angels train mightily to fly six planes in close formation without crashing, and we are thrilled at their results. However, hundreds of birds with no formal training launch themselves at the same time, twist and turn, change direction, stay with the flock, and don't bump into each other. How do they do it? Craig Reynolds (American computer graphics expert, 1953 –) wrote a computer program in 1986 ("Boids") that emulated bird flocks using only three basic rules about the other birds:[4]

- Stay close together.
- Follow the crowd.
- Don't crowd your neighbor.

We changed his wording a bit, because there is a clear parallel to three of our six social instincts. Panic Anxiety keeps people close together, Social Anxiety prompts people to keep their place in the crowd, and the rejection sensitivity of Atypical Depression helps us avoid crowding our neighbors. Oh, and the programmer also unwittingly built in at least two more basic rules: Carefully notice symmetry and arrangement (when the nest is in flight), and keep flapping. Our Obsessive-Compulsive traits make sure that we too pay attention to important physical distances and arrangements, and that we can walk without planning every step. That makes four of our social instincts. As an acute death-instinct syndrome, Melancholia would play little role in active bird flocks. Consciousness, if it had bird-flock value at all, would be most useful if it was needed to detect and respond to an oncoming eagle (or a surgeon with a shotgun)—raw instinct amidst lack of eagle awareness could be fatal. So, the instinctive "decisions" that allow birds to flock are not too different from four or five of the six emotional instincts that regulate the human herd.

Having learned division of labor from bees, and shipping from ants, birds have helped us make movies. In the film *The Lord of the Rings,* the computer-programmed Orc army followed the three Boid rules, as well as the pseudo-OCD automatic-behavior instructions to slice their human opponents in half.[4] Similarly, computer programs simulate lifelike crowds of robotic people in action for films, television and advertisements. By adding yet other human traits to the core instincts, the results look more and more like the herd, both on film and even with physical robots.

People (and other living creatures) aren't always free to follow their instincts, and some work has already been done on frustration of core herding behaviors. When computerized schools of fish (who follow the same basic rules as birds) are "enclosed" in too small a computer-designated ("virtual") space, they lose their coordination entirely. When the space gets a little larger, they swim in an endless circle. Only with enough virtual space do they behave like free-swimming schools of fish.[4] This opens up all sorts of future possibilities for robotic imitation of our first four anxiety and depressive disorders. If some fish are programmed to stay too close to the herd, will they look phobic of the larger world (or frantic if they can't get back)? If some follow the crowd leaders too faithfully, will they look more subordinate (or frantic for guidance if they are somehow put in "command")? If they steer too clear of their neighbors, will they look lonesome (and move even further apart if they do bump into someone)? If they pay way too much attention to symmetry and arrangement, will they miss the forest for the trees on some designated task (and never complete their assignment on time)? It would be easy to computer animate the corresponding verbal or facial expressions of human emotion, but not so easy to have robots feel real human angst.

A HERD OF HUMANS

Enough of birds, bees, ants and fish. What happens if you take as many human personality traits as you can think of, measure them all in large samples of people, and then ask a computer to sort it all out? This has been done many times, largely using the statistical technique of factor analysis. All those traits tend to group into the same five personality Factors. So, a major concept gaining strength in the study of human personality is the Big-Five personality model. Also known as the five-factor model (FFM), NEO, CANOE, and OCEAN—the acronym NECA(M)O would better reflect our six social instinct flavors in the order that we have introduced them here (the initials in the acronyms are spelled out below). It's not that there isn't more to us humans than six traits (not to mention their many Factor subcomponents—known as "facets," which are essential for more precise understanding of our diverse personalities), but those five major Factors match up with our major social instincts and diagnoses. Researchers are only starting to explore the relationships of NECA(M)O to anxiety and depressive disorders, but there is surface similarity worth exploring.

In the order that the corresponding social instincts were first discussed here, the Factors are:

- Neuroticism: Corresponding to our Panic Anxiety/separation instinct. This Factor is based on expressed experience of negative emotions, stress and emotional instability.
- Extraversion: Corresponding to an absence of our Social Anxiety/subordinate hierarchy instinct. It is based on expressed preferences for social leadership.
- Conscientiousness: Corresponding to our Obsessive-Compulsive/nesting instinct. It is based on expressed concern for orderliness, details, arrangement, and task completion.
- Agreeableness: Corresponding to our Atypical Depression/social harmony instinct. It is based on questions about expressed attention to other people's feelings.
- (Melancholia): Melancholia is not in the five-factor model. As an acute death instinct, you wouldn't expect it to show up in surveys of generally healthy people, and the presence of Melancholia would also discourage their participation. It might show up as a distinct sixth factor in a sample that included enough people with active Melancholia, as long as there were questions about the right symptoms.
- Openness to experience: Corresponds to our Consciousness instinct. The factor is based on expressed interests in ideas, understanding, art, and curiosity.

Although these linkages have strong face validity (they look good), there is also some supporting research. For example, Panic Anxiety is associated with high Neuroticism scores.[5] Social Anxiety is associated with low Extraversion scores.[6,7] Further research will need to better examine the Big-Five Factor subtypes, age and gender differences,[8] counter-instinctive behavior effects, interactions between Factors, and to better focus on our more specific anxiety and depressive diagnoses.

In our own experience, personality tests accompanied by careful interviews are good tools for assessing executive and leadership skills. However, when executives adopt new counter-instinctive skills through executive coaching, there is significant discordance between written personality tests and interview findings.[9] Their outward behaviors may change, but their inner instincts and personality structure do not. Yet another example of the law of unintended consequences is that when certain leadership skills improve on the surface, the underlying instincts emerge as new and sometimes worse problems,[10] or, of course, as angst. In one mild example, a southern executive learned to be more empathic toward employees, realized that it made him more effective, but found himself forever "nervous as a long-tailed cat in a room full of rocking chairs."

Although research comparing Big-Five Factors to clinical personality disorders has had limited and complex results, the Factors may offer new insight into the relationship of personality disorders to our core social instincts. On the genetic side, there are genetic factors that influence Big-Five Factors such as Extraversion (Social Anxiety). New research is also finding that personality Factors (and thus syndromes and social instincts) are influenced by large numbers of genes, and that using mathematically derived gene clusters (up to thousands of genes) does a much better job of predicting Big-Five Factors than does any one single gene.[11] As we also might expect, a decline in frontal-lobe function on a brain scan (fronto-temporal degeneration) releases instincts from conscious control, and thus results in significantly changed and mostly worsened expression of the Big-Five Factors.[12] Moreover, four of the Big Five are associated with specific areas of the frontal lobe.[13] Only Openness (Consciousness) is more expansively present throughout the frontal lobe.

It may well be that intricate interactions of four social instincts explain much of the complexity of personality disorders. One study examined 10 standard *DSM-IV-TR* personality disorders, and found that each had a different pattern of association with Neuroticism (Panic Anxiety), Extraversion (Social Anxiety), Conscientiousness (OCD) and Agreeableness (Atypical Depression) Factors.[14] Openness (Consciousness) doesn't appear in their model (nor does Melancholia). Delightfully, these Factor/personality associations correspond well with those same anxiety and depressive syndromes that we see clinically in the same personality disorders. For example, dependent personality disorder is strongly associated with Neuroticism (just like those folks with Panic Anxiety who are attached at the hip), whereas Obsessive-Compulsive Personality is strongly associated with conscientiousness (OCD, of course). Antisocial personality is a combination of low Agreeableness and low conscientiousness (perhaps counter-instinctive Atypical Depression, with too little OCD—we'll get to that later with help from our blues friends, The Who).

ANIMAL FACTORS

The presumption of certain "personality" traits allows computer modeling of bird flocks and schools of fish. However, if core biological personality factors can actually be measured in people, then how about in other animals? This has been looked at in our chimpanzee cousins (pan troglodytes—*troglodytes* is Greek for "cave-dweller"). They don't fill out questionnaires, but observers rate their observed behaviors in zoos, research populations, and wild sanctuaries, and then subject the new data to the same kind of personality factor analysis that is used for people data.

What drives the mind of a chimp? There are major Factors called Extraversion (Social Anxiety/social hierarchy), Conscientiousness (Obsessive-Compulsive/nesting), Agreeableness (Atypical Depression/social harmony) and one additional factor, dominance. adult chimps don't appear to have clear Factors for Neuroticism (Panic Anxiety/separation) or for Openness (Consciousness).[15] If these troglodyte findings pan out in the long run, they may suggest that chimps are less likely than humans to retain Panic Anxiety/separation issues into adulthood, and also less likely to become existential philosophers, university professors or novelists. As we will see, these last two Factors/instincts may well be an important part of what makes us more human than our cousins.

LITTLE CREATURES

Speaking of smaller creatures and humans, we might wonder when these instincts first appear in us, and whether they are all there from the start. Robert Fulghum (American author and minister,1937 –) famously wrote a book titled *All I Really Need to Know I Learned in Kindergarten.*[16] Although his list of 16 things to learn sounds so commonsensical as to be mundane, it is so intuitively profound that it resonates with readers and writers all over the world. Indeed, it is well worth looking up. And since we all should know the drill by now, we can find that all six of our social instincts are on his list (and thus also the Big Five). In fact, every item on his list corresponds to one of the six instincts. In addition, all four OCD subtypes are also there (if we assume that someone had to save up before handing out a stash of cookies and milk). Maybe in kindergarten we are just starting to become aware of what our instincts already tell us. From that point of view, kindergarten helps us become more conscious of what we have inside of our selves.

GRADE SCHOOL AND ABOVE

Unlike most other creatures, human "civilization" goes beyond inborn social instincts. Jared Diamond (American author and scientist, 1937 –) wrote a history of societies called *Guns, Germs and Steel.*[17] Among other things, he discusses six characteristics that made certain animals good candidates for human domestication. Three of them are important for production: omnivorous diet, rapid growth rate and successful breeding in captivity. The other three, though, are personality tendencies: to have social harmony with others, to have a strong social hierarchy, and to not Panic and flee. A reasonable guess is that most domesticated animals also have good nesting habits, that Melancholia is not common in a healthy population, and that significant Consciousness would be unlikely (except for the occasional talking farm animal on television).

The next obvious question, and an ongoing source of concern at cocktail parties, is whether humans can be domesticated. Some of us do have Diamond's first three physical criteria, but we vary at how much of the three social instincts we each have. Darwin noticed that wild animals have erect ears,[18] whereas domestic animals (even of the same species) have floppy ears (wild elephants excepted). Because most humans do not have floppy ears, maybe that answers that.

Still, some of us seek more highly domesticated herds than others. For example, we are well aware of the profound personality differences between dog people and cat people. Dog people are higher on Extraversion (more social leadership/lower Social Anxiety), Agreeableness (more social harmony/more Atypical Depression) and Conscientiousness (more nesting/OCD), but lower on Neuroticism (less moodiness/less Panic Anxiety) and lower on Openness (less Consciousness). So it is not surprising that dog people like socially companionable and floppy-eared domestic dogs. Cat people, on the other hand, prefer to keep more detached, independent, and pointy-eared felines as "wild" captives around the house.[19] Dog people just might feel frustrated if they tried to herd cats.

THE VARIETIES OF MORAL EXPERIENCE

Moral discussion seems to be raining down like cats and dogs these days. Should the courts show compassion to perpetrators, or should they follow the letter of the law? Should we provide for the needy, or should we enable them to succeed? Most people are somewhere in the middle on these kinds of issues, and where they stand has much to do with what they feel. Moral decisions, like most decisions, are profoundly influenced by emotions. As Matt Ridley summarizes the view of Antonio Damasio (Portuguese neuroscientist and author, 1944 –), "In short, if you lack all emotions, you are a rational fool."[1] So it is not surprising that where you stand on political issues may be a reflection of your personality style and social instincts.

Jonathan Haidt (American psychologist, 1963–) has developed a moral framework based on five types of ethical concern. His list includes: ingroup/loyalty, authority/respect, purity/sanctity, harm/care, and fairness/reciprocity.[20] His order has been changed here to correspond again to our own social instinct/diagnosis list (and to our NECA(M)O order of the Big Five). Face validity is again one place to start:

- Ingroup/loyalty morality sounds like separation/Panic Anxiety concerns.
- Authority/respect morality sounds like social hierarchy/Social Anxiety concerns.

- Purity/sanctity morality sounds like nesting/OCD concerns (including cleanliness, arrangement, and behavioral-control instincts).
- Harm/care morality sounds like social harmony/Atypical Depression concerns.
- (Melancholia, alas, is again missing in action).
- Fairness/reciprocity morality sounds like Consciousness and rational assessment.

When you look at real data, there is already some clear connection for these associations of moral dimensions with Big-Five Personality Factors (more so in Americans than in Brits for some reason), though this line of research is just beginning.[21]

As to the question of why we have political disagreements, part of the answer has to do with our individual personalities and social instincts. Political conservatives assign similar importance to each one of these five moral domains. Political liberals assign similarly high weights to the two individual-related domains (harm/care and fairness/reciprocity domains), but assign much lower weights to the three group-related domains (ingroup/loyalty, authority/respect, and purity/sanctity domains). In a fascinating way, both political groups have similar weightings on all five moral domains when subjects are distracted while completing the questionnaire ("whatever you do, do not think about white bears"). With their conscious mediation thus reduced, conservatives pay less heed to the group-related moral domains (ingroup/loyalty, authority/respect, and purity/sanctity).[22] All of this explains why the mental distractions of loud concerts, natural disasters and polar bear dens make for politically neutral zones.

RISING FROM THE HERD

Those of us still in the herd have instinctive, genetic and biological influences on our varied personalities. If ignorance is bliss, then species without Consciousness are happy in the herd. Indeed, the safety of a school of fish is greatest when most members follow instincts blindly, with very few leaders attending to lurking dangers.[23] If we assume that fish don't do much thinking, then those fish do not think of themselves as oppressed or constrained. However, our human personalities and behavior are far more shaped by culture, experience, family, education, and circumstances, and although all of these determinants play a role in shaping how we interact with other people, we also make conscious choices all by ourselves.

Effective leaders, for example, know how to modify their managerial personality style according to the circumstances and the personalities of their subordinates. Roger MacKinnon (American psychiatrist, 1927–) would make this point to psychiatrists in residency training. With a lengthy written psychotherapy project due on short deadline, he would go around the classroom to ensure timely completion by every resident. To some he would offer kind encouragement, to others he firmly restated the deadline (pointing out potential consequences), and to a few he would merely say, "I'm sure everything is fine." His social interactions in the class were consciously adapted to the personalities of each individual resident. Besides getting the projects done on time, this offered a dramatic demonstration of an essential teaching point. Adapting yourself to everyone's differences is essential for helping them. This lesson came in handy for coordinating the work of some 20 contributors to a medical textbook.[24] One bystander, overhearing editorial phone calls, quickly learned to identify the authors at the other end, just by the style of discussion.

This kind of essential learned behavior is difficult to learn, and it is sometimes discomfiting to use. Just as executive coaching can teach people to go against their instinctual grain, so too can this kind of momentary personality adjustment. Instinct is a driver of suitable herd behavior, and an impediment to learning new behaviors. The ability to move beyond (and sometimes against) basic social instincts is a uniquely human characteristic. We can use reason and Consciousness to decide what to do, but at an emotional cost. Deep on the inside, we experience those behaviors as transgressions against the herd. Therein lies the rub. We feel those costs, in greater and lesser degree, as the punishing angst of our anxiety and depressive disorders. We continue nonetheless because we are unwittingly willing to pay that price. This human ability to use reason to transcend instinct and to endure emotional pain also helped us develop civilization. Civilization, in turn, encourages us to maximize our Consciousness and reason and to stray yet further beyond our social herd instincts, but it also offers ways to ease that angst. One mechanism is rules of civilization that reinforce and retain core constraints of social instinct, sometimes in opposition to noble ideas. Other mechanisms assuage our angst even as it arises. Even with our civilized advances, and despite our best intentions, our inner core still wants our outer selves to follow the footsteps of the herd.

9

CLIMBING TO CIVILIZATION:
THE RISE OF REASON AND
THE ASCENT OF ANGST

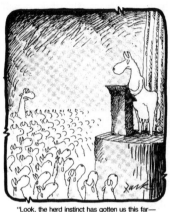

"Look, the herd instinct has gotten us this far—
why do we need parliamentary procedure now?"

"The history of the world is none other than the progress of the consciousness of freedom."
—Georg Wilhelm Friedrich Hegel (German philosopher; 1770–1831)

"What is peculiar in the life of a man consists not in his obedience, but his opposition, to his instincts. In one direction or another he strives to live a supernatural life."
—Henry David Thoreau (American Essayist, Poet and Philosopher; 1817–1862)

CONSCIOUSNESS, REASON AND CIVILIZATION

How has our happy human herd moved on to consciously reasoned behaviors and to advanced human civilization? How is it that some of us today have overcome our instinctual societal roles? Those who Panic can travel and fly these days, not all leaders are "born leaders," there is much room for civil disagreement, and the melancholic are seldom left alone to die. Our now less-instinctual selves have banded together to form societies and civilizations, with reason at their core. Freud in his *Civilization and Its Discontents* pointed out that rational behavior and advanced society require us to overlook instinctive concerns about others, though the instincts that he had in mind were more aggressive and sexual in nature than they were purely social.

How come our lurking social instincts don't bring on an overwhelming angst that brings reason and civilization tumbling down around our feet? It's certainly not that all anxiety and depression have disappeared. For that matter, how do we all get along in modern human society where our governing and limiting social instincts are so often overridden? Somehow, the rise of reason has allowed us to challenge our instincts, to cope with our angst, to develop civilizations that help protect us against angst and against the social discord of overruled instinct. With the protections of civilization, we may even have further evolved and intensified our social instincts.

TO THINK, PERCHANCE TO TEAM

From an historical, societal, and evolutionary perspective, there were many events that gradually reshaped our experience of these instinctive syndromes. Consciousness, where this process started, is a good place for us to start this reasoned contemplation. First of all, why did evolution bother to bless us with conscious thought? Given the importance of social interaction, an early benefit of Consciousness was to enhance our ability to sense the emotions and behaviors of others, to enable a Theory of Mind (ToM), and figure out what to do next. This is a major advantage not only for group solidarity, but also allows us to compete better against other creatures with lesser Consciousness.

We are not the only species with Consciousness, but we almost certainly have more of it. Dolphins may come pretty close. One memorable story is of a dolphin that was taught to perform a new trick every day. The idea was to see how many different tricks she could learn. One day, the dolphin arrived in the training pool, and proceeded to perform a brand new trick she had come up with all by herself. Because she had the presence of Conscious mind to realize that a new trick was needed each day, she made up her own (there a joke somewhere here about finding one's porpoise in life).[1] In another experiment, two dolphins learned one command to perform the same trick together, and another command to invent new tricks on their own. When the two dolphins were then asked to follow both commands at the same time, they promptly dove under water, surfaced on their backs, and came up with the new trick of slapping their tails in unison. Maybe we can't make this stuff up, but the dolphins did. In addition, they made it up in a social way—their newly invented trick was a result of conscious social interaction between themselves and their human handlers. Bird-brained pigeons, on the other hand, can't even teach themselves to peck out novel response patterns in order to get fed.[2]

We've learned only recently that modern humans (*Homo sapiens*) co-mingled with Neanderthals (*Homo neanderthalensis*) in Europe. Neanderthals probably had the ability to speak, so we no doubt communicated as we cooperated, fought and even interbred. However, we are still here, and they remain with us only as a tiny part of our largely *Homo sapiens* genome. How did they disappear? A good guess is that our more effective social groups helped us to out-compete them for food, shelter and other resources, and thus allowed us to go forth and out-multiply them.[3] The last Neanderthals died off a mere 28,000 years ago, their final members living in isolated and resource-poor pockets of the European continent, probably without any conscious clue about what hit them.

REASON AND ANGST

More advanced human Consciousness led to more sophisticated language, which in turn allowed yet more sophisticated Consciousness. This higher level of human Consciousness has allowed us to differentiate between our societal roles and those emotions that reinforce social instincts. Here's a question: Do our Consciousness and reason help us to recognize our own social instincts? Ancient ancestors were presumably too influenced by the unhappy feelings and cognitions that prompted our social instincts to do that. Melancholia, for example, would have been pretty near a death sentence back then. However, faced with Melancholia today, most of us do not actually curl up and die. Rather, many of us try to push forward and reinvent a meaningful new role for ourselves. Of course, this process becomes much easier and more effective once the Melancholia has been treated.

One possibility is that as Consciousness advanced, awareness of instinctual angst increased, and we used our reasoning skills to control or harness the distress. The more intelligent we are, the more we can develop coping skills, and so the less influence there is on our actual behavior. In addition, our brains have evolved to moderate the actual emotional experience of social angst. Along those lines, research suggests that clinical anxiety is diminished in those who have a thicker cortex in one particular part of the frontal lobe; this larger cortex gives them more brain power to subdue the anxiety of instinct.[4]

Consciousness has come to have far more value than social awareness and cooperation alone. It helped our ancestors and some other species better find food, develop and use tools, share information, and protect against predators. It is an essential underpinning for modern reason, language, art, music, science, religion, law, social structure, government—and, importantly, for angst awareness.

CLIMBING TO CIVILIZATION

Our ability to use Consciousness in order to transcend mere instinct is one factor that allowed the development of civilization. Civilization has many purported causes. The development of domestic grains that can be farmed and stored often gets much of the credit. Consequent easier living meant more free time for many people, and thus a greater opportunity to use intellect and cognition. Civilization relies on a membership with many different skills sets, and it also permits some individuals to move into new and more intellectual roles: artist, manufacturer, philosopher, and, eventually, even psychiatrist. However, those with superior technical skills may have found themselves in an elevated social role at odds with their inner social instincts, and thus struggling with a greater experience of anxiety and depressive disorders. Our alpha dog Bonnie thinks that civilization began when domesticated wolves became household dogs, but that may just be her wishful thinking.

FIGHTING THOSE HERD INSTINCTS

So, reason and civilization allow us to transcend social instincts, as long as we can cope with their persistent and painful reminders. Some people, though, take it a step further than mere coping. Emotionally painful instincts are a call to action, a challenge to overcome, a pathway to self-improvement. In each case the counter-instinctive approach yields practical advantages and emotional pain. We are no doubt more angst-ridden than ants, fish, birds, and apes—because they are all better than we are at toeing that instinctual line. This also puts us at greater risk for some physical illnesses (see chapter 10). Then again, we surpass other creatures at art, philosophy, manufacturing, farming, medicine, creativity and material success, not to mention warfare.

This notion of counter-instinctive behavior is not new. It is pretty close to the established psychoanalytic notion of behaving in a way that is opposite to your inclinations ("reaction formation"). Think of all those people who try to prove themselves, because inside they think that they are inferior. Or think of those stridently moralistic people who are fighting against their own dishonest impulses. Freud, in his *Instincts and Their Vicissitudes* wrote about sexual instincts: "Our inquiry into the various vicissitudes which instincts undergo in the process of development and in the course of life...shows us that an instinct may undergo the following vicissitudes: Reversal into its opposite, Turning round upon the subject's own self, Repression, Sublimation." Reversal into its opposite is our topic at hand.

Rational behavior and counter-instinctive behavior led us to civilization, made us need civilization, and are also what civilization and Consciousness require of us. Was counter-instinctive behavior initially a cause or consequence of civilization—or did they emerge together? For that matter, have some of us biologically evolved toward counter-instinctive behavior (one instinct making us feel like doing one thing, while an instinct for counter-instinctiveness tells us to do the opposite of what that feeling suggests)? The emotional rush of counter-instinctive angst is painful yet compelling. If those people so-inclined stop, or even pause, the resurgent angst pushes them forward again. The more they feel it, the more they seek it, and it can lead to unexpected and unconstrained destinations. "Always do what you are afraid to do" said Ralph Waldo Emerson (American essayist and poet, 1803–1882). If there are genes for counter-instinctiveness, they are there to promote civilization rather than to soothe our emotional state. We have seen these patterns with our core instinctive diagnoses.

A counter-instinctive response to Panic Anxiety leads some to wander far from home, ascend dangerous mountains, or rise to the frightening perceived isolation of intellectual, artistic and material heights. Because some people Panic in physically high places, they become terrified of falling off. However, rather than staying on the ground floor, some of them become skiers or climbers, determined to conquer the most frighteningly steep mountain slopes. More importantly, they are trying to conquer their Panic. And then there are those who try to conquer the Panic they feel at thoughts of scaling forbidden heights of success. Some reach the higher heights of bigwigs and renown, but Panic Anxiety persists. As William Styron (American novelist, 1925–2006) said, "Writing is a fine therapy for people who are perpetually scared of nameless threats...for jittery people."

A counter-instinctive response to Social Anxiety leads to outward extroversion, public performance, exquisite sensitivity to the emotions of others, or unceasing efforts to rise up the hierarchy. Are you afraid to speak up in class? Well, conquer that fear by speaking more or taking a Dale Carnegie course. In fact, anecdotes abound that some of the best performers and salesmen, (from the retail level to investment bankers) seem to have Social Anxiety. Think back to the words of The Band's "Stage Fright." Instead of avoiding self-embarrassment altogether, they use their anxiety to develop highly nuanced performance skills and sales approaches that minimize any chance of failure. They do sell more tickets and widgets, but they still worry about embarrassing themselves.

Counter-instinctive Atypical Depression leads to ongoing efforts to seek acceptance, or to a driven workaholic persona. Feeling lethargic? Push yourself at work, at the gym and in a marathon. Fearing rejection? Prove yourself worthy though accomplishments, possessions, and unceasing effort. Said Thomas Alva Edison (American inventor, 1847–1931) "Restlessness is discontent and discontent is the first necessity of progress." In the end, though, there is still a sense of isolation and fear of rejection, uncovered as torment when lying awake but not relaxed on a sunny beach.

COUNTER-INSTINCTIVENESS IS THE MOTHER OF INVENTION

So in light of Consciousness, civilization and counter-instinctiveness, the emotional symptoms of anxiety and depression can lend themselves to societal accomplishment. For those who use their symptoms as self-improvement signals, there are benefits for both society and the individual. Rather than just instinctual signals for societal roles, the symptoms can also lead to larger societal contributions. Society profits from ambition, creativity, and aspiration. It is easy to imagine that this kind of emotionally driven creativity led to advances in art, science, manufacture, technology, and commerce. When we meet or read about leaders in these fields, the presence and inner intensity of anxiety and depressive disorders is absolutely striking. There are many biographies that make this point about individual notables, and other tomes offer a broad overview of links tying creativity and leadership to emotional distress.[5] William Faulkner (American novelist, 1897–1962) pointed out, "An artist is a creature driven by demons. He doesn't know why they choose him and he's usually too busy to wonder why."

We are definitely left with the feeling that emotional symptoms are central motivators of individual accomplishment. Says Aristotle: "Great men are always of a nature originally melancholy" (no doubt the great philosopher meant *angst-ridden,* rather than *melancholic* in our sense). Because counter-instinctive behavior and angst have some adaptive value, evolution may have selected for them. So we might have an evolved tendency toward counter-instinctiveness—or at least some of us might have.

In addition, we might even have higher doses of social instinct biology than apes and other creatures, thus also making us prone to greater angst. We have been talking about some genetic factors that influence anxiety and depressive disorders. Despite the unpleasant distress, the genetic reduction in serotonin activity might well be an evolved adaptation that enhances creativity or productivity to improve the survival of our human DNA. Other genetic variants that increase the risk of common syndromes may likewise have adaptive value for our human lineage. Some of these variants are already known to be much more common in people than in our ape cousins.[6] Even the NRG 1 gene variant that predisposes to Schizophrenia has been shown to predict greater creativity.[7] Well, at least the human civilization we gain helps temper the human angst we endure.

PANIC MAKES THE MIND GO WONDER

Some of the most creative souls have Panic Anxiety as an ongoing motivator and tormentor. "Anxiety is the handmaiden of creativity," said T.S. Eliot (American playwright and poet, 1888–1965). For example, Panic is much more common in women writers than in matched nonwriters.[8] The intense distress of Panic Anxiety can drive people to seek new solutions and perspectives—in a desperate quest to exorcise their demons through new thoughts of home and symbolic reunion. "Necessity is the mother of taking chances," said Mark Twain (American author, 1835–1910). More specifically, counter-instinctive Panic Anxiety contributes to creativity by focusing on novel and thus emotionally alarming ideas that open new avenues of thought.

We are not alone. Dorothy Cheney and Robert Seyfarth observed that when Harley, a young wild baboon, became stranded alone on an island, he resourcefully "…joined a group of impala and foraged with them for two days. Then, perhaps tiring of the impalas' rather tedious company, he joined a group of vervets [monkeys], who tried but failed to chase him away. Throughout his separation, Harley gave contact barks [baboon panic calls]…"[9] Harley did finally have a happy reunion with his real family. His separation anxiety was mother to his desperate invention.

Panic is hardly the sole source of creative accomplishment, and neither is it sufficient by itself. Perseverance, luck and intelligence are necessary companions. As Louis Pasteur (French chemist; 1822–1895) points out, "Where observation is concerned, chance favors only the prepared mind." Dopamine (that neurotransmitter that motivates our appetites) encourages novelty-seeking behavior. The same sort of dopamine increases that predisposes people to psychosis also increase experimentally measured creative abilities.[10] Likewise, the increased size of dopamine-loaded brain areas is also associated with greater creativity measures.[11] So apparently, "mad geniuses" are anxious, desperate for home, brilliant, tenacious, and a bit daft.

DEVELOPMENTAL CIVILIZATION 101

Those mad geniuses have made essential contributions to civilization for untold millennia. Applying reason to instinct, conscious morality to social custom, and rational thought to problems at hand, they helped us move beyond incremental lifestyle changes to more dramatic paradigm shifts in human society.[12] Consciousness inclines us toward the search for knowledge and meaning, especially as it provides for greater mastery of ourselves, our societies, and our natural world. Civilization allows, encourages, and enables that quest. At the same time, it mitigates our angst, and provides conscious structures to support the weakened effects of our social instincts.

Our primeval ancestors, focused on their natural surroundings, developed novel tools and bona fide art. If we could hear their campfire discussions, there is little doubt we would have heard them philosophically musing about the workings of the world, the nature of higher powers, and the intricacies of social interactions. In historical times, Plato and his fellow Greeks separated out the "natural philosophy" of science from a more all-encompassing conception of philosophical inquiry. Mad or otherwise, ancient Greece may well have had more than its fair share of geniuses. The influence of Consciousness on social instinct allowed civilization and Greek philosophy, and civilization, in turn, helped lessen the personal angst and social disturbance that arose with disobeyance of social instinct.

TIME FOR A BEER

So if unpleasant angst has been around for so long, how did we deal with it way back when? Alcohol came along early on, and it may have been with us for as long as 100,000 years. The prevailing theory is that humans domesticated grain for food, and then discovered that stored grain can become beer. According to a more recent theory, we first domesticated grain for alcohol, and bread was only an afterthought.[13] At a human archaeological site some 11,500 years old, there is evidence of a society that farmed, despite a diet that contained little grain (and our Neanderthal cousins were pretty much pure carnivores). All that hard work planting, harvesting and preparing grain makes far more sense for a cold one than for mere bread, especially if fruit and game are plentiful.

Beer humor aside, why would beer be worth so much effort? Maybe ancient man found that alcohol calmed his (and her) instinctual angst, and, thus, allowed more freedom from social instinct. By allowing transcendence of biological angst, it played a role in allowing the development of civilization. Alcohol enabled us to dampen painful social instincts as we tried to follow rational thoughts about social roles. That would make it the first widely used psychopharmacological medication.

Psychiatrists know well that alcohol is used as self-medication for anxiety, especially for Social and Panic Anxiety. In common parlance, alcohol is a "social lubricant," "liquid courage," "happy juice," and "nectar of the gods." *Uisge Beatha*, or whiskey, translates as "water of life," and one beer was long marketed as "Guinness for Strength." At a Friday evening cocktail party many years ago, a seminary priest who was also a psychiatrist (really) noticed a young man sweating heavily. He went over and advised the Socially Anxious seminarian to "drink heavily." Today, the psychiatrist would know to suggest an SSRI and to drink only in moderation.

Alcohol is pretty popular among the depressed, too. It's not that good wine or cheap liquor will treat depression, but it offers an effective (if temporary and problematic) escape from depression and dismay. There is even a joke about that. A woman at a cocktail party sees a sad and drunken man with a glass in his hand. Feeling sorry for whatever sorrow he needs to drown, she asks him why he drinks so much.

"It's because of my problem," he says. "That's awful," she replies, "and what is your problem?" "I drink too much," says he.

We think of alcohol as "disinhibiting" because it relaxes our social graces and allows our hidden thoughts, wishes, and appetites to push forth. It actually has a more specific biological mechanism. The disinhibition comes from tamping down our protective social instincts. There is evidence that alcohol was used for feasting, celebration, and religious ritual for many thousands of years before the development of Christian communion; wine dates back at least to 4000 BCE.[14] Those early liquid refreshment events were opportunities that offered angst relief, promoted culinary and romantic excess, provided some chemical happiness, and, last but not least, helped to relax social interactions. In the words of Benjamin Franklin: "Beer is living proof that God loves us and wants us to be happy."

One way that alcohol may work its magic is through increased serotonin and its social comfort effect. So those people who have lower genetic levels of serotonin activity tend to drink more and to have more alcohol cravings.[15,16] When laboratory rats have a drink, their serotonin levels go up, especially if they have low levels resulting from childhood maternal separations.[17] Alcohol use may also increase dopamine levels, increasing our desire for novelty and tolerance for risk. Lest we forget, alcohol also affects the GABA neurotransmitter system, and thus dampens ordinary anxiety. That is no small comfort for those with anxious angst.

Social Anxiety

In this historical context, alcohol may have been most useful for relief of Social Anxiety and relaxation of social hierarchy. Imagine early man having drinks around a primeval campfire—so much easier to relax and mingle with the alpha males and females. There is a study in which volunteer college students were forced (forced!) to drink either alcohol or plain orange juice, and then shown images of threatening or nonthreatening faces. Not surprisingly, the sober subjects paid more attention to the threat posed by angrier faces, and even more attention if they had Social Anxiety to spare. On the other hand, the intoxicated subjects paid less attention to the angry faces, but the level of their Social Anxiety no longer made much of a difference. At least in college then, alcohol levels the social hierarchy playing field.[18] But most of us already knew that.

We also know that people with Social Anxiety are at higher risk for relying on alcohol to get them through social situations.[19] Among the symptoms of Social Anxiety, mere avoidance of social situations is not the best predictor of alcohol reliance. That honor goes to fear of scrutiny and embarrassment—in other words, the specific core social hierarchy mechanism.[20]

For these reasons, beer and other alcohol has been used as a way to enhance group decision making. Sufficiently intoxicated, people offer ideas more freely, and more freely consider the ideas of those lower on the totem pole. In Persia 2,500 years ago and in barbarian Germany 1,900 years ago, the affairs of state were deliberated and decided under the influence. Then they made sure to double check their decisions the next morning. Then again, other ancient societies worked it the other way around. They decided sober, then reconfirmed drunk.[21] You can't be too careful.

Modern Japan is still an example of a highly hierarchical society in which Social Anxiety is also common. As we learned, people follow strict social protocols at work, but then everyone (the men, anyway) goes off to drink after work. This is a way to level the social playing field and to better understand what co-workers are really like inside. We do a bit of the same in the States, as well as playing golf and watching sports. When social façades are down, inner traits, skills, and appetites show through, especially when beer is involved, and when sports commentary and golfing quirks are socially uninhibited. Misbehavior on the golf course is a telling hint of inner tendencies. Mulligan, anyone?

Panic

Sometimes people are desperate for a beer. This could be because they are hot, thirsty, finally off from work, or just plain dramatic. On the other hand, it could be because they have sudden Panic Anxiety (or ongoing anticipatory anxiety). Off the cuff, Panic seems to be the second most common instinctive promoter of alcohol consumption. Not only that, even when Panic patients don't drink too much themselves, there is a much higher likelihood that some of their family members do.[22] In the case of Panic, the benefits may come from a generalized anxiety dampening effect. Just like the benzodiazepines, alcohol acts on that GABA neurotransmitter system that regulates anxiety. Indeed, alcohol withdrawal is treated with benzodiazepines to prevent a too-sudden change in GABA activity levels.

MORE ON ALCOHOL AND CIVILIZATION

We have also found other uses for alcohol. A good stiff drink is a way to relax after a frightening encounter or a stressful day, and it is a way to prepare for military battle (or for an artistic performance). It was once used as a pain killer, for physical wounds after battle and emotional wounds after performance. Alcohol, of course, is still used as an antiseptic. In the Middle Ages, and even in post-Revolutionary America, the water supply was sufficiently contaminated that it was unfit to drink. For safety, most adults and children drank low alcohol beer sanitized by alcohol and the brewing process itself ("small beer"). Perhaps that helped us through some difficult times.

DRUNK AS A SKUNK

Yes, animals do drink alcohol in the wild, mostly in the form of naturally fermenting fruits and berries. Elephants, howler monkeys, chimpanzees, reindeer, and tree shrews imbibe great quantities when they can, sometimes at risk to their alertness and physical stability. Laboratory rats offered a 24-hour open bar tend to have a daily drink before dinner, a nightcap afterwards, and a party twice a week.[21] Despite their own drinking habits, researchers don't know why these other mammals drink—and the animals aren't talking—but perhaps a little angst relief is satisfying for anyone. Indeed, rats will run for the bottle after foot-shock stress (okay, electric shock isn't exactly social angst), but also after a drug that stimulates anxiety (yohimbine).[23]

ALCOHOL-FREE SOCIETIES

Most mammals drink only on rare occasion, and nearly all are polygamous. Historically, human mammals drank less than we do today, and they were often polygamous as well, (at least those at the top of the heap). King Solomon supposedly had 700 wives and 300 concubines. This didn't leave too many women left over for lesser men, nor much choice for the women. The arrival and greater use of alcohol allowed men a more level playing field in the competition for wives. Alcohol gives beta-dog men the courage to find a mate and gives alpha-dog men the grace to let them, or maybe it just makes the alpha-dog humans fall into a drunken and oblivious stupor (surely they would have had first dibs on the booze).

However, there are societies that don't allow alcohol, including traditional Muslims and fundamentalist Mormons. Both groups practice polygamy (religiously and politically allowed for some Muslims, but long-since prohibited by the mainstream Church of Jesus Christ of Latter Day Saints and by the state of Utah). Likewise, a study (by wine economists) of traditional societies on multiple continents found that alcohol use leads to greater monogamy.[24] In the absence of alcohol, some cultures embrace a marital playing field tilted toward the top-dog males, who collect a larger share of the women.

At least these societies are spared the ravages of alcohol itself. Although alcohol has helped civilization in many ways—reducing instinctual angst, promoting civilization, disinfecting pathogenic bacteria, replacing gasoline in cars, inspiring the cocktail party, and all of that culminating in the development of modern craft beers—the bad news is that alcohol has opened a Pandora's box of substance abuse, which we'll get to in chapter 10.

DARWIN'S REVENGE

Evolution has an opinion about alcohol, too. If alcohol helps us diminish our evolved social instincts, then beer is a counter-evolutionary force. Evolution fights back with a genetic mutation (of "acetaldehyde dehydrogenase"). For people with this mutation, alcohol is not fully metabolized into the chemical acetaldehyde, the acetaldehyde level increases, and that leaves them feeling quite ill. If you fool with Mother Nature, your genes will have their revenge. Ultimately, they have no choice but to reduce or avoid alcohol use.[25] This mechanism is essentially similar to the way that the medicine disulfiram (brand name Antabuse) is used to prevent drinking. Overall, evolved alcohol avoidance limits the problematic intoxication, physical illness,[26] and behavioral ravages of alcoholism, including suicide,[27] but it also makes it harder to achieve the benefits of alcohol for reducing instinctive angst. The genetic variant is most common in Asians, especially from China, Japan, and Korea,[28] but it is also found in some Jews.[29]

ANSWERING TO A HIGHER AUTHORITY

Once instinctual roles are diminished through Consciousness, culture and alcohol, then how is a society held together? Self-interest is one answer, but not enough. Religiously based moral and legal codes provided a more conscious mechanism for societal well-being, while still allowing some self-choice of societal roles and alleviation of angst. Many religious leaders of all faiths point out that religious practice is also an important and useful tool for the management of anxiety and depression. On the other hand, some people would counter that certain historical religious practices encouraged people to merely submit to their instinctual roles. When Karl Marx (German philosopher, 1818– 1883) said that "religion is the opiate of the masses," he may have meant that religion not only provided substitute pleasure, but that it kept the common man in his unpleasant place as well.

As we developed Consciousness, we began to think about how people and nature worked, and how things got that way. We quested for social belonging, for the status of socially paramount alpha male (or female), for purity and moral guidance, for social harmony, for acceptance of inevitable death, and for conscious meaning and understanding. These six quests, of course, mirror our six social instincts. Religion, in one theory, is a natural consequence of our evolutionary adaptation, with religiousness itself an evolved adaptation. To the faithful, this would mean we are born as believers because of God's will. To unbelievers, though, the existence of some evolutionary religious adaptation would prove that religion is a biological delusion. However, unbelievers could not assert that if God had wanted us to believe, we would have been born that way. Freud voiced a similar view of religion as delusion in *The Future of an Illusion*. Jean-Paul Sartre (French existentialist philosopher and playwright, 1905–1980) posed the religious quandary: "That God does not exist, I cannot deny. That my whole being cries out for God I cannot forget."

Our inborn religious needs can be satisfied by a traditional religion, a philosophical tradition, scientific understanding, or even by a firm reliance on atheism. Although there are many varieties of religious experience, they all utilize communality, priestly guidance (the Quaker Religious Society of Friends aspired to a leaderless congregation, but it ended up with pastors and lay leaders nonetheless), moral codes, ritual, faith, knowledge, prayer, and contemplation. Religion has been part of human society for millennia, and probably began with campfire discussions and shamans. Doctrine, practice, and edifice grew over time. Recent archaeological research has unearthed a massive temple dating back to 11,600 BCE.[30]

The much vaunted conflict of science and religion is better seen as a tension between differing religious domains. As Einstein pointed out, "Science without religion is lame, religion without science is blind." Indeed, when the brains of religious and nonreligious people are studied with fMRI (functional Magnetic Resonance Imaging), they are quite similar in a very important way. "True or false" questions about scientifically testable material facts activate centers for memory retrieval, but questions about religious belief activate frontal-lobe brain centers for emotion and self-perception.[31] Science and religion make their homes in separate parts of our brains.

The conscious moral valence of religion derives from our emotional social instincts. Moral codes without emotions are lame; emotions without moral codes are blind. Along these lines, studies using the Big-Five Personality Model show that religiousness is predicted by orderliness (conscientiousness, and our OCD/nesting instinct), and also by empathic sensitivity (Agreeableness, and our Atypical Depression/social harmony instinct).[32] These associations also fit with the often religious content of OCD (ritual behaviors and scrupulous attention to amorality) and of mania (a social harmony endeavor—that "mission from God").

So we can also look at religious practice through the lens of our six social instincts. Panic Anxiety is alleviated by group membership and activities, including rituals, holidays, feasts, and ceremonies. Prayer can alleviate Panic Anxiety by meditation and distraction, but also by offering feelings of personal closeness to counter fears of separation. Indeed, one study looked at psychiatric symptoms in the context of three particular components of religious comfort: close and loving, approving and forgiving, and creating and judging. It was primarily the close-and-loving component that was associated with fewer symptoms.[33] Similarly, the prayers of the religious activate brain areas for social cognition, as if they were communicating with someone.[34] Although it could well be that a sense of personal connection to God alleviates the separation anxiety of Panic, it could also be that people who feel closer are already those with fewer symptoms.

Religion offers comfort for those afflicted with Social Anxiety. Sigmund Freud in *Civilization and Its Discontents* said that "God is a projection of the human need for a father"[35]—a source of strength and direction. This ultimate alpha creature is variously called the King, the Lord, the Almighty, the Father, the Unified Field Theory and, of course, "God" and "Goddess," offering the comfort of a wise and omnipotent leader of the pack. The first five of the Ten Commandments are about recognition of and submission to this leader. Some religions, including some Eastern faiths, indeed emphasize passive acceptance of authorities, fate, and role. Accepting a submissive role prevents the angst of trying to move up the ranks.

Religion also offers something to those whose OCD traits leave them needing to clean, arrange, save, and behave. Many religions emphasize physical cleanliness, most emphasize clean living, science (as a quasi-religion) emphasizes methodological purity, and atheism advocates "washing away" superstition. Carefully arranged religious rituals and specific prayer routines are typical. Moral codes specify proper and prohibited behaviors, and this would be one view of the last five of the Ten Commandments of Judeo-Christian tradition. Compared to less religious research subjects, highly religious Protestants have more OCD symptoms such as washing, checking, need for certainty, and concern for their untoward thoughts.[36] Likewise, highly religious Jews are more likely to have true OCD than their less religious brethren. Two thousand years ago, the Jewish Essene sect led lives of pronounced ritual, religion, and asceticism. Reading the Dead Sea Scrolls they left behind suggests that they, too, were strongly guided by OCD instincts.

The Golden Rule is common to most major religions, and it is the embodiment of empathic concern: Do unto others as you would have them do unto you. This elegantly distilled recipe meets the concerns of Atypical Depression and social harmony. An alternate view of Commandments 6–10 is that they promote Conscious social harmony by prohibiting the most serious breaches of the Golden Rule. One study looked at brain activation while subjects viewed images of intentional and accidental harm to people and things. Younger research subjects viewing the images of deliberate harm showed increased activation of emotional brain centers, and they felt greater sadness, and the older (and presumably wiser) subjects also had increased activation of their frontal cortex. Armed with their socially informed cortex, the older subjects had heightened Conscious focus to supplement their visceral instinctive response.[37]

The melancholic death instinct is addressed by the many religious edicts to care for the sick and the dying and by the prohibition against suicide in some religions. Among caregivers of the dying, the more religious are less likely to become depressed themselves.[38]

Religions seem to vary in their view of Consciousness. On the one hand, some religions advocate moral codes that are actually a codified reflection of our social instincts.[39] Along those lines, Proverbs 3:7 seems to elevate Biblical instruction above conscious choices: "Be not wise in thine own eyes: fear the LORD, and depart from evil." On the other hand, some other religions, as well as science and atheism, emphasize a preference for rational choice, even though Consciousness itself seems to be a social instinct.

WE'RE FROM THE GOVERNMENT AND WE'RE HERE TO HELP

Early societies intermingled government, law, and religion, but secular government also assumed similar roles. With Consciousness and civilization, subtle democratic elements incrementally wove through social interactions. Alpha-dog leaders became more accountable to Everydog. Perhaps this started when majorities of a population group were able to influence their emotional and intellectual leaders, or perhaps when overwhelming numbers mandated their role in decision making. At some point, some mad genius introduced more formal democratic elements in ancient Greece (if not before), in Christianity (the Protestant Reformation), and in Revolutionary America. "We hold these truths to be self-evident, that all men are created equal, that they are endowed by their Creator with certain unalienable Rights" wrote Thomas Jefferson (American president, 1743–1826) in the Declaration of Independence, quite rationally trying to overrule instinctive, royal, and cultural hierarchies. However, "too much" democracy can have unexpected consequences. For example, a successful lawyer described grade school classes in which students were all called on in turn. Himself suffering from Social Anxiety, he dreaded the call, terrified that he would embarrass himself. Though still Socially Anxious even today, he has learned from his experience and is successful in meetings and presentations.

Laws codify the moral rules for a society. The Code of Urukagina from 2300 BCE is the oldest known formal legal system. Urakagina took office after a corrupt leader, and his Code emphasizes reason and equity over established hierarchy. For example, an aristocrat could no longer just commandeer the property of a lesser resident (a "shublugal"). Among other things, Urukagina also spells out quantities of both beer and bread for rations, payment, and funeral offerings. The later Code of Hammurabi, from 1700 BCE, reflects the judicial decisions of a leader, and it proposes specific punishments for crimes and offenses. Under Hammurabi, the Golden Rule applies only to others of equal status. His Code reinforces hierarchy by decisions that take into account the societal rank of the victim and perpetrator. Maybe a drink would have helped level the judicial playing field; wine is mentioned only as commerce, and there is nary a mention of beer.

Animals, of course, have neither legal codes nor formal governmental structures. Because everyone follows instinctual instructions and restrictions, their herds seem mostly to get along pretty well. It isn't that they are completely without crime, as any observer of subordinate apes stealing food would attest, but they do settle their differences without courts and lawyers. After our beta dog Cassidy grabbed and ate that apple pie, he hung his head, hid in the corner, and looked downright ashamed of himself. He knew he had exceeded his station, and no doubt was blushing under all that facial hair. When Bonnie the alpha dog ate a strawberry rhubarb pie, she held her head high, had a huge smile on her face, and tried to jump on the counter when the next pie was underway. Mark Twain may have overlooked guilty dogs when he said that "Man is the only animal that blushes—or needs to."

Alpha dog Bonnie may be a creature of advancing civilization. The changing rules of modern liberal civilization can be viewed as a quest to remove ancient social instincts from codified law. Hierarchical roles are diminished under law, (though not as much in the military and corporate worlds), in favor of consciously derived ethical constructs. "Progress" means overcoming social-instinct restrictions, even at the price of increasing angst and sometimes social disarray. Through culture and law, humans try to modify the instinctual social roles of themselves and of others. *Human rights* often means overcoming the dictates of instinct. To frame politicians in these terms, conservatives oppose the adverse consequences of heedless opposition to instinct. Liberals and progressives applaud a more mindful and pleasurable pursuit of freedom and free will, despite any resulting personal or societal angst.[40] At the risk of sounding optimistic, our society often manages to find the happy medium.

SPREADING THE WORDS

So far, we've talked about the roles of alcohol, religion and government in promoting civilization by moderating the angst-evoking effects of Consciousness on social instinct. Mass communication is another mechanism for advancing civilization and reducing angst. Our ancient ancestors no doubt talked about where and how to find food, but they also carried on oral histories over generations, with important implications for morality, society, family, and religion. Memorization and verbal transmission over time was enhanced by adaptation of these histories into musical rhyme. The invention of writing allowed oral traditions to be transcribed into documents such as the Old Testament. With the printing press invention of Johannes Gutenberg

(German inventor and blacksmith, 1398–1468), the Bible was a logical early publication. The printing revolution that followed was a founding stone of intellectual and social advancement of all kinds. "Spreading the word" is not limited to religion per se; it includes all kinds of intellectual and factual information that enhances civilization. And because no good deed goes unpunished, Gutenberg went bankrupt soon after his Bible was printed.

THE DECLINE OF BAD DEEDS

A lot of good things have happened over the last few thousand years. We have been able to use our Consciousness and reason to develop civilizations. Even as those civilizations expanded in size, so, too, did their ability to trade and communicate over great distances. Civilizations reached out to other civilizations, and we became more simpatico with humans from other families, villages, tribes, societies, and continents. More and more people became part of the same extended herd, subject to the same kindred social instincts. Those instincts were reinforced by the rise of religion, enlightened philosophical perspective, government, law, and democracy. As a result, over the long haul, there has been a dramatic and steady reduction in violent death, and in other forms of violence and "inhumane" behavior. Although there are some major recent exceptions, and violence isn't gone by any means, we *Homo sapiens* have managed to extend civilized in-herd behaviors to much of our global civilization. This process is detailed in *The Better Angels of Our Nature,* an extraordinary book by Steven Pinker (American psychologist; 1954 –).[41]

THE MOOD TUBE

Today we have many forms of mass media to help us deal with lurking social instincts. This happens in at least three ways: by discouraging violations of social instincts, by offering substitute gratifications, and by helping us to cope when those painful feelings do appear. Mass media offer a view of empathy, pain endurance, fantasied solutions, real solutions, coping tools, substitute comforts, consolation, and substitute companionship. Songs, books, newspapers, magazines, movies, radio, television, and Internet content all serve these purposes, but television is the most fun to talk about.

Struggling to find the comfort of social instincts under control? Learn from the approaches of the happy herds on immensely popular shows like *Father Knows Best, The Cosby Show, Friends, Seinfeld,* and *NCIS* (even crime shows can be about keeping the herd together). *NCIS* stands for Naval Criminal Investigative Service, but its vast audience appeal reflects a focus on what we might call Non Conscious Instinctive Sociality.

How about vicarious gratification of your desire to disobey your social instincts? Want to fantasize about far away travels, without fear of personal catastrophe? Watch *Lost* or pretty much any travel show. Want to become the leader of the pack, but without your own embarrassment angst? Watch the contestants competing on *American Idol,* or learn from Cesar Millan on *The Dog Whisperer* how to be the pack leader of your canine. Want help with nesting? Watch *This Old House* and other home repair and real-estate shows. Need reminders about good behavior in a civil society? How about *Dragnet* or *Law and Order*? Need to learn more about how to handle feelings of social rejection? Watch soap operas and romance reality shows like *The Bachelor.*

These shows are popular because they resonate with our social instincts. They offer not only a less frightening substitute for actual experiences, but they also offer a kind of rehearsal for real-life problems, with ideas for real-life solutions. Tell the truth now, hasn't Cesar's work with dogs ever made us think about how to deal with people? Cesar himself points out that his work is far more with the owners than with the dogs who are just trying to get along with them. And some of the people we find hard to deal with are merely responding to us: a tough nut for most of us to crack. Television and all of the other mass media are much safer venues for emotional rehearsal than the real world. With the help of that rehearsal, some shy people can sidle up to a karaoke bar to sing (most often after some beer, of course). People watch all that TV to help them with pesky social concerns, and not just for the news and weather.

THERE BUT NOT THERE

Modern communications allow us to stretch our social limits with less angst. Letters, telephone, e-mail, texting, Internet chat, Internet games—these inventions offer us progressively more detached and anonymous opportunities to be bravely connected. Just as Panic Anxiety patients feel reassured by traveling with a companion "phobic partner" they also feel better having a mobile phone with them.[42] Not only are they prepared for catastrophe (the chance predator, say), but they have a lifeline to home. Shy, Socially Anxious, and rejection-sensitive college students feel much more comfortable in online communication, which has neither visual nor auditory cues, than they do with someone in person.[43,44] As we might expect, those who most rely on detached online socializing are those who already feel uneasy in close social relationships.[45]

One problem, of course, as with television, is that, although these experiences feel safer, they are not the same as living in the real world. They may gain us online friends, but we must still make that leap to real friends, with the risk of real separations, hierarchies and rejections. That leap can be tough to make, as online-dating service users have learned. First, you just look around the Web site, then you fantasize, then you interact, and then maybe you meet, but hidden emotional angst bursts forth on first meeting, especially if you meet someone who at least resembles what you imagined. Even with computer-aided dating, the social instincts remain.

Perhaps we should think about a brave new world of romance and reproduction. Computer Aided Design has been linked now with Computer Aided Manufacturing (CAD/CAM) to provide a near seamless digital design and manufacturing process. Physical products can even be manufactured by a modified ink jet printer. They are actually printing out real aircraft parts. So are we on the road to a different kind of CAD/CAM: Computer Aided Dating linked to Computer Aided Mating? With the development of newer reproductive technologies, some more complete kind of escape from our pesky instincts is not farfetched at all. That would carry on the process of our DNA pretty well (except, of course, should we decide to use cloned or modified DNA), but it would present a whole new social construct to think about, and it is already underway.

HELP ME IF YOU CAN

Civilization has also come up with direct ways to relieve the angst of social instincts thwarted. No doubt, back on the African savanna and in the caves of Europe, there were healers of some sort—shamans perhaps, who tended to the distress of herd members. Formal credentialing was a later development. Emotional and practical support, advice and guidance, and prayer and philosophy can make some good progress against the pain. Even so, the main effort over the millennia was largely focused on surface manifestations, rather than evidence-based treatments for underlying causes. There wasn't much that could be done about adverse effects of the four humors or satanic influences, not that they didn't try.

As a society, we now recognize that anxiety and depressive disorders (and psychosis) are illnesses in our modern context, and that better treatments are available. This has developed from converging advances in psychiatric diagnosis, neuroscience, psychopharmacology, psychotherapy, and social psychology that point us in directions where our instincts do not want us to look. Remember the story of the man looking for his keys under the light of a street lamp? A passerby offered to help, and asked where he had lost them. "They are over there," said the man, pointing to a dimly lit corner, "but the light is better here." Well, the light of psychiatric inquiry has started pointing to those dimly lit spots where new therapies and theories await. With growing illumination, we even have public-service campaigns to increase awareness of

depression and other ills, not to mention incessant and sometimes misleading pharmaceutical advertisements.

LISTEN HERE

At its beginning, modern psychotherapy began to address motivations, behavior
choices and the unhappy emotions that can result. Although it is easy to imagine that
the ancient Greeks knew about this approach, recognition of this process in more
recent times started with Sigmund Freud and his contemporaries in the 19th century.
Psychotherapy also began to address the complex interactions of surface emotions,
biological emotions, perceptions, hidden expectations and fears, and relationships.
Although modern theory and technique has changed dramatically since Freud's day,
none of these purely psychotherapeutic approaches alter the underlying biology of
most anxiety and depressive disorders. All psychotherapies are means to help people
better endure, cope, understand, choose, prosper and enjoy life despite persistent biological instincts.

TIME HEALS ALL WOUNDS

As we age and accumulate experience and thought, we acquire wisdom. Although it
is not a replacement for (or impediment to) good psychotherapy, Consciousness plays
an increasing role with age, and instinct plays a decreasing one. Witness our older
research subjects who color their moral concerns with reason.[37] At the last, though,
when dementia sets in, we return to instinct sans Consciousness and sans learning.

ANGST VITAMINS

More recently, psychopharmacology has entered the battle against emotional distress. Psychiatry never actually relied on alcohol as a treatment; it tastes great, but
it is less fulfilling, and it has too many side effects. Over the past hundred years,
though, we have stumbled upon or designed useful medications for all five of our core
syndromes. Some have fallen by the wayside (cocaine), whereas others have become
celebrated mainstays of care (SSRIs). For the first time in history, we have the tools
to address the emotional core of biological instincts with medications that are relatively effective and safe. This does not mean that psychotherapy is unnecessary. On
the contrary, good therapy becomes that much more useful when combined with
effective medications. Aside from feeling less angst, there could be yet other benefits
of psychotherapy and medication. As we shall see, the slings and arrows of instinct in
civilization are many and varied.

10

ILLNESS AND INSTINCT:
CONSCIOUSNESS HAS CONSEQUENCES

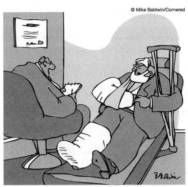

© Mike Baldwin/Cornered

"Took your advice and decided to face my fears. I still get panic attacks, but at least now there's a darn good reason."

"Man is the only creature that refuses to be what he is."
—Albert Camus (French philosopher; 1913–1960)

"Reasonable people adapt themselves to the world. Unreasonable people attempt to adapt the world to themselves. All progress, therefore, depends on unreasonable people."
—George Bernard Shaw (Irish playwright; 1856–1950)

CONSCIOUSNESS DOESN'T BUY HAPPINESS

Let's face it, the level and persistence of our angst is not normal. At least it wouldn't be for other primates, mammals, or creatures in general. No self-respecting marmot or goose would put up with it. They'd be running and hiding in their instinctual roles just as fast as they could. But we don't. On the contrary, we almost revel in angst. We definitely don't like it, but our conscious decisions overrule our instinctive ones, often with marvelous but emotionally painful results. Indeed, a focus on conscious thought and rational accomplishment is a hallmark of civilization. As we have seen, sometimes we succeed exactly because we defy those very instincts that cause our distress. As William Faulkner (American novelist, 1897–1962) pointed out, "Man will not merely endure: he will prevail." We may even have evolved to have higher levels of social instinct than our animal cousins, and we may have even evolved a human tendency for counter-instinctive adaptation. More than language, intellect, art, domesticated fire, tools, bipedalism, opposable thumbs, or anything else, our human ability to rise above and even against the angst of instinct is our most defining feature.

We humans are more able and often more willing to seek fulfillment of our appetitive and intellectual instincts, and rational enough to invent newer and more appealing super stimuli to satisfy them. Tree shrews drink fermented fruits, but not cabernet wines or margaritas made with fine tequila. An eagle might dine on duck, but not on duck à l'orange or on Peking duck. Rabbits may be romantically active, but they don't make themselves more sexually appealing through exercise, makeup, luxury cars, or personal charm, even if they do wear fur coats. All of our appetitive upgrades bring us reason, civilization, the finer things in life, laptop computers—and all sorts of angst-driven problems.

Appetitive, material, creative, intellectual and status accomplishments are enjoyable and rewarding (just thinking about a margarita is fun), but they don't necessarily bring inner happiness. "Wherever you go, there you are" said Thomas à Kempis (Dutch monk, 1380–1471). Even with material and cultural success, you still bring your instincts and angst with you. No matter how successful you are, those annoying social instincts are still there. One rational conceptualization of this situation (to repeat the point) is that while money doesn't buy happiness, if you are going to be unhappy anyway, you might as well be rich and successful. This is true enough, and this solution has also been called "affluenza"—an affliction of affluence that merely colors the darkness of angst.

EVERY SILVER LINING HAS A CLOUD

As we look at the downside of Consciousness and civilization, let's start with a smile. We all know that smiling is good thing; it eases social interaction, and the mere act of smiling even makes us feel momentarily better. However, bus drivers who consciously force courteous smiles all day, despite how they may actually be feeling, tend to feel sad and to withdraw from work (although it is different when their smiles are fed by actual happy thoughts).[1] Going against your emotions (counter-instinct) has unexpected and unhappy consequences. Similarly, conscious suppression of angry feelings also makes people unhappy.[2] Addressing a broader range of behaviors, executive coaching teaches managers to act in more effective ways, despite how their inner feelings and habits would guide them. Some management skills may improve, but the underlying instincts make fascinating new problems crop up in unexpected places.[3]

These relatively small clouds raise the question of still larger ones. Doctors have long mused about so-called diseases of civilization.[4] Our reasoned and counter-instinctive behaviors lead to problems largely unknown among the other animals: "mental illness," suicide, drug abuse, crime, common heart diseases, family dysfunction, and problems that amount to failures to clean, arrange, behave, and save.

DIAGNOSABLE ANGST

This being a psychiatry book, let's start with psychiatric problems. We've learned about how frustration of instinctive social roles leads to the emergence of painful and diagnosable anxiety and depressive syndromes. So what makes us human also puts us at risk for mental illness. Although some animals living in the wild can have similar syndromes, few seem to have our human propensity for intense or prolonged angst. We like to think of ourselves as people who merely suffer from adversity, rather than as people with disorders—much less as creatures who willfully violate innate social dictates. People with serious anxiety and depressive disorders usually have an exaggerated perception of the real difficulties in their world, or else they magnify the extent of their own practical limitations. They don't look for treatment at first, because consciously they see the problem as largely "out there," with little coming from their own inner world. In addition, and on a deep inner level, they may unwittingly take their angst as an expectable response to their social behaviors—an earned punishment for their hubris.

THEY ALL MOVED AWAY FROM ME

Jean-Paul Sartre, unable to look to a higher power or better theory to address people's social distress, cried out that "Hell is other people." In other words, we pull away from others because we are put off by their emotional pain and behaviors, and especially because it somehow resonates with our own emotional pain or fears. This process contributes to the stigma of mental illness. Angst is something that we neither like to address in other people nor openly describe about ourselves. In our evolutionary theory there is an added level of understanding. If people have the angst of anxiety or depressive disorders, that is *prima facie* evidence that they are breaching instinctive biological rules. So we unwittingly move away from them because we sense a disregard for the hidden norms of our social instincts.

Arlo Guthrie (American folk singer, 1947–) turns stigma on its head in "Alice's Restaurant," a talking blues song where he describes how his court conviction for littering leaves him seated with criminals at his draft-board screening:

He said "What were you arrested for, kid?" And I said, "Littering." And they all moved away from me on the bench there, and the hairy eyeball and all kinds of mean nasty things, till I said, "And creating a nuisance." And they all came back, shook my hand, and we had a great time on the bench, talking about crime...

If angst is evidence of biological misbehavior, then it is also evidence of a kindred spirit—if being a nuisance colors your particular flavor of angst. A study of modern-day hunter-gatherers in Tanzania suggests that when honey sticks are provided to group members, the small number of "free riders" who take more than their fair share do indeed tend to befriend their like-minded brethren.[5] Oh, and by the way, a blues song about stigmatization for a truly intimidating crime would not be as funny as one about littering (or honey hoarding).

Even so, many of us struggle with how best to respond to others' emotional despair. For example, in 1997 the Equal Employment Opportunity Commission issued well-meaning guidelines for "reasonable accommodation" of employees with mental illness. One suggestion was that a depressed employee with decreased concentration should be put into a private room. Solitary confinement for depression seems inhumane and unhelpful, although it does oddly resemble the hibernation-like response to rejection in Atypical Depression. Equally disturbing about the guidelines was the discouragement of proper diagnosis and effective treatment, the implicit stigmatization of afflicted employees, and the presumption that they would not get better.[6] Subsequent conversations with employment lawyers and human resource officials revealed that some had the initial thought not to hire anyone who seemed a little bit "off." Life is full of unintended consequences, but fortunately, most employers still hire more sensibly.

MORE BAD NEWS ABOUT GOOD NEWS

Even though psychiatry and mental health now have better diagnoses, more effective medication and psychotherapy treatments, and wider public acceptance, not all is yet well in the world. Psychiatric practice and research perhaps receives more critical attention than any other medical specialty. Diagnosis is where medical care starts. Yet, there are medical and mental-health practitioners who believe that diagnosis is a bad idea, "too difficult," too time consuming, or even that diagnoses should be ignored. This last stance comes from a view that distress should not be "medicalized," that the problems are due mostly to external circumstances, or that psychiatric diagnoses are a figment of pharmaceutical-company imagination (this last concern is only sometimes true). As a result, the quality of diagnosis out there is often modest, and the diagnoses on forms are often downright fictional.

This also brings us back to the diagnostic discussion that we started out with. Catch-all diagnoses in psychiatry, although legitimate, are easier to use than careful attention to their more specific subtypes. Diagnoses like Major Depressive Disorder (MDD), generalized anxiety disorder (GAD), and Post Traumatic Stress Disorder (PTSD) also focus less attention on the inner instinctual world of the patient, less on the real social concerns at issue, but more on those problematic outward circumstances that may at first seem to be the obvious cause of distress. Because these general diagnoses (and their nonspecific treatments) are more acceptable to many patients and some clinicians, this issue doesn't generate much public concern.

The problem is that simplistic diagnoses and easy fixes don't work very well in psychiatry or elsewhere in medicine. Imagine if people were routinely treated for leg pain disorder (LPD) rather than for an underlying fracture, laceration, muscle sprain, or cancer. Not just at a first office visit, but forever. Even though LPD is not a real diagnosis (doctors frown on lumping many syndromes with a common symptom into one category), most of us have experience with physical problems that get worse with nonspecific treatment until the right diagnosis is made.

Any possible problems with psychiatric treatment receive outsized media attention. Some years ago, a question was raised whether SSRI antidepressants raise suicide risk. Outrage! A media circus ensued, doctors were afraid to prescribe SSRIs, and patients were afraid to take them. For the period of time that SSRI prescriptions were avoided, people died as the completed suicide rate increased. Indeed, the child and adolescent suicide rate increased by 14% after 2003 in the U.S., and by 49% in the Netherlands.[7] Outrage? Not so much. When the dust finally settled, it turned out that SSRIs, unsurprisingly, reduce the risk of completed suicides.[8] There are other examples, but let's not dwell. Suffice it to say that civilization pays close attention to anything that threatens to quell or expose our hidden social instincts.

By way of comparison, it has long been suspected that some common back surgery procedures have less benefit than risk. When controlled studies were finally reported, it turned out that surgery did offer some low-back pain patients more rapid pain relief, but that pain and disability two years later were pretty much the same as in the nonsurgical patients.[9,10] Nonsurgical patients do have fewer surgical complications, of course. There was not so much outrage about this. Since these studies, there has been only modest change in the use of these surgical procedures.

There is a silver lining to this cloud of critical evaluation. With such alert public attention, psychiatric research has pioneered carefully defined diagnostic criteria and well-controlled treatment trials. Many years ago, for a study of psychological characteristics of patients with coronary artery disease, there was a standard assessment method for the psychological traits, but none for scoring an exercise stress test with cardiac imaging ("Thallium Stress Test"). The researchers devised their own method for the study.[11] Even so, there is still much room for improvement in research, diagnosis, and treatment in psychiatry, and greater independence from financial bias, just as there is in the rest of medicine.

SUICIDE IS PAINFUL

There are animals who do themselves in. Whales beach themselves, melancholic animals may curl up and die, some animals risk death from predators in protecting their kin, and salmon die after spawning. None of these is deliberate self-destruction. Animals don't do suicide. Lemmings don't follow each other in death dives off of cliffs. "Suicide is contrary to the inclination of nature," wrote Thomas Aquinas (Italian priest and philosopher, 1225–1274), meaning that man's natural inclination is to both survive and support his social community.

However, humans do kill themselves. Suicide is another downside of Consciousness and civilization. Exaggerated expression of social instincts is one reason. Panic Anxiety is increasingly recognized as a major risk factor for suicide.[12] The intense separation anxiety can leave some people with catastrophic fears accompanying a false belief that there is no hope of return to a comforting social home. In modern human society, it is all too easy to be apart from others, or to feel alone in the middle of a crowd. Melancholia, a death instinct after all, promotes a physiological death process. Some people, applying their Consciousness to the issue at hand, accelerate this instinctive feeling with deliberate self-destruction. Psychiatric lore teaches that the risk may actually be higher just after Melancholia resolves. The depressive lethargy is gone, but the thoughts have not yet changed.[13] Accidental suicides are not uncommon, especially with drug and alcohol abuse, which are commonly underpinned by anxiety disorders, as we shall see. Given a chance, a laboratory rat might overdose on cocaine, but not because it wants to die.

TOO MUCH IS NOT ENOUGH

Although the "nectar of the Gods" may go back as much as 100,000 years, and may well have helped spark civilization, enough is enough. But when painful instincts are strong, so is the inclination to alcoholism. Common parlance uses derivative words for people who are possessed by other coping methods: workaholic, wealthoholic, chocoholic, loveaholic, and shopaholic are just a few alternatives to try out. Alcohol and many drugs are physically addictive (you have withdrawal symptoms if you stop suddenly), but the real problem is psychological dependence on this coping method. Successful detoxification treatment of alcohol abuse all too often leads back to, well, alcohol abuse, especially if the underlying instinctive syndromes are not treated. After all, those symptoms will be worse after alcohol cessation. Even when the instincts are appeased with the right medications, the ingrained alcohol coping response persists for long afterward.

Alcohol can do some good things for us: It reduces painful instincts, makes us feel happy, makes us more social engaged (excepting those who drunkenly put a lampshade on their head), enables relaxed social interactions, and loosens the overly inhibited. However, while modest alcohol use is often more of a solution than a problem, we are faced today with an alcohol universe beyond the imaginings of our ancestors or of our genes. We have alcohol made from grapes, barley, wheat, rice, corn, agave, sugar cane, taro, potatoes, apples, plums, and almost any kind of plant material with sufficient sugar or carbohydrate. We craft our liquor carefully, taste test for consumer preferences, age for mellowing and aroma, add flavors, mix with fruit juice and other liquors, and add onions and olives and lime wedges. The result is a supremely enjoyable tasty alcohol for every taste and occasion, available in vast quantities almost everywhere in the world. There is no shortage of advertisement, cultural practice, and social pressure to indulge. Modern alcohol is a Supernormal Stimulus that evolution didn't prepare us for. That's not enough to make alcoholics out of most of us, but it makes overindulgence all that more tempting for those in need of angst relief.

It is true that some animals in the wild will get drunk, and maybe for similar reasons. However, although they may know the way to the bar (a tree of fermenting fruit, for example), few stay drunk for long, and none of them farm plants to have a fermentable crop for booze. Those laboratory rats may use cocaine to the death, but they drink alcohol largely in moderation.

Sermon: So What's the Harm?

Where do we begin? Let's start with some immediate problems of drinking too much. Social lubrication eases painful instinct and promotes civilization, but intoxication clouds the senses and prevents good judgment. This being a sermon, let's look to Proverbs 31 (4–7):

> It is not for kings, O Lemuel, it is not for kings to drink wine; nor for princes strong drink:
> Lest they drink, and forget the law, and pervert the judgment of any of the afflicted.
> Give strong drink unto him that is ready to perish, and wine unto those that be of heavy hearts.
> Let him drink, and forget his poverty, and remember his misery no more.

Angst relief is for the angst afflicted, not for those who need to preserve the best combination of their social instincts and conscious reasoning, and not for those who don't know when to stop.

Next problem in line for us modern types is driving. Animals leave the bar on foot; we leave by car. Alcohol reduces our biological reaction time, as well as our ability to rationally assess our fitness to drive. The result is disaster. Alcohol-related motor vehicle accidents are endemic, and alcohol is epidemic at accident scenes. Evolution did not anticipate Chevrolets, Hondas, Fords, BMWs, and Lamborghinis.

Then there is the nearly endless list of medical complications of long-term alcohol abuse. There is no need to dwell on graphic details, so suffice it to say that hearts, minds, livers, stomachs and more can suffer mightily from an ongoing onslaught of alcohol. Evolution didn't prepare us for six-packs of beer or 80-proof vodka at the corner store.

What Leads Us into This Temptation?

What leads us into alcohol abuse are some of the same social instincts that we self medicate with alcohol. Offhand clinical experience (anecdotal medicine is the worst kind of scientific data) suggests that alcoholism is most commonly a response to Social Anxiety, with Panic Anxiety a runner up. Fortunately, there is also real medical data to support this. In a large epidemiological study in the United States, social and Panic Anxieties were the two strongest predictors of alcohol problems (and of other drug problems).[14] Social Anxiety predicts alcohol problems better than other syndromes,[15] and alcohol abuse is often a reaction to preexisting anxiety.[16] Not everyone with Social Anxiety abuses alcohol, but among those who do there is also a tendency to use other drugs, gamble too much, break rules and laws, or become psychotic.[14] This could be because recklessly appetitive people also crave too much alcohol. In addition, too much alcohol also brings other appetitive behaviors to the fore. Indeed, dopamine activity (our appetitive neurotransmitter) may be increased by alcohol.[17]

Alcohol helps people cope with social situations, which they might otherwise avoid without some liquid courage.[18] What they are afraid of is not so much social interaction itself, but the possibility of scrutiny (the hairy eyeball from someone higher in rank).[19] Simple interventions to reduce excessive drinking in college students can effectively reduce alcohol consumption, but only for those students who don't have much Social Anxiety.[20] People, indeed, are using a tasty, time-tested, and dangerous psychopharmacological method to treat themselves (and to level the perceived social hierarchy). Alas, when safer and more effective medications are suggested to them, many would rather choose alcohol than submit to authoritative "drugs" for help.

Real science also comes to the rescue for the association of Panic and alcohol abuse. Not only do many alcoholics have Panic Anxiety, but their biological relatives also have more Panic and more alcohol use than other people.[21] Alcohol helps Panic in a more general way. Rather than through some specific reduction of social stress, overwhelming anxiety is blotted out by the antianxiety and sedative properties of alcohol. Anecdotal medicine tells us that at least one other of our five syndromes is linked to particular drugs of abuse. Atypical Depression seems to lead to alcohol and marijuana use (another natural drug that stretches back to antiquity),[22] if not also to heroin and opiates.

The bottom line is that we are still too attached to our alcohol, despite the health risks. We are entranced by stories about the history, culture, humor, and archaeology of alcohol.[23] Better treatment of substance abuse will come from closer attention to problematic social instincts, substance-abuse prevention, coping strategies, and self-understanding. Too much is too much. Enough is just right.

CRIME DOESN'T PLAY

Instincts lead us to alcohol and drugs, which lead in turn to crime, our next disease of civilization. A good deal of crime is directly related to substance abuse. People steal to get money for drugs, and the influence of drugs and alcohol can lead to both violence and to criminally impaired judgment. We can also run through our five social instinct syndromes and find more direct relationships between specific instincts and crime.

Panic Anxiety predicts future development of antisocial personality disorder (the word *antisocial* refers to some rule breakers and criminals, but not to loners).[24] Looking at middle-school and high-school students, Social Anxiety leads to early antisocial tendencies.[25] When you look at grown-ups with antisocial personality disorder (which begins in childhood) or adult antisocial behavior (which doesn't), both are associated with greatly increased rates of Panic Anxiety, Social Anxiety, and Dysthymia (probably meaning Atypical Depression).[26] People do not like feeling as if they are stuck at the bottom of the hierarchy, or subject to rejection everywhere they go—and that even includes some people born at the top of the heap. So if that's how life feels to them, it isn't surprising that some would try to beat the system.

The Who (British electric blues band) long ago wrote about managing the tension between beating the system and following the rules, in these selected verses from their "Behind Blue Eyes:"

No one knows what it's like
To be the bad man

To be the sad man
Behind blue eyes

No one knows what it's like
To be hated
To be fated
To telling only lies

But my dreams
They aren't as empty
As my conscience seems to be

No one bites back as hard
On their anger
None of my pain and woe
Can show through

If I swallow anything evil
Put your finger down my throat
If I shiver, please give me a blanket
Keep me warm, let me wear your coat

Some of us missed the title pun for 40 years. With Atypical Depression, fighting to toe the line can't be easy with your eyes full of blues.

There is another piece to the story of social crime. Not all victims of criminal violence are known to the offender. Ancient humans were no doubt concerned about members of their own tribes, but warred often against other tribes that might happen by. Along these lines, the actual wording of the Ten Commandments tells us "Thou shalt not murder," rather than the more humanitarian, more modern, and better known "Thou shalt not kill." In our modern world we have much greater contact with people outside our families, social networks, communities, and nations. This can initially lead to encounters in which instinctual rules don't come into play (different gene pool, after all), and appetitive or protective violence ensues. On the other hand, the increasing contact across cultures and continents over time has led to a world in which battle deaths are gradually and gratifyingly decreasing.[27]

Real Animals

Is the concept of "crime" uniquely human? Certainly other primates are more violent to outsiders than to their own troop members. They probably experience the results as battle casualties and war booty more than as violent assault, murder, or theft. Within the troop, however, they are likely to obey their instincts and avoid transgression. Baboons are alarmed when researchers fool them into hearing what sounds like social rank disobedience. When coyotes play too hard, they apologize. Do those transgressions feel like crimes to them? How about a junior baboon that steals food, or a coyote that doesn't apologize? Animals have no written criminal code, but social instincts are sometimes reinforced by aggressive responses or by exile from play. If you mistreat your dog, it may come back to bite you. Is that their crime, or is it their natural response to your misbehaving instincts?

THE HEART IS HUNTED BY LONELINESS

Coronary artery disease (CAD) and heart attacks (myocardial infarction; MI) have long been thought of as diseases of civilization. They are less common in more traditional societies, and downright rare in other animals. Human CAD was probably common even in ancient civilization. Despite an average death at only about forty years, some 44 of 52 ancient Egyptian mummies had evidence of CAD, some of them from nearly four thousand years ago.[28] Civilization and heart disease are about social roles, not about laptops, greasy French fries, high-speed driving, or even chariot racing. Through mighty struggle, medical science has significantly reduced CAD illness and death, but it has had less success in pinning down the underlying causes with any certainty. So what is it about civilization that might predispose people to heart disease?

Robert Sapolsky (American anthropologist, 1957–) points out that while zebras have a stress response to the occasional lion, we humans have stress responses to everyday traffic jams and more, thus leading to physical illness.[29] However, our strongest stresses are those mediated by our social instincts, and only a few of us actually see traffic (or chariot) jam perpetrators as determined leonine predators. Indeed, recent research has increasingly shown the importance of our anxiety and depressive syndromes as risk factors for heart disease. Healthy people with more long term psychological distress have more CAD (for example, calcium in the coronary arteries on CAT scan evaluation).[30] One way or another, long-term activation of angst is bad for the heart.

HOME IS WHERE THE HEART IS

Once again, let's review our social instincts in our same order (NECA(M)O in Big-Five terms). Each instinct/syndrome/personality factor plays a role in CAD, and Panic Anxiety is where we start. Healthy military veterans with Panic are more likely to develop new CAD later.[31] Just having Panic Anxiety probably means more heart disease risk for anyone.[32] There are several ways that Panic might increase risk. Although it could be that people with Panic have higher rates of such conventional risk factors as smoking, high blood pressure, or high cholesterol blood levels, that probably doesn't explain it all.[32]

Another possibility is that people with Panic Anxiety have big hearts—(too big, in fact). When heart size gets large, it is called hypertrophic (most often left ventricular hypertrophy, or LVH). And when LVH gets really big (cardiomegaly) there can be problems with the heart muscle itself (cardiomyopathy). The cause of cardiomyopathy is usually not known, but it can be fatal, and it is one of the most common reasons people need a heart transplant. If we interview people facing the prospect of a heart transplant, 83% of those with end-stage cardiomyopathy have Panic Anxiety, as compared to only 16% of those with other kinds of end-stage heart disease.[33] This finding appears on careful interview[34] but not when just simple screening tools are used. When we then look at healthy Panic patients, they turn out to have more heart enlargement (previously unsuspected) than healthy control subjects.[35,36] Panic is also more common with the more newly described Takotsubo cardiomyopathy (Japanese for "octopus pot"), which is mostly a temporary syndrome in older women.

When enlarged, the heart muscle not only needs more blood for extra oxygen, but it is also less effective at pumping blood. With CAD added into the large heart picture, the narrow arteries also reduce blood supply to the heart itself. This combination of a large heart and a reduced blood supply is a recipe for a heart attack.[37]

So how could the heart enlarge in some minority of Panic patients? How could grown-up separation anxiety lead to heart disease? Separation makes the heart beat harder. Increased amounts of neurotransmitters like adrenaline are released into the bloodstream, especially in those prone to anger with their Panic,[38] and in those with prolonged Panics that look like agitation.[39] We know that a similar kind of cardiomyopathy is seen when the body itself makes too much adrenaline ("pheochromocytoma") and when people activate adrenaline systems through use of amphetamines in excess. There is also another possibility. During an actual heart attack (MI), some people are especially afraid of dying. Those same people have more evidence of new inflammation and tissue damage, and worse outcomes in the long run. Maybe real Panic makes a real heart attack that much worse.[40]

EAT YOUR HEART OUT

Next in our line-up is Social Anxiety. This fits nicely with Sapolsky's observation that lower-ranking (Socially Anxious) baboons have higher levels of the stress hormone cortisol—evidence that it isn't easy being low down on the baboon totem pole. Some even have high blood pressure.[41] This could be because they are low on the totem pole, or it could be because they would rather move up. Just like baboons, we humans see danger in social hierarchy.

There is a long and complex history to this research. To examine the relationship of Social Anxiety and heart disease, we look to the concepts of Type A behavior (Coronary Prone) and Type D behavior (Distressed). Type A behavior was described in the 1950s by cardiologists Ray Rosenman and Meyer Friedman. Type A's are intense, driven and hostile. In cardiologists' offices, they wear out the front edge of the waiting-room-chair seat fabric as they prepare to spring into the examining room. When they turn up in a psychiatric office, they seem to have counter-instinctive versions of Social Anxiety and Atypical Depression. Indeed, at least one study suggests that some are shy yet extroverted, and that another group are hard-driving workaholics.[42]

More recently, the Type A concept has been updated to the Type D concept, and when Type D was closely examined, it likewise broke down into one component that looks like Social Anxiety (social inhibition), and another one that looks like Atypical Depression (negative affectivity).[43] Both the older Type A and the newer Type D are good predictors of CAD risk in a wide variety of settings, and both can be manifested by inner anger and sometimes by outward irritability. Anger, especially when kept inside by civilized people trying to look civilized, may be a strong predictor of CAD risk.[44] "Anger-in" as it is sometimes called, may intensify the biological effects of Type A and Type D and their component anxiety and depressive syndromes. Shakespeare voiced this in Macbeth: "The grief that does not speak, whispers the overfraught heart and bids it break." Although evolution prepared us biologically for counter-instinctive behavior, it didn't prepare our hearts for a lengthy lifetime of going against the emotional grain.

PUTTING YOUR HEART INTO IT

This brings us to OCD. The demands of nest keeping include perseverance in the face of adversity, and we use that perseverance in the face of our other sources of angst. It gets us through the tough spots and lets us counter instincts we don't like, but it leaves us with ongoing biological arousal and its effects on our hearts. Not only that, but OCD increases CAD risk when excessive endurance of other aroused social instincts feeds into the biological consequences of hostility and anger.[45]

HEARTACHE

Time now to turn to Atypical Depression. Recent decades have seen considerable interest in depression as a risk factor for CAD. The focus though, has been on broadly defined Major Depressive Disorder, or on even less well-defined depression-rating scales. The best you can say from those studies is that ongoing distress (which can be from any of our five syndromes, not to mention other influences) does predict heart disease, but that the specifics are unknown. One study did look at the relationship between Major Depression subtypes and serum cholesterol levels. The clearest finding by far was that Atypical Depression (but not global Major Depression) is associated with higher bad cholesterol levels, even after adjusting for other factors.[46]

The more specifically defined Atypical Depression shows up counter-instinctively as the hard-driving components of Type A and Type D behavior. Although blues musicians are especially adept at reflecting Atypical Depression, the laid-back bluesman looks quite different from the driven but similarly depressed workaholic. Combining inner lethargy, sadness and withdrawal with a strong need to overcome them, Atypical Depressives sometimes become driven workaholics. Fighting to keep Atypical Depression at bay has productivity advantages for civilized people. Driven workaholics need to keep working, no matter what. Time off is a problem for them, typically solved by extra work, or by overinvolvement in hobbies and other activities. They don't see this activity level as a problem; they just like to stay busy, and they do get a whole lot done.

Counter-instinctively, they pursue a lifestyle and role at odds with their personal biological natures. The outward workaholic is constantly fighting to stay interactive and awake, even though his inner Atypical Depression generally wants to withdraw and take a nap. Consistent with emerging research, this sort of counter-instinctive role can be highly stressful. A forced smile can be a dangerous thing. The more you fight to smile, the more you feel your angst, and the more you take it to your heart.

FAINT OF HEART

Here, as elsewhere, Melancholia is not a chronic syndrome that gradually contributes to other problems. It comes suddenly into play when CAD has us on our last legs, and it may even help trigger a sudden cardiac event. As the urge to give in to death emerges, HDL ("good cholesterol") levels go down as we prepare for the end.[46] Fortunately, the evolutionary death instinct is easy to treat, and our bodies and minds can be pleasantly surprised by the benefits of modern cardiac care.

HEARTS AND MINDS

Consciousness, along with OCD nesting, is what helps us to overcome instincts, and encourages us to endure the slings and arrows of enduring angst that follow. As we've noted, that can mean enduring more biological instinct, as well as the adverse biological consequences. Evolution gives us the tool to decide what we want, but it isn't yet prepared for what we choose.

THE MATTER WITH THE HEART

So our six instincts and five syndromes all play some role in the heart disease of civilization. In particular, they subject us to physiological stresses that somehow cause our arteries to clog with atherosclerosis to the point of clinical CAD. What fools these instincts be. By countermanding social instincts we run the risk of feeling more detached from our herd. Neither the depressed workaholic nor the Social Anxious extrovert feels well connected to other people. Subjective social isolation is a predictor of markers for stress and heart disease.[47] Zebra cortisol levels are raised by the presence of lions; ours are raised by feeling alone in a crowd.

There are many theories of CAD. One simple version has it that if our coronary arteries clamp down too hard or too often ("vasospasm"),[48] the result will be damage to the arterial lining, inflammation as it tries to heal,[49] gradual formation of atherosclerotic thickening, and eventually narrowing and reduced flexibility of the scarred artery. Cholesterol plays a role in the scarring and healing process. Healthy medical students with Type A behavior show evidence that they habitually clamp down their coronary arteries, as compared to mellower Type B classmates with more relaxed arteries.[50]

In the laboratory, students with lower self-esteem have more evidence of inflammation in response to mental stress procedures such as giving a speech, or trying say the right color name when the word green is printed in blue.[51] And if you make people feel socially rejected in the laboratory, they have higher levels of inflammation markers in their blood.[52] Atypical Depression leads to more feelings of social rejection, and with a counter-instinctive coping response, those rejection feelings are further intensified. Not good for the heart. In healthy adults, if psychological stress induces higher levels of inflammation markers, those people will have more stiffness of the carotid artery three years later (the carotid artery in the neck is much easier to study than the arteries attached to the heart itself).[53]

Any ongoing stress to the lining of the arteries leads ultimately to less responsiveness and more damage,[54] and that process is hastened by harsher physical stresses associated with the fight against civilization angst. Eventually, the arteries are damaged and thickened enough that they are poorly responsive to oxygen needs and have a narrowed passageway for blood. Clinical CAD is not far behind. A major new study showed that the maximal thickness of the carotid artery wall predicts CAD events above and beyond all other cardiac risk factors.[55] Size matters for coronary arteries.

RISKY BUSINESS

Modern civilization is not defined just by counter-instinctive behavior. The modern diet has been influenced by the supernormal taste and availability of food. Ancient man had plenty of cholesterol, but he did not feast on the refined sugars and high carbohydrate pasta that we do, and he doubtless had more exercise and less obesity. Could this be a cause of civilized CAD? Less than a century ago, the town of Roseto, Pennsylvania was settled by Italian immigrants who brought their culture with them. Their diet was heavy on pasta and fat, they exercised little, they weighed too much, and they were too fond of tobacco. Despite that, their CAD levels were mysteriously lower than surrounding communities.

The answer to this mystery came from studies of the next generation in Roseto. With little change in anything else, the traditionally supportive Italian society gave way to a more independent-minded American society. New CAD levels were now close to those of neighboring towns.[56] The early Rosetans were less likely than their children to adopt American counter-instinctive habits. The children had greater access to the benefits of individualism in American civilization, but at a price.[57]

It isn't that the well-documented conventional cardiac risk factors don't count, but for too long we have assumed that statistical predictors of risk must be causing CAD. Male gender, family heart-disease history, serum cholesterol levels, high blood pressure, diabetes, smoking, Type A (or D) behavior, and lack of exercise are all worrisome predictors of CAD, but we don't actually know that they cause CAD. We only know that they alert us to CAD risk. Some of them are important to remediate for various other medical reasons, but we don't know that reduced CAD follows as well. Less well known is that a diagonal earlobe crease is a strong predictor of CAD.[58] Fortunately, no one has yet suggested earlobe removal as a prevention strategy for heart disease.

Although dietary cholesterol reduction does little for CAD illness and death (the modern statin class of anticholesterol drugs do help), there may be other dietary factors that should be looked at. For example, people who eat the most chocolate have a 37% reduction in their risk for CAD.[59] This reminds us of the idea that Atypical Depression contributes to CAD, and that its chocolate cravings could be an attempt to raise serotonin levels.

Anyway, we should get back to beer. Moderate drinkers have the least risk for heart disease—one drink a day for women, two drinks a day for men. People who drink either less or more than that have greater risk for CAD. Could it be that alcohol has some directly protective effect on the heart? Maybe, but it also could be that alcohol dampens the stress of social instincts (perhaps a serotonin effect), and reduces their effects on the heart. It is also possible that those who drink moderately are exactly those with less instinctual stress, so that a drink a day is merely the mark of a less distressed person (less in need of serotonin), who happens to be less prone to heart disease.

LOSING YOUR OCD

Under the rationality of Consciousness, the demands of civilization and the temptations of our appetitive instincts, many of us overlook our basic nesting instincts. In our infinite wisdom, we cut corners with evolution-tested methods of protecting home, family, and tribe. Clean, arrange, save, and behave.

A Messy Nest

Keeping the nest neat, clean, and sanitary is a primary purpose of those OCD instincts that we civilized humans have sometimes overlooked. Recorded history is full of infectious diseases, plagues, and epidemics that could have been avoided or diminished through the elementary sanitation methods practiced by other species. Our modern ancestors have let sewage contaminate drinking water in a way that no other mammal would tolerate. Drinking "small beer" reduced only some of the infectious risks. Wild pigs are actually quite clean animals, but domesticated farm pigs live in grubby pigsties. They suffer the porcine consequences of our Conscious conquest of our human instincts.

Doing It Right the Second Time

We don't always arrange things as well as our instincts might teach us. A good carpenter measures twice and cuts once, and then checks her results, but there is more badly built furniture out there than badly built bird's nests. Part of this is human capacity for complexity. No bird would ever try to write the vastly detailed operating system for a personal computer (the digital nest for our computer application programs), yet we humans manage to produce a product that works rather well. On the other hand, we sometimes take shortcuts in the name of efficiency, financial cost, time constraints, triviality, indifference, or even antipathy. So some consumer products are poorly made and subject to expensive repairs and recalls. Before online banking, most of us didn't check our checking accounts. Some software programmers even have messy apartments.

THE ORIGIN OF DEBT

Saving is not what it used to be. The invention of money was a milestone in the advance of civilization. It facilitated commerce, investment and savings, and the invention of financial mismanagement followed promptly thereafter. With so many tantalizing Supernormal Stimuli to spend our money on, it is a wonder that anyone saves anything at all. Indeed, product development is based on the idea of making products as appetizing as possible. The good news, of course, is that our society produces good food, good housing, good televisions, good cars, and good entertainment. The more money you spend, the better stuff gets, and the more satisfied you are with that stuff.

Even so, as long as you have at least a basic level of financial security, more money and better stuff doesn't actually make you a happier person.[60] Worse, conscious reasoning tempts us to think that better stuff is the royal road to happiness. Contrary to our nesting nature (and despite those backyard rodents squirreling away acorns for the winter), we don't always save for the future as we should. People can find themselves owing more money on their enjoyable homes than those houses are even worth, yet few self-respecting chipmunks would ever find their burrows "underwater." Governments and pension funds, being run by people, often have the same shortcomings. Rather than saving for a rainy day, they wait until a rainy day to bemoan their lack of savings.

Because evolution did not prepare us for so many ways to satisfy our appetitive instincts, we are led into the temptations of a path that leads to material satisfaction without social satisfaction. The New Testament reminds us of this: "But they that will be rich fall into temptation and a snare, and into many foolish and hurtful lusts, which drown men in destruction and perdition. For the love of money is the root of all evil: which while some coveted after, they have erred from the faith, and pierced themselves through with many sorrows"(1 Timothy 6:9–10). Too much attention to our appetites leads us away from a more socially satisfying middle path.

WHERE DID EVERYONE GO?

We don't behave like our ape cousins, and probably not like our primeval ancestors either. This change has brought us civilization, intellectual advancement, personal autonomy, personal satisfaction, and beer. On the other hand, the weakening of instinctual social structures has its downsides. If we are more independent from the family or tribe, then we may have less support and assistance when we need it. Similarly, we lose something when societal traditions, functions, and roles are diminished. Divorce allows exit from a painful or unsatisfying marriage, but it decreases the sense of social stability for both parents and children. Flattening of social hierarchies makes the world fairer for Everyman, but it may increase in-fighting and hostile peer competition. Our instincts have a harder time telling us to behave ourselves in the nest.

WHAT'S A POOR PRIMATE TO DO?

So, we have moved from single-cell bacteria to collective single-cell slime molds, to multicellular organisms, to groups of many individuals, to instinctually structured social organisms, to multiple semi-autonomous individuals in modern civilization. With Consciousness increasingly ascendant over social instincts, an ultimate triumph of reason over instincts could lead us some day to a curious situation. We would then be a collection of individuals without instinctual cues to guide our social behaviors. We would finally lose all shackles of the herd, but find ourselves de-evolved to something like brilliant communal slime molds.[61] Socially minded behaviors would come only from the complexities of reason, law, religion and self-interest. Although this day may never come, it is one of many questions that lead us to wonder what our options are. What's a poor primate to do?

11

FREE TO CHOOSE:
HOW TO BALANCE YOUR
REASON AND INSTINCT

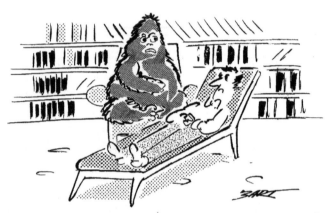

"Nothing to be ashamed of, you know-after, all, we're primates."

"Nothing in biology makes sense, except in the light of evolution"
—Theodosius Dobzhansky (Russian geneticist; 1900–1975)

"The final mystery is oneself."
—Oscar Wilde (English playwright; 1854–1900)

WHO ARE YOU?

Under this evolutionary theory, an essential part of our human exceptionalism is our enhanced ability to use reason to overcome and transform biologically evolved social instincts. Although other animals have some basic tools, language, and society, we are the leading edge of earthly art, science, civilization, and rationality. Our emotional lives are the sum total of the effects of our minds: childhood and adult experiences, reason, and culture, along with the sum total effects of our brains: social, appetitive, and protective instincts, and the occasional effects of medical illness, alcohol, and medication. In real life, it is nigh impossible to sort out any discrete influences of mind and brain. Even the line hidden inside us is blurred, because the biological brain effects of instinct can change with experience and with mindfully chosen medication, not to mention that all of the data from our minds is encoded in biological memory.

THE CALCULUS OF BRAIN AND MIND

So you have to ask yourself: Are you feeling yourself today? What is the real you, anyway? Maybe it is the brain behind your native social instincts. Social instincts alone would make us play nice with each other, but they limit our individuality, accomplishment and free will. Or maybe it is the mind behind your conscious reasoning. Consciousness and reason alone would let us choose our own paths, experience free will, and foster advanced civilization, but they carry certain risks to ourselves and our communities. This brain-and-mind issue mirrors the age-old philosophical issue of determinism and free will. If physicists are to be believed, everything in the future is determined by the present (quantum randomness aside), and we have no actual free will. At the very least, though, some of us find enormous comfort in the illusion of free will.

SUFFERING AND SUCCORANCE

Relief from suffering is a primary goal of civilization. Our ancestors were motivated to develop advanced human society by their interest in making the human world a better, safer, happier and more abundant place for themselves and their communities. Thomas Jefferson (American politician, 1743–1826) wrote in the Declaration of Independence, "Life, Liberty and the Pursuit of Happiness" are inalienable rights, and central to our human identity. As an outgrowth of civilization, medicine is focused on the reduction of suffering and the improvement of well-being. As the medical motto goes, *Primum non nocere* (Latin for "First, do no harm"), but doctors also try to do some good. Modern medicine uses careful diagnosis to prescribe medication, life-style changes, and other treatments toward that end.

Psychiatric treatment is likewise a tool toward the goal of succorance for suffering, and for making possible a better life. We need to think of this, though, in the contexts of brain and mind, and of determinism and free will. From an evolutionary perspective, does medication deflate biological instincts? Well, yes, but maybe those instincts are painful and counterproductive in today's society. Does humane relief of those biological symptoms make us less authentic to our true selves? In small part yes, but our rational minds are a more important part of the illusion of free will. Moreover, treatment typically offers a lot less angst, better personal relationships, and more productive careers.

So then what are the advantages of not treating anxiety and depressive syndromes in modern society? Good news first: One advantage for society is that these primeval emotional instincts still nudge people into social harmony. This may be better or worse for the individual, but it does help form a cohesive, successful, and mutually supportive society. Too many people unfettered by either biological instinct or moral code can lead to unpleasant conflict and societal dysfunction. The last thing we want is a society in which it is every man and woman for him- or herself.

WAS MURPHY AN OPTIMIST?

Though we now have better and more useful diagnoses than ever before, "Everything that can go wrong, will go wrong" as says Murphy's Law. Even researchers often fail to distinguish between important anxiety and depressive subtypes. In the clinical realm, careful diagnoses are often not even attempted. Instead, there is that preference for simpler, broader and less time- and skill-intensive categorical diagnoses. Major Depression and Generalized Anxiety Disorder (to name just those two), and even subjective complaints of "depression" or "stress" are everywhere. Even within the broader diagnoses, some clinicians pay little attention to the actual symptoms of those syndromes. In addition, this nonspecific approach is appealing to practitioners who view angst as due solely to life problems, and to those who choose to protect insurance-claim-form confidentiality with the least specific diagnosis possible.

With the decline of stigma, there is a growing inclination to take inappropriate advantage of the diagnostic schema. Some high-income families are more likely to use psychiatric diagnoses to gain special academic accommodations for their children.[1] This is not because the kids in high-income districts are necessarily more afflicted, but because special accommodations are a way to give them a leg up in society. Writers have noted that the improvement of psychiatric diagnosis and treatment in recent years has paradoxically coincided with a surging increase in psychiatric disability claims. Although most claimants really do have diagnoses, they feel freer to proclaim need for disability status. On evaluation, many have not been offered or have not accepted effective treatment, and few are eager to risk their entitlement payments for the possibility of clinical improvement. In this realm, also, there are clinicians who prefer to see employment disability as solely a consequence of on-the-job injury, or of employer mistreatment. When you think about it, however, only a minority of people with a bona fide bad boss or a genuine physical illness is overwhelmed to the point of angst. There is more to the picture than mere circumstance.

Effective medications are here to stay, better ones are in the offing, and who knows what genetic and other treatments hold for the future. Some have argued for the complete medical elimination of the "mental illness" that we are calling social instinct. However, if we treated "everything," would that open Pandora's box (letting evil treatment effects run wild), or let the genie out of the bottle, (setting magical treatment forces free under untrustworthy control)?

For example, the recently developed of drugs for male erectile dysfunction are clearly magical genies to many. They have been a boon for sexless marriages and for unhappy men and their partners. They have even helped rhinoceros conservation efforts a bit, because these effective modern drugs have reduced the demand for traditional but less-effective ground rhinoceros horn. When older men have more sex with their older partners, however, a new problem emerges: The women are prone to bladder infections.

Keeping Your Head in a Helmet

There is also something called the helmet effect. Wearing a bicycle helmet protects us against head injury, except that passing motorists who spot the helmet will actually drive closer to us.[2] Not only that, but our own helmet hubris may cause us to take greater risks on our own because we feel more protected. This isn't limited to bicycles. Helmets in American professional football have cut down on skull fractures and neck injuries, but they have also led to more aggressive head-butting tactics that cause concussions and possible brain damage. Ski helmets similarly feed thoughts of invulnerability and thus inevitable collisions with people and trees. Nor is this limited to actual helmets. In a heavy snowstorm, it seems like the cars that fly off the road most are massive SUVs. Too much awareness of any protection against danger or discomfort leads us to offset the reduced risk by recalibrating our safely instincts. Because too much protection against social instinct angst could have similar consequences, psychiatric treatment warrants thoughtful attention.

SIX HELMET FLAVORS

We can use psychiatric helmets to protect us from the angst of our six instincts and five diagnoses. Panic Anxiety keeps us in close geographic and behavioral proximity to the herd. Panic treatment clearly has its advantages, but runs the risk of allowing fearless and feckless wandering. Not all who wander from the herd are lost, but some find themselves herdlessly hoping for a better day. Since angst (especially the Panic flavor) also feeds creativity and innovation, you have to wonder whether untreated syndromes are nonetheless painfully advantageous for individuals and society.[3] Anecdotal impression suggests that creativity is learned early, and that treatment doesn't slow down the creative process. If anything, it helps creative people be more productive, confident and content. However, there are some who prefer to retain their angst as food for their muse. Still, if we had some way of heading off Panic from the get-go, we might have fewer creative people. Similarly, if early Panic prevention headed off thrill-seeking behavior at the pass, society would lose the contributions of adventurers and daredevils. Life would be a bit blander.

What if social-anxiety instincts were eliminated early on? Everyone could be a purebred SSRI alpha dog. Cesar Millan would think it bad for canine societal harmony if every dog tried to be the alpha leader. If every human felt like the top dog, we might have more problems with competitive disappointment (when alpha dogs join together as the freshman class at Harvard, many have to grudgingly lower their sights). Individuals would be less weighted down by shyness, but there would be less respect for hierarchical structures and harmony.

And OCD instincts? If they were somehow erased from our genomes, we'd have a much harder time keeping our nests clean, neat, well stocked and friendly. Some of us have enough trouble with these things already.

If we completely lost the social harmony of Atypical Depression, we would feel less guilt and less guilty depression. What a relief, except that we would suffer a loss of social harmony and altruism, and find more people angry at us for our transgressions (not that that would bother us). We would also suffer the loss of those workaholics who labor long and hard to fight off their depression—and get so much done for everyone.

Lastly, we are already in a position to eliminate the acute effects of Melancholia, even though much needs to be done to improve diagnosis and treatment. There is little downside for the individual, and society benefits from the knowledge and wisdom of older members. However, the downside for society is in the financial costs of keeping elderly and seriously ill people alive longer. Many will fully recover from their physical illness, but others will need substantial and expensive ongoing medical care. This issue is already politically prominent now, even without considering the effects of better Melancholia treatment.

Consciousness is not something that many of us would want to see disappear. It is an instinct not per se linked to angst. Consciousness causes problems when there is not enough of it (as in psychosis), when we omit it ("uncortically"), or when we misuse it. Uncritical and shortsighted thinking in the guise of ostensibly rational decision-making about any kind of issue is the risk here. Consciousness aside, even the most rational of psychiatric diagnoses and psychopharmacology for our other syndromes still run the theoretical risk of unintended consequences.

WISHFUL THINKING AND UNINTENDED CONSEQUENCES

Overcoming our social instinct angst through treatment (or even alcohol) carries great benefits and some potential for risk. Robert K. Merton (American sociologist, 1910–2003) listed five possible causes of unexpected consequences[4]:

1. Ignorance: Who can know in advance what happens when social instinct and angst are lost?

2. Error: Who can know the effects of mistaken diagnosis, nonspecific medication use, or absence of psychotherapy benefits?

3. Immediate interest: Are there longer-term advantages to enduring angst, or of reverting to more primal instinctive roles?

4. Basic values: Does medication erode or obviate such traditional approaches as rational problem solving or steadfast resolve?

5. Self-defeating prophecy: Does too much medication, too soon or for too long, limit our social experience of the world and our ability to learn from experience?

BULLS AND BEARS

It is tempting to look at the financial world of Wall Street through the lens of unexpected psychopharmacological consequences. A reporter's question, "Why are there so many nervous people on Wall Street?" was once answered, "Because that is where nervous people like to work." It does seem that anxiety disorders are more common in finance, especially at higher echelons and in certain specialties. Those who seek appropriate treatment with medication and formal psychotherapy typically play by the rules at work, maintain or improve their performance and personal life, and feel a whole lot better about it. What they are less likely to do is experience symptom relief as license to solely look out for number one.

However, there are many Wall Street workers who get through the day with casually prescribed legal medications, similar medications from the street, illegal cocaine, and too much alcohol. These substances are sometimes utilized to feel happier, or for momentary symptom relief. Effective treatment of syndromes is infrequent, and combination with effective psychotherapy less frequent still. What kind of effect does this have on decisions and judgment? Do SSRIs encourage rule-breaking in the Wall Street culture? Do people feel like shameless top dogs, without even risk of guilty feelings? Do antianxiety drugs reduce ordinary fear that people should heed? Does cocaine give people strength to do things that they shouldn't? At the end of the day, this may be one part of what turns finance away from socially greasing the wheels of commerce, and toward a more solitary focus on self-reward. The most enduring figures on Wall Street are those that do well by doing good.

FINDING YOURSELF

The monk on the mountaintop (and the Buddha himself) might say that the secret to life is finding a happy middle path. Too much angst is too much, but with no social instinct at all there are too many potential risks and losses. Would we even want to be shiny, happy people in an angst-free society? Too much reason can go astray, but with none we are mere members of a herd. Formal psychotherapy can help find that balance. Judicious medication should reduce syndromal angst without inducing some false happiness. In an acute crisis, supportive ("hand-holding") psychotherapy and good advice is very useful. Beyond that, therapy should help us sort out our emotions, our behaviors, our goals, and our relationships. This rudimentary description sounds simple, but this discerning task requires clinicians with broad training, well-honed skill, careful attention, and patience.

SOCIETAL ETHICS OF EVOLUTIONARY PERSPECTIVE

Concern about the ethical risks of psychiatric diagnosis and treatment is not new. Diagnoses can be and too often are abused in personal relationships and in hiring (and firing) decisions. Decisions to mandate treatment should be done with extraordinary care, and only in the interests of a patient who poses significant risk to himself or to others. For financial, geographic, and cultural reasons, the best treatment is more available to those already on the top of the socioeconomic ladder. This gives added disadvantage to those further down who may need more help, and who may even have more angst. Remember that Social Anxiety, for example, is more common among the less well heeled.

The evolutionary perspective raises new questions. Is it ethical to encourage treatment that may reduce social instincts? Could greater evolutionary understanding lead to more effective manipulation by advertising agencies (actually, that is kind of what they try to do), or by governments? Even if the social biology is adjusted with medication, mind-set and habits may lag far behind. Absent good psychotherapy, some would find themselves in uneasy noninstinctual roles. At the risk of stretching for an analogy, think of the lottery winners who gleefully gain millions of dollars, only to find themselves financially bankrupt a few years later.

Then again, there are greater opportunities for ethical advancement. Barring the unforeseen consequences, who could argue with reduced misunderstanding, diminished violence, and a whole lot less angst? It is even possible that we can achieve greater synergism of religion, law, and ethics with our individual and societal goals. Of course, that isn't a new thought.

FREE TO CHOOSE

At the same time, anxiety and depressive symptoms can be painfully useful clues to our own social needs. They are worth thinking about. However, where reason says that we should override instinctual symptoms, good treatment can help reconcile the two. Panic about being trapped is not so useful in modern elevators and planes.

Fears of social embarrassment should not give such pause to a student called on in class, and they certainly shouldn't relegate him or her to the bottom of a social pecking order. All this leaves us with a central question to ponder: How can we reconcile our inborn biological instincts and angst with our rational decisions and with the circumstances and demands of modern society? Most of us like to choose our own paths (or at least feel like we do). Understanding the instinctual cues that influence our choices is a first step to making those choices on our own.

TO BEGIN WITH

You've gotta ask yourself one question: Do you feel yucky? If your angst is intense, prolonged, self-defeating or ill-timed, it's worth talking with friends, relatives, physicians, or religious leaders about your feelings and options. A next step is for a thorough consultation, looking at the common syndromes, but also at your life and relationships, recent life changes for better and for worse, medical issues, and blood tests.[5] All this might seem like too much information, but the problems you are already aware of aren't usually the whole picture. The most problematic concerns are often too painful or frightening to think about at first. Somewhere along the line, gradual recognition of those underlying issues is a big help.

The best way to view a consultation is as a professional opinion about sources of your angst and about treatment suggestions that you can consider. As we have talked about, a careful and specific diagnosis is very important both for considering medication and for anticipating issues in psychotherapy. Hopefully, a well-trained and attentive clinician will offer an accurate diagnosis and good suggestions, but you should ask questions, too, and you can still take a pass. You are free to choose.

For most people with common anxiety and depressive syndromes, treatment usually starts with an emotional crisis. In evolutionary terms, there is heightened tension between hidden social instincts on the one hand, and rational choices or altered circumstances on the other. Aside from educating the psychiatrist about you, the evaluation is a chance to start addressing some of the crisis through medication and clarification. If things go well, the crisis-management phase might last a month or three, and life might settle back toward normal within several months. By that point, you might start to have a grasp of which instincts ("behavior patterns") may be on your problem list. Better understanding of your instincts, self, family and relationships, root-cause problems, goals, and all the complex hidden interactions between these factors ("conflict") takes longer. After all, you are trying to figure out not only your hidden instincts and fears, but also many layers of social learning and mental compromise superimposed over decades. You are repairing Mother Nature, and repairing the effects of civilization and reasoned coping, if you will. Needless to say, treatment that threatens to look at what is really bothering you will make you uneasy at times. At the same time, any treatment that lasts too long and yet provides little benefit is worth discussing, and maybe worth a second professional opinion.

Treatments that work on surface symptoms and behaviors are appealing, partly because they don't trigger our innate caution about socially instinctive rules, and similarly because they imply that the problems are due largely to our circumstances or coping styles. Be cautious about treatment approaches that use surface approaches yet promise immediate or prolonged benefit. Meditation, for example, is very helpful for many people, but it isn't sufficient for real angst and real-life problems. There is little evidence of deep and lasting benefit from approaches such as most vitamins, homeopathy, herbal treatments, exercise, and other simple fixes that ignore the role of instincts, syndromes, and coping responses. Akin to supportive psychotherapy, they may only help coping because they offer real or symbolic companionship. Likewise, mistaken use or overuse of modern psychiatric medication raises questions about efficacy and appropriateness. Peter Kramer writes about the lure of "cosmetic psychopharmacology" to enhance social skills in the absence of prior distress.[6] At least in the psychiatric office, though, most folks turn up with real and significant emotional distress.

PSYCHOTHERAPY IN A NUTSHELL

Just in case you missed it, psychotherapy works best when combined with the right medication. On occasion, people require psychotherapy for a life crisis unrelated to exacerbation of their instinctive syndromes. Sometimes people have an undiagnosed medical problem that either worsens or causes the emotional distress. All that being said, conventional psychotherapy has the greatest benefit when patients say more and therapists say less. That keeps the focus on people's own worlds and concerns, and it gives the therapist a clearer view of the issues at issue. Every person is different, but there are many similarities among people, too.

Directly or indirectly, psychotherapy is primarily about those very social relationships that turn up in our theory. As Carl Jung said, "Man's task is to become conscious of the contents that press upward from the unconscious." At the end of the day, that helps people feel more comfortable in now closer relationships, and more at ease in often successful careers. Reaching that goal takes time, effort, patience, and skill. Treatment must not miss either the forest of underlying issues and instincts, or the trees of daily events. Other life issues, including work and career issues, often derive from core evolutionary concerns. Frequently, people focus on fears of failure—the flip side of their concerns about success. Our instincts may power hidden fears that success will force us to choose between social abandonment and relinquishing achievement, or between shame and renewed submission, or between suffering guilt and offering repentance. Relationship concerns can thus lead even the most talented amongst us to self-defeating behaviors in family, romance, social life, and the workplace. For these reasons, executives who are adept at managing other's emotions' in addition to their own ("emotional intelligence") are likely to find greater career success.[7]

Closeness issues turn up not only in the topics and events discussed in psychotherapy, but in the treatment relationship as well. If someone has a view of people colored by their instincts, coping methods, and conflicts, then this will inevitably show up in their thoughts and feelings about the therapist ("transference" as we say). This is an invaluable up-close opportunity for the therapist to understand how life looks to the patient. Dreams, too, can be useful. Dreams occur for biological purposes, most likely to store and revise memory. In the process, they reflect how our worlds look to us. Often, they are about interests in moving experiences: physical motion, emotionally close relationships, and career advancement. As people make progress in therapy, that progress shows up in new dreams in which the impediments to moving experience have diminished. People gradually unlearn some of the entrenched behavior patterns that had, in primeval times, eased the angst triggered by aspirations that were in conflict with instinct and social circumstance.

Our instincts turn up in particular ways in our dreams. Panic Anxiety feeds concerns about separations and fears of catastrophe. Dreams are often about catastrophe (sometimes narrowly averted): earthquakes, confinement, terrorists, and lost bearings. Social Anxiety informs dreams about hierarchical standing, often at times of perceived advancement in the real world. A dream of being naked in public reflects thoughts of shameful exposure for your true aspirations. A dream about failing a college exam long ago is an attempt at angst-reducing self-demotion to the ranks of the unqualified. Atypical Depression can appear in dreams as protections against social rejection. For example, a relationship dream in which the companion is separated by distance or technology shows self-protection against the possibility of rejection. All dreams of course, are personal, and must be looked at in the right context at the right time. If one of these generalities strikes a chord, keep in mind that, by itself, the benefit of recognizing that chord is modest. There is much more work required to really understand and utilize the processes shown in a dream.

Stephen Kucera (American evolutionary geneticist; 1965–) has even wondered whether effective psychotherapy might involve a gene-by-environment interaction.[8] The emotional, linguistic, and rational aspects of psychotherapeutic process might trigger epigenetic changes over time, thus diminishing the genetic expression of our angst-ridden instinctive syndromes. All this makes one wonder whether the "corrective emotional experience" of some psychotherapies could include a medication-like effect. Now, that is something to ponder and explore.

With any luck, psychotherapy (and actual medication) can relieve angst, reduce self-defeating behaviors, increase self-awareness, improve relationships, and allow greater purpose in work and life. At some point, the potential value of even the best treatment is outweighed by the need for more investment of time, money, and emotional effort. Look for improvement, not complete resolution or total cure.

WHAT HAS EVOLUTION DONE FOR US LATELY?

Evolution is an ongoing process. Humans will not forever be the same as they are now. We will change in ways that help our genes survive, and the forces that shape genetic selection are not the same as they were eons ago on the African savanna. Even in recorded history, novel selection factors have been introduced. Perhaps the wide use of alcohol allowed some instincts to intensify over generations. Retaining childhood separation anxiety as adult Panic Anxiety has societal advantages for creativity, especially if the worst distress can be moderated by alcohol. Civilization itself may have fostered a climate in which enhanced Consciousness may have had a personal reproductive advantage, as well as societal advantages through greater understanding of our social and physical worlds. If anything, modern culture has increasingly applied the Golden Rule of Atypical Depression for social harmony even with outside and distant tribes. Back in high school we all knew the different student cliques, the members of which were no doubt attracted to each other by common instincts. So has evolution increasingly selected for a diverse and complementary mixture of jocks, nerds, artists and technology buffs?

Much has been written about the effects of civilization on our physical evolution over the past 10,000 years or so.[9] On the social side, this later evolution may have varied by circumstance and culture. Somehow, there is a lower genetic level of serotonin (the "social director") activity in Japan, China, and Korea. Although this may put people at greater risk for Social Anxiety or Atypical Depression, they are also protected by a more "collectivist" culture. Did the genes evolve because they allowed people to better fit into that particular kind of society? Or did the culture evolve to correct for increased genetic risk of angst? Whichever it was, culture and biology no doubt evolved together.[10,11] Ethnic Japanese in America live in a more individualistic and multicultural society than their relatives in the old country. So, as with the second generation Italian-Americans of the Roseto study, it is not surprising that Japanese-Americans have a higher rate of coronary artery disease than their relatives in Japan.[12]

WHAT HAPPENS TO US NOW?

Intriguingly, how will the nature of these biological instincts further evolve over future generations? Niels Bohr (Danish physicist; 1885–1962) pointed out that "Prediction is very difficult, especially about the future." Even so, there is endless speculation about what path evolution will take our genome down in the future. We don't really know much about what makes some people have more children in a given society (especially those children who survive to have their own children, in turn). In those countries in which the reproduction rate is low (such as Italy and Japan), the future population will increasingly reflect the characteristics of those who do have the most children. Human reproductive choices can also have effects. One study looked at reproduction rates in a polygamous society in Senegal, using Big-Five personality factors. Not surprisingly, men with high Extraversion (alpha dogs with precious little Social Anxiety) had more children. Among women, those with more Neuroticism (stay close to home instincts with more Panic Anxiety) had more children.[13] Needless to say, these patterns might be quite different in other cultures. In China and India, parents commonly use prenatal testing to abort female children, leaving a population that is increasingly male.

Some people avoid having children, either to give preference to their careers, because they are socially isolated, or because they fear passing on their own angst. However, this may also have the adverse effect of reducing the prevalence of, say, Atypical Depression and its social harmonizing effects. With modern technology, some people may spend more time online and less time finding a mate. Improved treatment, on the other hand, may reduce angst, social isolation, and possibly ambivalence about having children. Whatever changes may happen, evolution may someday swing us back in the opposite direction toward some instinctive equilibrium conducive to a sustainable balance of rational civilization and herd instinct. We should also wonder what would happen if the drug companies should suddenly shut down next week or 500 years from now. Let's leave these predictions to Niels Bohr.

SUMMING UP

So maybe much of common psychopathology amounts to alarm about being separated from the group, beta-dog anxious submission, obsessive overnesting, painful rejection sensitivity in the service of social harmony, culling of the unproductive, and limitations of our Consciousness. When we add in family, circumstances, and culture, we have some deeply personal variations on angst. Not all of this theory is new. This overview brings together pieces from ancient literature, modern science, other theorists, well-known quotes, music, and cartoons. There is plenty of room for elaboration and improvement of this theory.

For science, there are questions to consider. How can we better understand, challenge, modify, detail, and document an evolutionary conceptual framework? Can psychiatry incorporate new knowledge to better help individuals enjoy and succeed at life? Can this theory gain further detail and support from additional research?

We've touched on some unanswered questions along the way. Useful research could better document the presence, significance, severity continuum, prevalence, familiality, and genetics of our six instincts and five core diagnoses (and possibly others). The social-instinct functions (both in patient populations and normal controls) would benefit by more examination through social psychology and psychoanalytic theory. The prospect of more detailed explication of clinical psychiatric phenomenology, diagnostic specificity, neuroimaging, psychopharmacological effects, and biological tests (carbon dioxide challenges and tryptophan-depletion studies, to name just two) is exciting. Similar work could address the corresponding five proposed psychosis subtypes. The Big-Five personality model seems to correspond well to this diagnostic model, but complex further work is needed to confirm that resemblance, including careful attention to counter-instinctive adaptations. Similarly, more of all this work in other species would support the primeval evolutionary origins and purposes of our six social instincts. In the words of William Faulkner, "The past is never dead. It's not even past."[14] To a greater extent than we have imagined, we still live today in an emotional world designed on that ancient African savanna.

APPENDIX OF DIAGNOSTIC CRITERIA: STANDARD DIAGNOSTIC STANDARDS AND SYMPTOMS FOR FIVE INSTINCTIVE SYNDROMES (AND FIVE RELATED PSYCHOSES)

CHAPTER 2: PANIC ANXIETY

Panic Attack

A. A discrete period of intense fear or discomfort, in which four (or more) of the following symptoms developed abruptly and reached a peak within 10 minutes:

1. Palpitations, pounding heart, or accelerated heart rate.
2. Sweating.
3. Trembling or shaking.
4. Sensations of shortness of breath or smothering.
5. Feeling of choking.
6. Chest pain or discomfort.
7. Nausea or abdominal distress.
8. Feeling dizzy, unsteady, lightheaded, or faint.
9. Derealization (feelings of unreality) or depersonalization (being detached from oneself).
10. Fear of losing control or going crazy.
11. Fear of dying.
12. Paresthesias (numbness or tingling sensations).
13. Chills or hot flushes.

CHAPTER 3: SOCIAL ANXIETY

Social Anxiety

A. A marked and persistent fear of one or more social or performance situations in which the person is exposed to unfamiliar people or to possible scrutiny by others. The individual fears that he or she will act in a way (or show anxiety symptoms) that will be humiliating or embarrassing.

B. Exposure to the feared social situation almost invariably provokes anxiety.

C. The person recognizes that the fear is excessive or unreasonable.

D. The feared social or performance situations are avoided or else are endured with intense anxiety or distress.

E. The avoidance, anxious anticipation, or distress in the feared social or performance situation(s) interferes significantly with the person's normal routine, occupational (academic) functioning, or social activities or relationships, or there is marked distress about having the phobia.

F. In individuals under age 18 years, the duration is at least 6 months.

CHAPTER 4: OBSESSIVE-COMPULSIVE DISORDER

Obsessive-Compulsive Disorder

A. Either obsessions or compulsions:

Obsessions as defined by 1, 2, 3, and 4:

1. Recurrent and persistent thoughts, impulses, or images that are experienced, at some time during the disturbance, as intrusive and inappropriate and that cause marked anxiety or distress.

2. The thoughts, impulses, or images are not simply excessive worries about real-life problems.

3. The person attempts to ignore or suppress such thoughts, impulses, or images, or to neutralize them with some other thought or action.

4. The person recognizes that the obsessional thoughts, impulses, or images are a product of their own mind (not imposed from without as in thought insertion).

Compulsions as defined by 1 and 2:

1. Repetitive behaviors (e.g., hand washing, ordering, checking) or mental acts (e.g., praying, counting, repeating words silently) that the person feels driven to perform in response to an obsession, or according to rules that must be applied rigidly.

2. The behaviors or mental acts are aimed at preventing or reducing distress or preventing some dreaded event or situation; however, these behaviors or mental acts either are not connected in a realistic way with what they are designed to neutralize or prevent or are clearly excessive.

B. At some point during the course of the disorder, the person has recognized that the obsessions or compulsions are excessive or unreasonable. *Note:* This does not apply to children.

C. The obsessions or compulsions cause marked distress, are time consuming (take more than 1 hour a day), or significantly interfere with the person's normal routine, occupational (or academic) functioning, or usual social activities or relationships.

The Florida Obsessive-Compulsive Inventory (FOCI) is a concise but more descriptive summary of OCD symptoms:

Florida Obsessive-Compulsive Inventory Part A

A. Have you been bothered by unpleasant thoughts or images that repeatedly enter your mind, such as:
   1. Concerns with contamination (dirt, germs, chemicals, radiation) or acquiring a serious illness such as AIDS?
   2. Overconcern with keeping objects (clothing, tools, etc.) in perfect order or arranged exactly?
   3. Images of death or other horrible events?
   4. Personally unacceptable religious or sexual thoughts?
B. Have you worried a lot about terrible things happening, such as:
   1. Fire, burglary or flooding of the house?
   2. Accidentally hitting a pedestrian with your car or letting it roll down a hill?
   3. Spreading an illness (giving someone AIDS)?
   4. Losing something valuable?
   5. Harm coming to a loved one because you weren't careful enough?
C. Have you worried about acting on an unwanted and senseless urge or impulse, such as:
   1. Physically harming a loved one, pushing a stranger in front of a bus, steering your car into oncoming traffic; inappropriate sexual contact; or poisoning dinner guests?
D. Have you felt driven to perform certain acts over and over again, such as:
   1. Excessive or ritualized washing, cleaning, or grooming?
   2. Checking light switches, water faucets, the stove, door locks, or the emergency brake?
   3. Counting, arranging; evening-up behaviors (making sure socks are at same height)?
   4. Collecting useless objects or inspecting the garbage before it is thrown out?
   5. Repeating routine actions (in/out of chair, going through doorway, relighting cigarette) a certain number of times or until it feels just right?

6. Needing to touch objects or people?

7. Unnecessary rereading or rewriting; reopening envelopes before they are mailed?

8. Examining your body for signs of illness?

9. Avoiding colors (*red* means blood), numbers (13 is unlucky) or names (those that start with D signify death) that are associated with dreaded events or unpleasant thoughts?

10. Needing to "confess" or repeatedly asking for reassurance that you said or did something correctly?

The Yale-Brown Obsessive-Compulsiv e Scale (YBOCS) includes an even more complete OCD symptom list. Neither should be used for self-diagnosis of OCD.

CHAPTER 5: ATYPICAL DEPRESSION

Atypical Features

(A form of major depression or of dysthymia)

A. Mood reactivity (*i.e., mood brightens in response to actual or potential positive events*).

B. At least two of the following:

1. Significant weight gain or increase in appetite.

2. Hypersomnia (*sleeping too much*).

3. Leaden paralysis (i.e., heavy, leaden feelings in arms or legs).

4. Long-standing pattern of interpersonal rejection sensitivity (not limited to episodes of mood disturbance) that results in significant social or occupational impairment.

C. Criteria are not met for melancholic depression or catatonic depression during the same episode.

CHAPTER 6: MELANCHOLIC DEPRESSION

Melancholic Features

(A form of major depression)

A. At least one of the following:

1. Loss of pleasure in all, or almost all, activities.

2. Lack of reactivity to usually pleasurable activities (does not feel much better, even temporarily, when something good happens).

B. Three (or more) of the following:

1. Distinct quality of depressed mood (i.e., the depressed mood is experienced as distinctly different from the kind of feeling experienced after the death of a loved one).
2. Depression regularly worse in the morning.
3. Early morning awakening (at least 2 hours before usual waking time).
4. Marked psychomotor retardation or agitation.
5. Significant anorexia (*appetite loss*) or weight loss.
6. Excessive or inappropriate guilt.

CHAPTER 7: SCHIZOPHRENIA AND PSYCHOSIS

Panic Anxiety Related Psychosis

Schizophrenia (Paranoid/Persecutory Subtype)

A. Characteristic Symptoms

Two (or more) of the following, each present for a significant portion of time during a 1-month period (or less if successfully treated):

1. Delusions.
2. Hallucinations.
3. Disorganized speech (e.g., frequent derailment or incoherence).
4. Grossly disorganized or catatonic behavior.
5. Negative symptoms, i.e., affective flattening, alogia, or avolition.

B. Social/Occupational Dysfunction

For a significant portion of the time since the onset of the disturbance, one or more major areas of functioning such as work, interpersonal relations, or self-care are markedly below the level achieved prior to the onset.

C. Duration

Continuous signs of the disturbance persist for at least 6 months. This 6-month period must include at least 1 month of symptoms (or less if successfully treated) that meet Criterion A (i.e., active phase symptoms) and may include periods of prodromal or residual symptoms.

D. Schizoaffective and Mood-Disorder Exclusion

Schizoaffective disorder and mood disorder with psychotic features have been ruled out because either (a) no major depressive, manic, or mixed episodes have occurred concurrently with the active-phase symptoms; or (b) if mood episodes have occurred during active-phase symptoms, their total duration has been brief relative to the duration of the active and residual periods.

E. Substance/General-Medical-Condition Exclusion

The disturbance is not due to the direct physiological effects of a substance or a general medical condition.

F. Relationship to a Pervasive Developmental Disorder

If there is a history of autistic disorder or another pervasive developmental disorder, the additional diagnosis of Schizophrenia is made only if prominent delusions or hallucinations are also present for at least a month.

Paranoid Subtype

A. Preoccupation with one or more delusions or frequent auditory hallucinations.
B. None of the following is prominent: disorganized speech, disorganized or catatonic behavior, or flat of inappropriate affect.

Social Anxiety Related Psychosis

Delusional Disorder (Paranoid/Persecutory Subtype)

A. Nonbizarre delusions (i.e., involving situations that occur in real life, such as being followed, poisoned, infected, loved at a distance, or deceived by spouse or lover, or having a disease) of at least 1 month's duration.
B. Criterion A for schizophrenia has never been met. *Note:* Tactile and olfactory hallucinations may be present in delusional disorder if they are related to the delusional theme.
C. Apart from the impact of the delusion(s) or its ramifications, functioning is not markedly impaired and behavior is not obviously odd or bizarre.
D. If mood episodes have occurred concurrently with delusions, their total duration has been brief relative to the duration of the delusional periods.

E. The disturbance is not due to the direct physiological effects of a substance (e.g., a drug of abuse, a medication) or a general medical condition.

Persecutory subtype: delusions that the person (or someone to whom the person is close) is being malevolently treated in some way.

Obsessive-Compulsive Disorder Related Psychosis

Schizo-Obsessive Disorder (Proposed Diagnostic Criteria*)

A. Symptoms are present that meet Criterion A for Obsessive-Compulsive Disorder at some time point during the course of the schizophrenia.

B. If the content of the obsessions and/or compulsions is interrelated with the content of delusions and/or hallucinations (e.g., compulsive hand washing due to command auditory hallucinations), additional typical OCD obsessions and compulsions recognized by the person as unreasonable and excessive are required.

C. Symptoms of Obsessive-Compulsive Disorder are present for a substantial portion of the total duration of the prodromal, active, and/or the residual period of schizophrenia.

D. The obsessions and compulsions are time-consuming (more than 1 hour a day), cause distress or significantly interfere with the person's normal routine, in addition to the functional impairment associated with schizophrenia.

E. The obsessions and compulsions in the patient with schizophrenia are not due to the direct effect of antipsychotic agents, a substance of abuse (e.g., cocaine), or an organic factor (e.g., head trauma).

Atypical Depression-Related Psychosis

Manic Episode

A. A distinct period of abnormally and persistently elevated, expansive, or irritable mood, lasting at least 1 week (or any duration if hospitalization is necessary).

B. During the period of mood disturbance, three (or more) of the following symptoms have persisted (four if the mood is only irritable) and have been present to a significant degree:
    1. Inflated self-esteem or grandiosity.
    2. Decreased need for sleep (e.g., feels rested after only three hours of sleep).

---

* Poyurovsky, M., Zohar, J., Glick, I., Koran, L.M., Weizman, R., Tandon, R., Weizman, A. (in press). Obsessive-Co mpulsive symptoms in Schizophrenia: implications for future psychiatric classifications. *Comprehensive Psychiatry.*

3. More talkative than usual or pressure to keep talking.

4. Flight of ideas or subjective experience that thoughts are racing.

5. Distractibility (i.e., attention too easily drawn to unimportant or irrelevant external stimuli).

6. Increase in goal-directed activity (either socially, at work or school, or sexually) or psychomotor agitation.

7. Excessive involvement in pleasurable activities that have a high potential for painful consequences (e.g., engaging in unrestrained buying sprees, sexual indiscretions, or foolish business investments).

C. The symptoms do not meet criteria for a mixed episode.

D. The mood disturbance is sufficiently severe to cause marked impairment in occupational functioning or in usual social activities or relationships with others, or to necessitate hospitalization to prevent harm to self or others, or there are psychotic features.

E. The symptoms are not due to the direct physiological effects of a substance (e.g., a drug of abuse, a medication, or other treatment) or a general medical condition (e.g., hyperthyroidism).

Melancholia-Related Psychosis
(a form of Major Depressive Disorder)

Psychotic Depression (Mood-Congruent Subtype)

Delusions or hallucinations whose content is entirely consistent with the typical depressive themes of personal inadequacy, guilt, disease, death, nihilism, or deserved punishment.

Diagnostic criteria are used with permission from the Diagnostic and Statistical Manual of Mental Disorders, Fourth Edition, Text Revision. © 2000 American Psychiatric Association. The FOCI is used with permission from Wayne Goodman (mountsinaiocd.org).

NOTES

Chapter 1: Angst Is the Modern Echo of Evolved Social Instincts

1 Darwin, C. (2008). *The descent of man, and selection in relation to sex*. London: Folio Society.

2 Darwin, C. (2007). *The expression of the emotions in man and animals*. Minneapolis, MN: Filiquarian Publishing.

3 Kinnally, E., Tarara, E., Mason, W., Mendoza, S., Able, K., Lyons, L., et al. (2010). Serotonin transporter expression is predicted by early life stress and is associated with disinhibited behavior in infant rhesus macaques. *Genes, Brain, and Behavior, 9*(1), 45–52.

4 Lyko, F., Foret, S., Kucharski, R., Wolf, S., Falckenhayn, C., & Maleszka, R. (2010). The honey bee epigenomes: Differential methylation of brain DNA in queens and workers. *PLoS Biology, 8*(11), e1000506.

5 Elliott, E., Ezra-Nevo, G., Regev, L., Neufeld-Cohen, A., & Chen, A. (2010). Resilience to social stress coincides with functional DNA methylation of the Crf gene in adult mice. *Nature Neuroscience, 13*(11), 1351–1353.

6 Freud, S. (1957). On narcissism: An introduction (1914). In *Complete Psychological Works, Standard Ed* (Vol. 14). London: Hogarth Press.

7 Freud, S. (1987). *A phylogenetic fantasy*. Cambridge, MA: The Belknap Press of Harvard University Press.

8 Modrell, M., Bemis, W., Northcutt, R., Davis, M., & Baker, C. (2011). Electrosensory ampullary organs are derived from lateral line placodes in bony fishes. *Nature Communications, 2*, 496. doi: 10.1038/ncomms1502

9 Freud, S. (2010). *Civilization and its discontents*. Mansfield Centre, CT: Martino.

10 Freud, S. (1976). *Instincts and their vicissitudes*. In *The Standard Edition of the Complete Psychological Works of Sigmund Freud* (Vols. XIV, 1914–1916). New York: W. W. Norton..

11 Jung, C. (1964). *Civilization in transition: The collected works of C. G. Jung* (Vol. 10). London: Routledge & Kegan Paul.

12 Stevens, A. (1993). *The two million-year-old self*. College Station, TX: Texas A&M University Press.

13 Jung, C. G., Baynes, H. G., & Baynes, C. F. (1928). *Contributions to analytical psychology*. London: Routledge & Kegan Paul.

14 Gilbert, P. (2006). Evolution and depression: Issues and implications. *Psychological Medicine, 36*(3), 287–297.

15 Allen, N., & Badcock, P. (2006). Darwinian models of depression: A review of evolutionary accounts of mood and mood disorders. *Progress in Neuropsychopharmacology and Biological Psychiatry, 30*(5), 815–826.

16 Andrews, P., & Thomson, J. J. (2009). The bright side of being blue: Depression as an adaptation for analyzing complex problems. *Psychological Review, 116*(3), 620–654.

17 Watson, P., & Andrews, P. (2002). Toward a revised evolutionary adaptationist analysis of depression: The social navigation hypothesis. *Journal of Affective Disorders, 72*(1), 1–14.

18 Nesse, R., & Ellsworth, P. (2009). Evolution, emotions, and emotional disorders. *American Psychologist,* 129–139.

19 Shultz, S., Opie, C., & Atkinson, Q. D. (2011). Stepwise evolution of stable sociality in primates. *Nature, 479*(7372), 219–222.

20 Mueller, C., & Dweck, C. (1998). Praise for intelligence can undermine children's motivation and performance. *Journal of Personality and Social Psychology, 75*(1), 33–52.

21 Skipper, Y., & Douglas, K. (2011). Is no praise good praise? Effects of positive feedback on children's and university students' responses to subsequent failures. *Bristish Journal of Educational Psychology, 82*(2), 327–339.

22 Alicke, M. D., & Sedikides, C. (Eds.). (2011). *Self-enhancement and self-protection in interpersonal, relational, and group contexts.* New York: Guildford Press.

23 American Psychiatric Association. (1994). *Diagnostic and statistical manual of mental disorders, 4.* Washington, DC: American Psychiatric Association.

24 Kahn, J. (2008). Diagnosis and referral of workplace depression. *Journal of Occupational and Environmental Medicine, 50*(4), 396–400.

25 Davidson, J., Woodbury, M., Zisook, S., & Giller, E. J. (1989). Classification of depression by grade of membership: A confirmation study. *Psychological Medicine, 19*(4), 987–998.

26 Hahn, M., Blackford, J., Haman, K., Mazei-Robison, M., English, B., Prasad, H., et al. (2008). Multivariate permutation analysis associates multiple polymorphisms with sub-phenotypes of major depression. *Genes, Brain, and Behavior, 7*(4), 487–495.

27 Xie, P., Kranzler, H., Poling, J., Stein, M., Anton, R., Brady, K., et al. (2009). Interactive effect of stressful life events and the serotonin transporter 5-HTTLPR genotype on post-traumatic stress disorder diagnosis in 2 independent populations. *Archives of General Psychiatry, 66*(11), 1201–1209.

28 Jensen, C., Keller, T., Peskind, E., McFall, M., Veith, R., Martin, D., et al. (1997). Behavioral and neuroendocrine responses to sodium lactate infusion in subjects with posttraumatic stress disorder. *The American Journal of Psychiatry, 154*(2), 266–268.

29 Muhtz, C., Yassouridis, A., Daneshi, J., Braun, M., & Kellner, M. (2011). Acute panicogenic, anxiogenic and dissociative effects of carbon dioxide inhalation in patients with post-traumatic stress disorder (PTSD). *Journal of Psychiatric Research, 45*(7), 989–993.

30 Hinton, D., Nickerson, A., & Bryant, R. (2011). Worry, worry attacks, and PTSD among Cambodian refugees: A path analysis investigation. *Social Science and Medicine, 72*(11), 1817–1825.

31 Brown, T., & McNiff, J. (2009). Specificity of autonomic arousal to DSM-IV panic disorder and posttraumatic stress disorder. *Behavioral Research and Therapy, 47*(6), 487–493.

32 Kahn, J., Gorelick, D., & Bridger, W. (1974). Mescaline facilities retention of passive avoidance in rats. *Physiological Psychology, 2,* 120–122.

33 Zheng, X., Liu, F., Wu, X., & Li, B. (2008). Infusion of methylphenidate into the basolateral nucleus of amygdala or anterior cingulate cortex enhances fear memory consolidation in rats. *Science in China, Series C, Life Sciences, 51*(9), 808–813.

34 Tye, K., Tye, L., Cone, J., Hekkelman, E., Janak, P., & Bonci, A. (2010). Methylphenidate facilitates learning-induced amygdala plasticity. *Nature Neuroscience, 13*(4), 475–481.

35 Fava, M., Rankin, M., Wright, E., Alpert, J., Nierenberg, A., Pava, J., et al. (2000). Anxiety disorders in major depression. *Comprehensive Psychiatry, 41*(2), 97–102.

36 Cassano, G., Perugi, G., Musetti, L., & Akiskal, H. (1989). The nature of depression presenting concomitantly with panic disorder. *Comprehensive Psychiatry, 30*(6), 473–482.

37 Beesdo, K., Bittner, A., Pine, D., Stein, M., Höfler, M., Lieb, R., et al. (2007). Incidence of social anxiety disorder and the consistent risk for secondary depression in the first three decades of life. *Archives of General Psychiatry, 64*(8), 903–912.

38 Matza, L., Revicki, D., Davidson, J., & Stewart, J. (2003). Depression with atypical features in the National Comorbidity Survey: Classification, description, and consequences. *Archives of General Psychiatry, 60*(8), 817–826.

39 Parker, G., Fink, M., Shorter, E., Taylor, M., Akiskal, H., Berrios, G., et al. (2010). Issues for DSM-5: Whither Melancholia? The case for its classification as a distinct mood disorder. *The American Journal of Psychiatry, 167*(7), 745–747.

40 Goodwin, R., Lieb, R., Hoefler, M., Pfister, H., Bittner, A., Beesdo, K., et al. (2004). Panic attack as a risk factor for severe psychopathology. *The American Journal of Psychiatry, 161*(12), 2207–2214.

41 Kinley, D., Walker, J., Enns, M., & Sareen, J. (2011). Panic attacks as a risk for later psychopathology: Results from a nationally representative survey. *Depression and Anxiety, 28*(5), 412–509.

42 Kramer, P. D. (1993). *Listening to Prozac.* New York: Penguin Books.

43 Attenborough, D. (2009, January 29). The swarm-maker molecule: How serotonin transforms solitary locusts into social ones. *Discover Magazine.* Retrieved from http://blogs.discovermagazine.com/notrocketscience/2009/01/29/the-swarm-maker-molecule-how-serotonin-transforms-solitary-locusts-into-social-ones

44 Miller, P. (2010). *The smart swarm: How understanding flocks, schools, and colonies can make us better at communicating, decision making, and getting things done.* New York: Avery.

45 Bilderbeck, A., McCabe, C., Wakeley, J., McGlone, F., Harris, T., Cowen, P., et al. (2011). Serotonergic activity influences the cognitive appraisal of close intimate relationships in healthy adults. *Biological Psychiatry, 69*(8), 720–725.

46 Trut, L. N. (1999). Early canid domestication: The farm-fox experiment. *American Scientist, 87*, 160–169.

47 Trut, L., Oskina, I., & Kharlamova, A. (2009). Animal evolution during domestication: The domesticated fox as a model. *Bioessays, 31*(3), 349–360.

48 Ratliff, E. (2011, March). Animal Domestication. *National Geographic.*

49 Meyer-Lindenberg, A., Hariri, A., Munoz, K., Mervis, C., Mattay, V., Morris, C., et al. (2005). Neural correlates of genetically abnormal social cognition in Williams syndrome. *Nature Neuroscience, 8*(8), 991–993.

50 Knutson, B., Wolkowitz, O., Cole, S., Chan, T., Moore, E., Johnson, R., et al. (1998). Selective alteration of personality and social behavior by serotonergic intervention. *The American Journal of Psychiatry, 155*(3), 373–379.

51 Moore, E. A. (1997). Effects of serotonin-specific reuptake inhibitors on intimacy. Dissertation Abstracts International: Section B: The sciences and engineering. *U.S. ProQuest Information & Learning,* California School of Professional Psychology, Alameda.

52 Marazziti, D., Akiskal, H., Rossi, A., & Cassano, G. (1999). Alteration of the platelet serotonin transporter in romantic love. *Psychological Medicine, 29*(3), 741–745.

53 Crockett, M., Clark, L., Lieberman, M., Tabibnia, G., & Robbins, T. (2010). Impulsive choice and altruistic punishment are correlated and increase in tandem with serotonin depletion. *Emotion, 10*(6), 855–862.

54 Caspi, A., Hariri, A., Holmes, A., Uher, R., & Moffitt, T. (2010). Genetic sensitivity to the environment: The case of the serotonin transporter gene and its implications for studying complex diseases and traits. *The American Journal of Psychiatry, 167*(5), 509–527.

55 Bell, C., Abrams, J., & Nutt, D. (2001). Tryptophan depletion and its implications for psychiatry. *The British Journal of Psychiatry, 178,* 399–405.

56 Spain, W., Schwindt, P., & Crill, W. (1991). Two transient potassium currents in layer V pyramidal neurones from cat sensorimotor cortex. *The Journal of Physiology, 434,* 591–607.

57 Ogliari, A., Spatola, C., Pesenti-Gritti, P., Medda, E., Penna, L., Stazi, M., et al. (2010). The role of genes and environment in shaping co-occurrence of DSM-IV defined anxiety dimensions among Italian twins aged 8–17. *Journal of Anxiety Disorders, 24*(4), 433–439.

Chapter 2: Panic Anxiety

1 MacLean, P. (1985). Brain evolution relating to family, play, and the separation call. *Archives of General Psychiatry, 42*(4), 405–417.

2 Cheney, D. L., & Seyfarth, R. M. (2007). *Baboon metaphysics: The evolution of a social mind.* Chicago: University of Chicago Press.

3 Overall, K. L., Hamilton, S. P., & Chang, M. L. (2006). Understanding the genetic basis of canine anxiety: Phenotyping dogs for behavioral, neurochemical, and genetic assessment. *Journal of Veterinary Behavior, 1,* 124–141.

4 Parthasarathy, V., & Crowell-Davis, S. L. (2006). Relationship between attachment to owners and separation anxiety in pet dogs (Canis lupus familiaris). *Journal of Veterinary Behavior: Clinical Applications and Research, 1*(3), 109–120.

5 Barrett, D. (2010). *Supernormal stimuli: How primal urges overran their evolutionary purpose.* New York: W. W. Norton.

6 Klein, D. (1964). Delineation of two drug-responsive anxiety syndromes. *Psychopharmacologia, 5,* 397–408.

7 Meuret, A., Rosenfield, D., Wilhelm, F., Zhou, E., Conrad, A., Ritz, T. & Roth, W. T. (2011). Do unexpected panic attacks occur spontaneously? *Biological Psychiatry, 70*(10), 985–991.

8 Kessler, R., Chiu, W., Jin, R., Ruscio, A., Shear, K., & Walters, E. (2006). The epidemiology of panic attacks, panic disorder, and agoraphobia in the National Comorbidity Survey Replication. *Archives of General Psychiatry, 63*(4), 415–424.

9 Kahn, J. P., & Sodikoff, C. *Unpublished Data.*

10 Pema, G., Dario, A., Caldirola, D., Stefania, B., Cesarani, A., & Bellodi, L. (2001). Panic disorder: The role of the balance system. *Journal of Psychiatric Research, 35*(5), 279–286.

11 Kahn, J., Stevenson, E., Topol, P., & Klein, D. (1986). Agitated depression, alprazolam, and panic anxiety. *The American Journal of Psychiatry, 143*(9), 1172–1173.

12 Katerndahl, D. A., & Realini, J. (1997). Quality of life and panic-related work disability in subjects with infrequent panic and panic disorder. *Journal of Clinical Psychiatry, 58*(4), 153–158.

13 Kinley, D., Walker, J., Enns, M., & Sareen, J. (2011). Panic attacks as a risk for later psychopathology: Results from a nationally representative survey. *Depression and Anxiety, 28*(5), 412–419.

14 Beitman, B. D., Thomas, A. M., & Kushner, M. G. (1992). Panic disorder in the families of patients with normal coronary arteries and non-fear panic disorder. *Behaviour Research and Therapy, 30*(4), 403–406.

15 Gros, D., Frueh, B., & Magruder, K. (2011). Prevalence and features of panic disorder and comparison to posttraumatic stress disorder in VA primary care. *General Hospital Psychiatry, 33*(5), 482–488.

16 Panksepp, J., Normansell, L., Siviy, S., Rossi, J., & Zolovick, A. (1984). Casomorphins reduce separation distress in chicks. *Peptides, 5*(4), 829–831.

17 Bandelow, B., Sojka, F., Broocks, A., Hajak, G., Bleich, S., & Ruther, E. (2006). Panic disorder during pregnancy and postpartum period. *European Psychiatry, 21*(7), 495–500.

18 Mauri, M., Oppo, A., Montagnani, M., Borri, C., Banti, S., Camilleri, V., et al. (2010). Beyond "postpartum depressions": Specific anxiety diagnoses during pregnancy predict different outcomes: Results from PND-ReScU. *Journal of Affective Disorders, 127*(1–3), 177–184.

19 Rambelli, C., Montagnani, M., Oppo, A., Banti, S., Cortopassi, C., Ramacciotti, D., et al. (2010). Panic disorder as a risk factor for post-partum depression: Results from the Perinatal Depression-Research & Screening Unit (PND-ReScU) study. *Journal of Affective Disorders, 122* (1–2), 139–143.

20 Bernstein, I., Rush, A., Yonkers, K., Carmody, T., Woo, A., McConnell, K. & Trivedi, M. H. (2008). Symptom features of postpartum depression: Are they distinct? *Depression and Anxiety, 25*(1), 20–26.

21 Wickramante, P., Gameroff, M., Pilowsky, D., Hughes, C., Garber, J., Malloy, E., et al. (2011). Children of depressed mothers 1 year after remission of maternal depression: Findings from the STAR*D-Child study. *The American Journal of Psychiatry, 168*(6), 593–602.

22 Yates, W. (2009). Phenomenology and epidemiology of panic disorder. *Annals of Clinical Psychiatry, 21*(2), 95–102.

23 Toru, I., Aluoja, A., Vohna, U., Raaq, M., Vasar, V., Maron, E., et al. (2010). Associations between personality traits and CCK-4-induced panic attacks in healthy volunteers. *Psychiatry Research, 178*(2), 342–347.

24 Kaplan, H. S., & Klein, D. F. (1987). *Sexual aversion, sexual phobias, and panic disorders.* New York: Brunner/Mazel.

25 Eaton, W., Kessler, R., Wittchen, H., & Magee, W. (1994). Panic and panic disorder in the United States. *The American Journal of Psychiatry, 151*(3), 413–420.

26 Zaider, T., Heimberg, R., & Iida, M. (2010). Anxiety disorders and intimate relationships: A study of daily processes in couples. *Journal of Abnormal Psychology, 119*(1), 163–173.

27 Kahn, J. P., & Langlieb, A. M. (2003). *Mental health and productivity in the workplace: A handbook for organizations and clinicians* . San Francisco: Jossey-Bass.

28 Erickson, S., Guthrie, S., Vanetten-Lee, M., Himle, J., Hoffman, J., Santos, S., et al. (2009). Severity of anxiety and work-related outcomes of patients with anxiety disorders. *Depression and Anxiety, 26*(12), 1165–1171.

29 Linden, M., & Muschalla, B. (2007). Anxiety disorders and workplace-related anxieties. *Journal of Anxiety Disorders, 21*(3), 467–474.

30 Schumacher, J., Kristensen, A., Wendland, J., Nother, M., Mors, O., & McMahon, F. (2011). The genetics of panic disorder. *Journal of Medical Genetics, 48*(6), 361–368.

31 Ogliari, A., Tambs, K., Harris, J., Scanini, S., Maffei, C., Reichborn-Kjennerud, T. & Battaglia M. (2010). The relationships between adverse events, early antecedents, and carbon dioxide reactivity as an intermediate phenotype of panic disorder: A general population study. *Psychotherapy and Psychosomatics, 79*(1), 48–55.

32 Spatola, C., Scaini, S., Pesenti-Gritti, P., Medland, S., Moruzzi, S., Ogliari, A., et al. (2011). Gene-environment interactions in panic disorder and CO(2) sensitivity: Effects of events occurring early in life. *American Journal of Medical Genetics: Part B: Neuropsychiatric Genetics, 156B*(1), 79–88.

33 Battaglia, M., Pesenti-Gritti, P., Medland, S., Ogliari, A., Tambs, K., & Spatola, C. (2009). A genetically informed study of the association between childhood separation anxiety, sensitivity to CO(2), panic disorder, and the effect of childhood parental loss. *Archives of General Psychiatry, 66*(1), 64–71.

34 Kendler, K., Myers, J., Maes, H., & Keyes, C. (2011). The relationship between the genetic and environmental influences on common internalizing psychiatric disorders and mental well-being. *Behavioral Genetics, 41*(5), 641–650.

35 Stein, M., Schork, N., & Gelernter, J. (2008). Gene-by-environment (serotonin transporter and childhood maltreatment) interaction for anxiety sensitivity, an intermediate phenotype for anxiety disorders. *Neuropsychopharmacology, 33*(2), 312–319.

36 Preter, M., & Klein, D. (2008). Panic, suffocation false alarms, separation anxiety and endogenous opioids. *Progress in Neuropsychopharmacology and Biological Psychiatry, 32*(3), 603–612.

37 Preter, M., Lee, S., Petkova, E., Vanucci, M., Kim, S., & Klein, D. (2011). Controlled cross-over study in normal subjects of naloxone-preceding-lactate infusions, respiratory and subjective responses: Relationship to endogenous opioid system, suffocation false alarm theory and childhood parental loss. *Psychological Medicine, 41*(2), 385–393.

38 Klein, D. F. (1993). False suffocation alarms, spontaneous panics, and related conditions. An integrative hypothesis. *Archives of General Psychiatry, 50*(4), 306–317.

39 Groopman, J. (1999, May 10). Pet Scan. *The New Yorker, 46*.

40 D'Amato, F. R., Zanettini, C., Lampis, V., Coccurello, R., Pascucci, T., Ventura, R., et al. (2011, April). Unstable maternal environment, separation anxiety, and heightened CO2 sensitivity induced by gene-by-environment interplay. *PLoS One, 4*, e18637.

41 Corsci, F., Gooyer, T., Schruers, K., Faravelli, C., & Griez, E. (2005). The influence of ethanol infusion on the effects of 35% CO2 challenge. A study in panic disorder patients and healthy volunteers. *European Psychiatry, 20*(3), 299–303.

42 Schruers, K., Esquivel, G., van Duinen, M., Wichers, M., Kenis, G., Colasanti, A., Knuts, I., Goossens, L., Jacobs, N., van Rozendaal, J., Smeets, H., van Os, J., & Griez, E., (2011). Genetic moderation of CO2-induced fear by 5-HTTLPR genotype. *Journal of Psychopharmacology, 25* (1), 37–42.

43 van Megen, H., Westerberg, H., den Boer, J., Slaap, B., & Scheepmakers, A. (1997). Effect of the selective serotonin reuptake inhibitor fluvoxamine on CCK-4 induced panic attacks. *Psychopharmacology (Berl), 129*(4), 357–364.

44 Shlik, J., Aluoja, A., Vasar, V., Vasar, E., Podar, T., & Bradwejn, J. (1997). Effects of citalopram treatment on behavioural, cardiovascular and neuroendocrine response to cholecystokinin tetrapeptide challenge in patients with panic disorder. *Journal of Psychiatry & Neuroscience, 22*(5), 332–340.

45 Fava, M., Rappe, S., Pava, J., Nierenberg, A., Alpert, J., & Rosenbaum, J. (1995). Relapse in patients on long-term fluoxetine treatment: Response to increased fluoxetine dose. *Journal of Clinical Psychiatry, 56*(2), 52–55.

46 Fyer, A., Liebowitz, M., Gorman, J., Davies, S., & Klein, D. (1985). Lactate vulnerability of remitted panic patients. *Psychiatry Research, 14*(2), 143–148.

47 Liebowitz, M., Coplan, J., Martinez, J., Fyer, A., Dillon, D., Campeas, R., et al. (1995). Effects of intravenous diazepam pretreatment on lactate-induced panic. *Psychiatry Research, 58*(2), 127–138.

48 Sanderson, W., Wetzler, S., & Asnis, G. (1994). Alprazolam blockade of CO2-provoked panic in patients with panic disorder. *The American Journal of Psychiatry, 151*(8), 1220–1222.

49 Nardi, A. E., Freire, R. C., Mochcovitch, M. D., Amrein, R., Levitan, M. N., King, A. L., et al. (2012). A randomized, naturalistic, parallel-group study for the long-term treatment of panic disorder with clonazepam or paroxetine. *Journal of Clinical Psychopharmacology, 32*(1), 120–126.

50 Milrod, B., Leon, A., Busch, F., Rudden, M., Schwalberg, M., Clarkin, J., et al. (2007). A randomized controlled clinical trial of psychoanalytic psychotherapy for panic disorder. *The American Journal of Psychiatry, 164*(2), 265–272.

51 Gorman, J., Martinez, J., Coplan, J., Kent, J., & Kleber, M. (2004). The effect of successful treatment on the emotional and physiological response to carbon dioxide inhalation in patients with panic disorder. *Biological Psychiatry, 56*(11), 862–867.

Chapter 3: Social Anxiety

1 Weisman, O., Aderka, I., Marom, S., Hermesh, H., & Gilboa-Schechtman, E. (2011). Social rank and affiliation in social anxiety disorder. *Behaviour Research and Therapy, 49*(6–7), 399–405.

2 Stein, D., & Vythilingum, B. (2007). Social anxiety disorder: Psychobiological and evolutionary underpinnings. *CNS Spectrums, 12*(11), 806–809.

3 Cheney, D. L., & Seyfarth, R. M. (2007). *Baboon metaphysics: The evolution of a social mind*. Chicago: University of Chicago Press.

4 Feinberg, M., Willer, R., & Keltner, D. (2012). Flustered and faithful: Embarrassment as a signal of prosociality. *Journal of Personality and Social Psychology, 102*(1), 81–97.

5 Ruscio, A. M., Brown, T. A., Chiu, W. T., Sareen, J., Stein, M. B., & Kessler, R. C. (2008). Social fears and social phobia in the USA: Results from the National Comorbidity Survey Replication. *Psychological Medicine, 38*(1), 15–28.

6 Fehm, L., Beesdo, K., Jacobi, F., & Fiedler, A. (2008). Social anxiety disorder above and below the diagnostic threshold: Prevalence, comorbidity and impairment in the general population. *Social Psychiatry and Psychiatric Epidemiology, 43*(4) 257–265.

7 Weeks, J. W., Rodebaugh, T. L., Heimberg, R. G., Norton, P. J., & Jakatdar, T. A. (2008). "To avoid evaluation, withdraw": Fears of evaluation and depressive cognitions lead to social anxiety and submissive withdrawal. *Cognitive Therapy and Research, 33*, 375–389.

8 Liebowitz, M., Gorman, J., Fyer, A., & Klein, D. (1985). Social phobia. Review of a neglected anxiety disorder. *Archives of General Psychiatry, 42*(7), 729–736.

9 Stein, M., & Stein, D. (2008). Social anxiety disorder. *Lancet, 371*(9618), 1115–1125.

10 Burstein, M., Ameli-Grillon, L., & Merikangas, K. (2011). Shyness versus social phobia in US youth. *Pediatrics, 128* (5), 917–925.

11 Cougle, J., Keough, M., Riccardi, C., & Sachs-Ericsson, N. (2009). Anxiety disorders and suicidality in the National Comorbidity Survey-Replication. *Journal of Psychiatric Research, 43* (9), 825–829.

12 Sherbourne, C., Sullivan, G., Craske, M., Roy-Byrne, P., Golinelli, D., Rose, R., et al. (2010). Functioning and disability levels in primary care out-patients with one or more anxiety disorders. *Psychological Medicine, 40*(12), 2058–2068.

13 Filho, A., Hetem, L., Ferrari, M., Trzesniak, C., Martín-Santos, R., Borduqui, T., et al. (2010). Social anxiety disorder: What are we losing with the current diagnostic criteria? *ActaPsychiatrica Scandinavica, 121*(3), 216–226.

14 Schneier, F., Blanco, C., Antia, S., & Liebowitz, M. (2002). The social anxiety spectrum. *The Psychiatric Clinics of North America, 25*(4), 757–774.

15 Tse, W., & Bond, A. (2002). Serotonergic intervention affects both social dominance and affiliative behaviour. *Psychopharmacology, 161*(3), 324–330.

16 Fang, A., & Hofmann, S. (2010). Relationship between social anxiety disorder and body dysmorphic disorder. *Clinical Psychology Review, 30*(8), 1040–1048.

17 Kelly, M., Walters, C., & Phillips, K. (2010). Social anxiety and its relationship to functional impairment in body dysmorphic disorder. *Behavior Therapy, 41*(2), 143–153.

18 Liao, Y., Knoesen, N., Deng, Y., Tang, J., Castle, D., Bookun, R., et al. (2010). Body dysmorphic disorder, social anxiety and depressive symptoms in Chinese medical students. *Social Psychiatry and Psychiatric Epidemiology, 45*(10), 963–971.

19 Tignol, J., Martin-Guehl, C., Aouizerate, B., Grabot, D., & Auriacombe, M. (2006). Social phobia and premature ejaculation: a case-control study. *Depression and Anxiety, 23*(3), 153–157.

20 Vythilingum, B., Stein, D., & Soifer, S. (2002). Is "shy bladder syndrome" a subtype of social anxiety disorder? A survey of people with paruresis. *Depression and Anxiety, 16*(2), 84–87.

21 Gawande, A. (2001, Feburary 12). Crimson tide: What is blushing? No one knows for sure, but it can ruin your life. *The New Yorker.* http://www.newyorker.com/archive/200 1/02/12/2001_02_12_050_TNY_LIBRY_000022696

22 Schneier, F., Johnson, J., Hornig, C., Liebowitz, M., & Weissman, M. (1992). Social phobia. Comorbidity and morbidity in an epidemiologic sample. *Archives of General Psychiatry, 49*(4), 282–288.

23 Van Roy, B., Kristensen, H., Groholt, B., & Clench-Aas, J. (2009). Prevalence and characteristics of significant social anxiety in children aged 8–13 years: A Norwegian cross-sectional population study. *Social Psychiatry and Psychiatric Epidemiology, 44*(5), 407–415.

24 Dalrymple, K., & Zimmerman, M. (2011). Age of onset of social anxiety disorder in depressed outpatients. *Journal of Anxiety Disorders, 25*(1), 131–137.

25 Mather, A., Stein, M., & Sareen, J. (2010, Oct). Social anxiety disorder and social fears in the Canadian military: Prevalence, comorbidity, impairment, and treatment-seeking. *Journal of Psychiatric Research, 44*(14), 887–893.

26 Kashdan, T. (2007). Social anxiety spectrum and diminished positive experiences: Theoretical synthesis and meta-analysis. *Clinical Psychology Review, 27*(3), 348–365.

27 Weisman, O., Aderka, I. M., Marom, S., Hermesh, H., & Gilboa-Schechtman, E. (2011, June). Social rank and affiliation in social anxiety disorder. *Behaviour Research and Therapy, 49*(6–7), 399–405.

28 Kashdan, T., & Collins, R. (2010). Social anxiety and the experience of positive emotion and anger in everyday life: An ecological momentary assessment approach. *Anxiety, Stress, and Coping, 23*(3), 259–272.

29 Van Leeuwen, E. J., Zimmermann, E., & Ross, M. D. (2011). Responding to Inequities: Gorillas try to maintain their competitive advantage during play fights. *Biology Letters, 7*(1), 39–42.

30 Laidlaw, A. H. (2009). Social anxiety in medical students: Implications for communication skills teaching. *Medical Teacher, 31*(7), 649–654.

31 Acarturk, C., Smit, F., de Graaf, R., van Straten, A., Ten Have, M., & Cuijpers, P. (2009). Economic costs of social phobia: A population-based study. *Journal of Affective Disorders, 115*(3), 421–429.

32 Stein, M. B., & Kean, Y. M. (2000). Disability and quality of life in social phobia: Epidemiologic findings. *The American Journal of Psychiatry, 157*(10), 1606–1613.

33 Hunter, L. R., Buckner, J. D., & Schmidt, N. B. (2009). Interpreting facial expressions: The influence of social anxiety, emotional valence, and race. *Journal of Anxiety Disorders, 23*(4), 482–488.

34 Garner, M., Clarke, G., Graystone, H., & Baldwin, D. S. (2011). Defensive startle response to emotional social cues in social anxiety. *Psychiatry Research, 186*(1), 150–152.

35 Moukheiber, A., Rautureau, G., Perez-Diaz, F., Soussignan, R., Dubal, S., Jouvent, R., & Pelissolo, A. (2010). Gaze avoidance in social phobia: Objective measure and correlates. *Behaviour Research and Therapy, 48*(2), 147–151.

36 Gamer, M., Hecht, H., Seipp, N., & Hiller, W. (2011). Who is looking at me? The cone of gaze widens in social phobia. *Cognition & Emotion, 25*(4), 756–764.

37 Schneier, F. R., Kent, J. M., Star, A., & Hirsch, J. (2009). Neural circuitry of submissive behavior in social anxiety disorder: A preliminary study of response to direct eye gaze. *Psychiatry Research, 173*(3), 248–250.

38 Weeks, J. W. (2009). Exploring the role of submissiveness in social anxiety: Testing an evolutionary model of social anxiety disorder. *Dissertation Abstracts International, 69.* Retrieved from PsycINFO. EBSCO.

39 Chiao, J. Y., & Blizinsky, K. D. (2010). Culture-gene coevolution of individualism-collectivism and the serotonin transporter gene. *Proceedings: Biological Sciences: The Royal Society, 277*(1681), 529–537.

40 Schreier, S. S., Heinrichs, N., Alden, L., Rapee, R. M., Hofmann, S. G., Chen, J., et al. (2010). Social anxiety and social norms in individualistic and collectivistic countries. *Depression and Anxiety, 27*(12), 1128–1134.

41 Wenzel, A., & Emerson, T. (2009). Mate selection in socially anxious and nonanxious individuals. *Journal of Osicla and Clinical Psychology, 28,* 341–363.

42 Wenzel, A., Graff-Dolezal, J., Macho, M., & Brendle, J. R. (2005). Communication and social skills in socially anxious and nonanxious individuals in the context of romantic relationships. *Behaviour Research Therapy, 43*(4), 505–519.

43 Kashdan, T., Adams, L., Savostyanova, A., Ferssizidis, P., McKnight, P., & Nezlik, J. (2011). Effects of social anxiety and depressive symptoms on the frequency and quality of sexual activity: A daily process approach. *Behaviour Research Therapy, 49*(5), 352–360.

44 Kashdan, T. (2004). The neglected relationship between social interaction anxiety and hedonic deficits: Differentiation from depressive symptoms. *Journal of Anxiety Disorders, 18*(5), 719–730.

45 DeVoe, S., & Pfeffer, J. (2011). Time is tight: How higher economic value of time increases feelings of time pressure. *The Journal of Applied Psychology, 96*(4), 665–676.

46 Weeks, J., Heimberg, R., Rodebaugh, T., & Norton, P. (2007). Exploring the relationship between fear of positive evaluation and social anxiety. *Journal of Anxiety Disorders, 22*(3), 386–400.

47 Cox, B., Fleet, C., & Stein, M. (2004). Self-criticism and social phobia in the US national comorbidity survey. *Journal of Affective Disorders, 82*(2), 227–234.

48 Blair, K., Geraci, M., Hollon, N., Otero, M., DeVido, J., Majestic, C., et al. (2010). Social norm processing in adult social phobia: Atypically increased ventromedial frontal cortex responsiveness to unintentional (embarrassing) transgressions. *The American Journal of Psychiatry, 167*(12), 1526–1532.

49 Mather, A., Stein, M., & Sareen, J. (2010). Social anxiety disorder and social fears in the Canadian military: Prevalence, comorbidity, impairment, and treatment-seeking. *Journal of Psychiatric Research, 44*(14), 887–893.

50 Dijk, C., Koenig, B., Ketelaar, T., & de Jong, P. (2011). Saved by the blush: Being trusted despite defecting. *Emotion, 11*(2), 313–319.

51 Prehn-Kristensen, A., Wiesner, C., Bergmann, T., Wolff, S., Jansen, O., Mehdorn, H., et al. (2009). Induction of empathy by the smell of anxiety. *PLoS One, 4*(6), e5987.

52 Pause, B., Ohrt, A., & Ferstl, R. (2004). Positive emotional priming of facial affect perception in females is diminished by chemosensory anxiety signals. *Chemical Senses, 29*(9), 797–805.

53 Pause, B., Adolph, D., Prehn-Kristensen, A., & Ferstl, R. (2009). Startle response potentiation to chemosensory anxiety signals in socially anxious individuals. *International Journal of Psychophysiology, 74*(2), 88–92.

54 Onishi, N. (2007, July 16). Japan learns dreaded task of jury duty. *The New York Times*.

55 Stevens, S., Rist, F., & Gerlach, A. (2008). Influence of alcohol on the processing of emotional facial expressions in individuals with social phobia. *The British Journal of Clinical Psychology, 48*(2), 125–140.

56 Lublin, J. (2011, April 14). *Introverted execs find ways to shine.* The Wall Street Journal . Retrieved from http://online.wsj.com/article/SB100014240527487039831045762630537 75879800.html?mod=WSJ_newsreel_careers%29

57 Van Kleef, G. A., Homan, A. C., Finkenauer, C., Gündemir, S., & Stamkou, E. (2011). Breaking the rules to rise to power: How norm violators gain power in the eyes of others. *Social Psychological and Personality Science, 2*(5), 500–507.

58 Kashdan, T. B., & McKnight, P. E. (2010). The darker side of social anxiety: When aggressive impulsivity prevails over shy inhibition. *Current Directions in Psychological Science, 19*(1), 47–50.

59 Stein, M., Yang, B., Chavira, D., Hitchcock, C., Sung, S., Shipon-Blum, E., & Gelernter, J. (2011). A common genetic variant in the neurexin superfamily member CNTNAP2 is associated with increased risk for selective mutism and social anxiety-related traits. *Biological Psychiatry, 69*(9), 825–831.

60 Ogliari, A., Spatola, C., Pesenti-Gritti, P., Medda, E., Penna, L., Stazi, M., et al. (2010). The role of genes and environment in shaping co-occurrence of DSM-IV defined anxiety dimensions among Italian twins aged 8–17. *Journal of Anxiety Disorders, 24*(4), 433–439.

61 Mosing, M., Gordon, S., Medland, S., Statham, D., Nelson, E., Heath, A., et al. (2009). Genetic and environmental influences on the co-morbidity between depression, panic disorder, agoraphobia, and social phobia: A twin study. *Depression and Anxiety, 26*(11), 1004–1011.

62 Stein, M., Seedat, S., & Gelernter, J. (2006). Serotonin transporter gene promoter polymorphism predicts SSRI response in generalized social anxiety disorder. *Psychopharmacology, 187*(1), 68–72.

63 University of California – San Francisco. (2011, April 15). Neurological basis for embarrassment described. *ScienceDaily*.

64 Watson, K., Ghosdasra, J., & Platt, M. (2009). Serotonin transporter genotype modulates social reward and punishment in rhesus macaques. *PLoS One, 4*(1), e4156.

65 Raleigh, M., McGuire, M., Brammer, G., Pollack, D., & Yuwiler, A. (1991). Serotonergic mechanisms promote dominance acquisition in adult male vervet monkeys. *Brain Research, 559*(2), 181–190.

66 Domschke, K., Stevens, S., Beck, B., Baffa, A., Hohoff, C., Deckert, J., & Gerlach, A. L. (2009). Blushing propensity in social anxiety disorder: Influence of serotonin transporter gene variation. *Journal of Neural Transmission, 116*(6), 663–666.

67 Lecrubier, Y. (1998). Comorbidity in social anxiety disorder: Impact on disease burden and management. *Journal of Clinical Psychiatry, 59*(17), 33–38.

68 Melas, P., Rogdaki, M., Lennartsson, A., Bjork, K., Witasp, A., Werme, M., et al. (2012). Antidepressant treatment is associated with epigenetic alterations in the promoter of P11 in a genetic model of depression. *International Journal of Neuropsychopharmacology, 15*(5), 169–179.

69 Tse, W., & Bond, A. (2002). Serotonergic intervention affects both social dominance and affiliative behaviour. *Psychopharmacology, 161*(3), 324–330.

70 Lipsitz, J., Markowitz, J., Cherry, S., & Fyer, A. (1999). Open trial of interpersonal psychotherapy for the treatment of social phobia. *American Journal of Psychiatry, 156*(11), 1814–1816.

Chapter 4: Obsessive-Compulsive Disorder

1 Polimeni, J., Reiss, J. P., & Sareen, J. (2005). Could obsessive-compulsive disorder have originated as a group-selected adaptive trait in traditional societies? *Medical Hypotheses, 65* (4), 655–664.

2 Alperson-Afil, N., Sharon, G., Kislev, M., Melamed, Y., Zohar, I., Ashkenazi, S., et al. (2009). Spatial organization of hominin activities at Gesher Benot Ya'aqov, Israel. *Science, 326*(5960), 1677–1680.

3 Moon-Fanelli, A. A., & Dodman, N. H. (1998). Description and development of compulsive tail chasing in terriers and response to clomipramine treatment. *Journal of the American Veterinary Medical Association, 212*(8), 1252–1257.

4 Cheney, D. L., & Seyfarth, R. M. (2007). *Baboon metaphysics: The evolution of a social mind.* Chicago: University of Chicago Press.

5 Hirata, S., Watanabe, K., & Kawai, M. (2008). "Sweet-potato washing" revisited. In T. Matsuzawa (Ed.), *Primate origins of human cognition and behavior* (pp. 487–507). Tokyo, Berlin, Heidelberg & New York: Springer.

6 Overall, K. L., & Dunham, A. E. (2002). Clinical features and outcome in dogs and cats with obsessive-compulsive disorder: 126 cases (1989–2000). *Journal of the American Veterinary Medical Association, 221*(10), 1445–1452.

7 Greene-Schloesser, D. M., Van der Zee, E. A., Sheppard, D. K., Castillo, M. R., Gregg, K. A., Burrow, T., et al. (2011). Predictive validity of a non-induced mouse model of compulsive-like behavior. *Behavioural Brain Research, 221*(1), 55–62.

8 Greene, M., & Miller, P. (2010). *The smart swarm: How understanding flocks, schools, and colonies can make us better at communicating, decision making, and getting things done.* New York: Avery.

9 Gordon, D. (1996). The organization of work in social insect colonies. *Nature, 380,* 121–124.

10 Storch, E. A., Rasmussen, S. A., Price, L. H., Larson, M. J., Murphy, T. K., & Goodman, W. K. (2010). Development and psychometric evaluation of the Yale-Brown Obsessive-Compulsive Scale—Second Edition. *Psychological Assessment, 22*(2), 223–232.

11 Ruscio, A. M., Stein, D. J., Chiu, W. T., & Kessler, R. C. (2010). The epidemiology of obsessive-compulsive disorder in the National Comorbidity Survey Replication. *Molecular Psychiatry, 15*(1), 53–63.

12 Mataix-Cols, D., Rosario-Campos, M. C., & Leckman, J. F. (2005). A multidimensional model of obsessive-compulsive disorder. *The American Journal of Psychiatry, 162*(2), 228–238.

13 Bloch, M. H., Landeros-Weisenberger, A., Rosario, M. C., Pittenger, C., & Leckman J. F. (2008). Meta-analysis of the symptom structure of obsessive-compulsive disorder. *The American Journal of Psychiatry, 165*(12), 1532–1542.

14 Matsunaga, H., Hayashida, K., Kiriike, N., Maebayashi, K., & Stein, D. J. (2010). The clinical utility of symptom dimensions in obsessive-compulsive disorder. *Psychiatry Research, 180*(1), 25–29.

15 Goodman, W. K., Price, L. H., Rasmussen, S. A., Mazure, C., Fleischmann, R. L., Hill, C. L., et al. (1989). The Yale-Brown Obsessive Compulsive Scale. I. Development, use, and reliability. *Archives of General Psychiatry, 46*(11), 1006–1011.

16 Barrett, D. (2010). *Supernormal stimuli: How primal urges overran their evolutionary purpose.* New York: W. W. Norton.

17 Liljenquist, K., Zhong, C. B., & Galinsky, A. D. (2010). The smell of virtue: Clean scents promote reciprocity and charity. *Psychological Science, 21*(3), 381–383.

18 Zhong, C. B., & Liljenquist, K. (2006). Washing away your sins: Threatened morality and physical cleansing. *Science, 313*(5792), 1451–1452.

19 Kuhn, T. S. (1996). *The structure of scientific revolutions.* Chicago: University of Chicago Press.

20 Diaferia, G., Bianchi, I., Bianchi, M. L., Cavedini, P., Erzegovesi, S., & Bellodi, L. (1997). Relationship between obsessive-compulsive personality disorder and obsessive-compulsive disorder. *Comprehensive Psychiatry, 38*(1), 38–42.

21 Feusner, J. D., Hembacher, E., & Phillips, K. A. (2009). The mouse who couldn't stop washing: Pathologic grooming in animals and humans. *CNS Spectrums, 14*(9), 503–513.

22 Calikuşu, C., Yücel, B., Polat, A., & Baykal, C. (2003). The relation of psychogenic excoriation with psychiatric disorders: A comparative study. *Comprehensive Psychiatry, 44*(3), 256–261.

23 Gupta, M. A., & Gupta, A. K. (1993). Fluoxetine is an effective treatment for neurotic excoriations: Case report. *Cutis; Cutaneous Medicine for the Practitioner, 51*(5), 386–387.

24 Leckman, J. F., Bloch, M. H., & King, R. A. (2009). Symptom dimensions and subtypes of obsessive-compulsive disorder: A developmental perspective. *Dialogues in Clinical Neuroscience, 11*(1), 21–33.

25 Leonard, H. L., Goldberger, E. L., Rapoport, J. L., Cheslow, D. L., & Swedo, S. E. (1990). Childhood rituals: Normal development or obsessive-compulsive symptoms? *Journal of the American Academy of Child and Adolescent Psychiatry, 29*(1), 17–23.

26 Wenzel, A., Gorman, L. L., O'Hara, M. W., & Stuart, S. (2001). The occurrence of panic and obsessive compulsive symptoms in women with postpartum dysphoria: A prospective study. *Archives of Women's Mental Health, 4*(1), 5–12.

27 Forray, A., Focseneanu, M., Pittman, B., McDougle, C. J., & Epperson, C. N. (2010). Onset and exacerbation of obsessive-compulsive disorder in pregnancy and the postpartum period. *Journal of Clinical Psychiatry, 71*(8), 1061–1068.

28 Uguz, F., Kaya, V., Gezginc, K., Kayhan, F., & Cicek, E. (2011). Clinical correlates of worsening in obsessive-compulsive symptoms during pregnancy. *General Hospital Psychiatry, 33*(2), 197–199.

29 Chaudron, L. H., & Nirodi, N. (2010). The obsessive-compulsive spectrum in the perinatal period: A prospective pilot study. *Archives of Women's Mental Health, 13*(5), 403–410.

30 Feygin, D. L., Swain, J. E., & Leckman, J. F. (2006). The normalcy of neurosis: Evolutionary origins of obsessive-compulsive disorder and related behaviors. *Progress in Neuro-psychopharmacology and Biological Psychiatry, 30*(5), 854–864.

31 Scheper-Hughes, N. (1985). Culture, scarcity, and maternal thinking: Maternal detachment and infant survival in a Brazilian shantytown. *Ethos, 13*(4), 291–317. Retrieved from http://www.jstor.org/stable/640147

32 LaPlante, M. D. (2011, November 5). Is the tide turning against the killing of 'cursed' infants in Ethiopia? CNN.com.

33 Culot, L., Lledo-Ferrer, Y., Hoelscher, O., Muñoz Lazo, F. J., Huynen, M. C., & Heymann, E. W. (2011). Reproductive failure, possible maternal infanticide, and cannibalism in wild moustached tamarins, Saguinus mystax. *Primates, 52*(2), 179–186.

34 Leslie, D. L., Kozma, L., Martin, A., Landeros, A., Katsovich, L., King, R. A., & Leckman, J. F. (2008). Neuropsychiatric disorders associated with streptococcal infection: A case-control study among privately insured children. *Journal of the American Academy of Child and Adolescent Psychiatry, 47*(10), 1166–1172.

35 Gabbay, V., Coffey, B. J., Guttman L. E., Gottlieb, L., Katz, Y., Babb, J. S., et al. (2009). A cytokine study in children and adolescents with Tourette's disorder. *Progress in Neuro-psychopharmacology and Biological Psychiatry, 33*(6), 967–971.

36 Miman, O., Mutlu, E. A., Ozcan, O., Atambay, M., Karlidag, R., & Unal, S. (2010). Is there any role of Toxoplasma gondii in the etiology of obsessive-compulsive disorder? *Psychiatry Research, 177*(1–2), 263–265.

37 Grabe, H. J., Meyer, C., Hapke, U., Rumpf, H. J., Freyberger, H. J., Dilling, H., & John, U. (2000). Prevalence, quality of life and psychosocial function in obsessive-compulsive disorder and subclinical obsessive-compulsive disorder in northern Germany. *European Archives of Psychiatry and Clinical Neuroscience, 250*(5), 262–268.

38 Berney, A., Leyton, M., Gravel, P., Sibon, I., Sookman, D., Rosa Neto, P., et al. (2011). Brain regional α-[11C]methyl-L-tryptophan trapping in medication-free patients with obsessive-compulsive disorder. *Archive of General Psychiatry, 68*(7), 732–741.

39 Marazziti, D., Akiskal, H. S., Rossi, A., & Cassano, G. B. (1999). Alteration of the platelet serotonin transporter in romantic love. *Psychological Medicine, 29*(3), 741–745.

40 Abbey, R. D., Clopton, J. R., & Humphreys, J. D. (2007). Obsessive-compulsive disorder and romantic functioning. *Journal of Clinical Psychology, 63*(12), 1181–1192.

41 Ferrari, J. R., & McCown, W. (1994). Procrastination tendencies among obsessive-compulsives and their relatives. *Journal of Clinical Psychology, 50*(2), 162–167.

42 Tallis, F., Rosen, K., & Shafran, R. (1996). Investigation into the relationship between personality traits and OCD: A replication employing a clinical population. *Behaviour Research and Therapy, 34*(8), 649–653.

43 Mancebo, M. C., Greenberg, B., Grant, J. E., Pinto, A., Eisen, J. L., Dyck, I., & Rasmussen, S. A. (2008). Correlates of occupational disability in a clinical sample of obsessive-compulsive disorder. *Comprehensive Psychiatry, 49*(1), 43–50.

44 Huppert, J. D., Simpson, H. B., Nissenson, K. J., Liebowitz, M. R., & Foa, E. B. (2009). Quality of life and functional impairment in obsessive-compulsive disorder: A

comparison of patients with and without comorbidity, patients in remission, and healthy controls. *Depression and Anxiety, 26*(1), 39–45.

45 Powers, T. A., Koestner, R., & Topciu, R. A. (2005). Implementation intentions, perfectionism, and goal progress: Perhaps the road to hell is paved with good intentions. *Personality and Social Psychology Bulletin, 31*(7), 902–912.

46 Pauls, D. L. (2010). The genetics of obsessive-compulsive disorder: A review. *Dialogues in Clinical Neuroscience, 12*(2), 149–163.

47 Bloch, M. H., Landeros-Weisenberger, A., Sen, S., Dombrowski, P., Kelmendi, B., Coric, V., et al. (2008). Association of the serotonin transporter polymorphism and obsessive-compulsive disorder: Systematic review. *American Journal of Medical Genetics. Part B, Neuropsychiatric Genetics, 147B*(6), 850–858.

48 Landau, D., Iervolino, A. C., Pertusa, A., Santo, S., Singh, S., & Mataix-Cols, D. (2011). Stressful life events and material deprivation in hoarding disorder. *Journal of Anxiety Disorders, 25*(2), 192–202.

49 Bloch, M. H., McGuire, J., Landeros-Weisenberger, A., Leckman, J. F., & Pittenger, C. (2010). Meta-analysis of the dose-response relationship of SSRI in obsessive-compulsive disorder. *Molecular Psychiatry, 15*(8), 850–855.

50 Rabinowitz, I., Baruch, Y., & Barak, Y. (2008). High-dose escitalopram for the treatment of obsessive-compulsive disorder. *International Clinical Psychopharmacology, 23*(1), 49–53.

51 Pampaloni, I., Sivakumaran, T., Hawley, C. J., Al Allaq, A., Farrow, J., Nelson, S., & Fineberg, N. A. (2010). High-dose selective serotonin reuptake inhibitors in OCD: A systematic retrospective case notes survey. *Journal of Psychopharmacology, 24*(10), 1439–1445.

52 Külz, A. K., Meinzer, S., Kopasz, M., & Voderholzer, U. (2007). Effects of tryptophan depletion on cognitive functioning, obsessive-compulsive symptoms and mood in obsessive-compulsive disorder: Preliminary results. *Neuropsychobiology, 56*(2–3), 127–131.

53 Zitterl, W., Aigner, M., Stompe, T., Zitterl-Eglseer, K., Gutierrez-Lobos, K., Wenzel, T., et al. (2008). Changes in thalamus-hypothalamus serotonin transporter availability during clomipramine administration in patients with obsessive-compulsive disorder. *Neuropsychopharmacology, 33*(13), 3126–3134.

54 Stengler-Wenzke, K., Müller, U., Barthel, H., Angermeyer, M. C., Sabri, O., & Hesse, S. (2006). Serotonin transporter imaging with [123I]beta-CIT SPECT before and after one year of citalopram treatment of obsessive-compulsive disorder. *Neuropsychobiology, 53*(1), 40–45.

55 Zohar, J., Kennedy, J. L., Hollander, E., & Koran, L. M. (2004). Serotonin-1D hypothesis of obsessive-compulsive disorder: An update. *Journal of Clinical Psychiatry, 65*(14), 18–21.

Chapter 5: Atypical Depression

1 Brosnan, S. F. (2008). How primates (including us!) respond to inequity. *Advances in Health Economics and Health Services Research, 20*, 99–124.

2 Bekoff, M., & Pierce, J. (2009). *Wild justice: The moral lives of animals.* Chicago: University Of Chicago Press.

3 Hayden B. Y., Pearson, J. M., & Platt, M. L. (2009). Fictive reward signals in the anterior cingulate cortex. *Science, 324*(5929), 948–950.

4 Pearson, K. A., Watkins, E. R., & Mullan, E. G. (2011). Rejection sensitivity prospectively predicts increased rumination. *Behavior Research and Therapy, 49*(10), 597–605.

5 Billah, T., Catovic, I., Siddique, R., & Siddique, M. (2011). Carbohydrate cravings associated with sleep. *Journal of Sleep and Sleep Disorders Research, 34*(Abstract Supplement), A292.

6 Kahn, J. P., & Sodikoff, C. *Unpublished Data.*

7 Blanco, C., Vesqa-Lopez, O., Stewart, J., Liu, S., Grant, B., & Hasin, D. (2012). Epidemiology of major depression with atypical features: Results from the National Epidemiologic Survey on Alcohol and Related Conditions (NESARC). *Journal of Clinical Psychiatry, 73*(2), 224–232.

8 Davidson, J. R. (2007). A history of the concept of atypical depression. *Journal of Clinical Psychiatry, 68*(3), 10–5.

9 Klein, D. F., & Davis, J. M. (1969). *Diagnosis and drug treatment of psychiatric disorders.* Baltimore, MD: Williams & Wilkins.

10 Romero-Canyas, R., Downey, G., Reddy, K. S., Rodriquez, S., Cavanaugh, T. J., & Pelayo, R. (2010). Paying to belong: When does rejection trigger ingratiation? *Journal of Personality and Social Psychology, 99*(5), 802–823.

11 Trull, T. J., Lippman, L. G., Tragesser, S. L., & Barre, K. C. (2008). Borderline personality disorder features and cognitive, emotional, and predicted behavioral reactions to teasing. *Journal of Research in Personality, 42*(6), 1512–1523.

12 Booker, J. M., & Hellekson, C. J. (1992). Prevalence of seasonal affective disorder in Alaska. *The American Journal of Psychiatry, 149*(9), 1176–1182.

13 Rosen, L. N., Tarqum, S. D., Terman, M., Bryant, M. J., Hoffman, H., Kasper, S. F., et al. (1990). Prevalence of seasonal affective disorder at four latitudes. *Psychiatry Research, 31*(2), 131–144.

14 Harrison, W. M., Sandberg, D., Gorman, J. M., Fyer, M., Nee, J., Uy, J., & Endicott, J. (1989). Provocation of panic with carbon dioxide inhalation in patients with premenstrual dysphoria. *Psychiatry Research, 27*(2), 183–192.

15 Alvergne, A., & Lummaa, V. (2010). Does the contraceptive pill alter mate choice in humans? *Trends in Ecology and Evolution, 25*(3), 171–179.

16 Uphouse, L. (2000). Female gonadal hormones, serotonin, and sexual receptivity. *Brain Research: Brain Research Reviews, 33*(2–3), 242–257.

17 Lerch-Haner, J., Frierson, D., Crawford, L., Beck, S., & Deneris, E. (2008). Serotonergic transcriptional programming determines maternal behavior and offspring survival. *Nature Neuroscience, 11*(9), 1001–1003.

18 Kochanska, G., Barry, R., Jiminez, N., Hollatz, A., & Woodard, J. (2009). Guilt and effortful control: Two mechanisms that prevent disruptive developmental trajectories. *Journal of Personality and Social Psychology, 97*(2), 322–333.

19 Campbell-Meiklejohn, D., Bach, D., Roepstorff, A., Dolan, R., & Frith, C. (2010). How the opinion of others affects our valuation of objects. *Current Biology, 20*(13), 1165–1170.

20 Woodford, R. (2003, September). Lemming suicide myth: Disney film faked bogus behavior. *Alaska Fish & Wildlife News.*

21 Levitan, R. D., Atkinson, L., Pedersen, R., Buis, T., Kennedy, S. H., Chopra, K., et al. (2009). A novel examination of atypical major depressive disorder based on attachment theory. *Journal of Clinical Psychiatry, 70*(6), 879–887.

22 Harkness, K., Washburn, D., Theriault, J., Lee, L., & Sabbaqh, M. (2011). Maternal history of depression is associated with enhanced theory of mind in depressed and nondepressed adult women. *Psychiatry Research, 189*(1), 91–96.

23 Surowiecki, J. (2005). *The wisdom of crowds.* New York: Anchor.

24 Bastian, B., Jetten, J., & Fasoli, F. (2011). Cleansing the soul by hurting the flesh: The guilt-reducing effect of pain. *Psychological Science, 22*(3), 334–335.

25 Gray, H. M., Ishii, K., & Ambady, N. (2011). Misery loves company: When sadness increases the desire for social connectedness. *Personality and Social Psychology Bulletin, 37*(11), 1438–1448.

26 Tan, H. B., & Forgas, J. P. (2010). When happiness makes us selfish, but sadness makes us fair: Affective influences on interpersonal strategies in the dictator game. *Journal of Experimental Social Psychology, 46*(3), 571–576.

27 Galliher, R. V., & Bentley, C. G. (2010). Links between rejection sensitivity and adolescent romantic relationship functioning: The mediating role of problem solving behaviors. *Journal of Aggression, Maltreatment, and Trauma, 19*, 1–21.

28 Harper, M. S., Dickson, J. W., & Welsh, D. P. (2006). Self-silencing and rejection sensitivity in adolescent romantic relationships. *Journal of Youth and Adolescence, 35*(3), 435–443.

29 Tops, M., Riese, H., Oldehinkel, A., Rijsdijk, F., & Ormel, J. (2008). Rejection sensitivity relates to hypocortisolism and depressed mood state in young women. *Psychoneuroendocrinology, 33*(5), 551–559.

30 Blackhart, G., Eckel, L., & Tice, D. (2007). Salivary cortisol in response to acute social rejection and acceptance by peers. *Biological Psychology, 75*(3), 267–276.

31 Downey, G., Freitas, A., Michaelis, B., & Khouri, H. (1998). The self-fulfilling prophecy in close relationships: Rejection sensitivity and rejection by romantic partners. *Journal of Personality and Socical Psychology, 75*(2), 545–560.

32 Park, L. E., Calogero, R. M., Harwin, M. J., & DiRaddo, A. M. (2009). Predicting interest in cosmetic surgery: Interactive effects of appearance-based rejection sensitivity and negative appearance comments. *Body Image, 6*(3), 186–193.

33 Calogero, R. M., Park, L. E., Rahemtulla, Z. H., & Williams, K. C. (2010). Predicting excessive body image concerns among British university students: The unique role of appearance-based rejection sensitivity. *Body Image,7*(1), 78–81.

34 Rose, N., Koperski, S., & Golomb, B. A. (2010). Mood food: Chocolate and depressive symptoms in a cross-sectional analysis. *Archives of Internal Medicine, 170*(8), 699–703.

35 Bruinsma, K., & Taren, D. L. (1999). Chocolate: Food or drug? *Journal of the American Dietetic Association, 99*(10), 1249–1256.

36 Dhir, A., Malik, S., Kessar, S. V., Sinqh, K. N., & Kulkarni, S. K. (2011). Evaluation of antidepressant activity of 1-(7-methoxy-2-methyl-1,2,3,4-tetrahydro-isoquinolin-4-YL)-cyclohexanol, a β-substituted phenylethylamine in mice. *European Neuropsychopharmacology, 21*(9), 705–714.

37 Brahmachary, R. L., & Dutta, J. (1979). Phenylethylamine as a biochemical marker of tiger. *Zeitschrift für Naturforschung: Section C: Biosciences, 34*(7–8), 632–633.

38 Bredy, T., & Barad, M. (2008). Social modulation of associative fear learning by pheromone communication. *Learning & Memory, 16*(1), 12–18.

39 Frederickson, J. (2010). "I'm sorry, please don't hurt me": Effectiveness of apologies on aggression control. *The Journal of Social Psychology, 150*(6), 579–581.

40 Thase, M. (2007). Recognition and diagnosis of atypical depression. *Journal of Clinical Psychiatry, 68*(8), 11–16.

41 Hellerstein, D., Aqosti, V., Bosi, M., & Black, S. (2010). Impairment in psychosocial functioning associated with dysthymic disorder in the NESARC study. *Journal of Affective Disorders, 127*(1–3), 84–88.

42 Twenge, J. M., & Campbell, W. K. (2003). "Isn't it fun to get the respect that we're going to deserve?" Narcissism, social rejection, and aggression. *Personality and Social Psychology Bulletin, 29*(2), 261–272.

43 Bergstrom, R. D., Vought, T., Dulin, M., & Stimers, M. (2009). The spatial distribution of the seven deadly sins within Nevada. *Association of American Geographers Annual Meeting*. Las Vegas, NV.

44 Janka, Z. (2003). [Serotonin dysfunctions in the background of the seven deadly sins]. *Ideggyógyászati Szemle, 56*(11–12), 376–385.

45 DeBaise, C. (2011, June 2). Can you handle rejection? *The Wall Street Journal*. http://blogs.wsj.com/in-charge/2011/06/02/can-you-handle-rejection/

46 Virtanen, M., Stansfeld, S. A., Fuhrer, R., Ferrie, J. E., & Kivimäki, M. (2012). Overtime work as a predictor of major depressive episode: A 5-year follow-up of the Whitehall II Study. *PLoS ONE, 7*(1), e30719.

47 Bibancos, T., Jardim, D., Aneas, I., & Chiavegatto, S. (2007). Social isolation and expression of serotonergic neurotransmission-related genes in several brain areas of male mice. *Genes, Brain, and Behavior, 6*(6), 529–539.

48 Kross, E., Berman, M., Mischel, W., Smith, E., & Wager, T. (2011). Social rejection shares somatosensory representations with physical pain. *Proceedings of the Nationall Academy of Sciences of the United States of America, 108*(15), 6270–6275.

49 Dewall, C. N., Macdonald, G., Webster, G. D., Masten, C. L., Baumeister, R. F., Powell, C., et al. (2010). Acetaminophen reduces social pain: Behavioral and neural evidence. *Psychological Science, 21*(7), 931–937.

50 Terracciano, A., Tanaka, T., Sutin, A. R., Sanna, S., Deiana, B., Lai, S., et al. (2010). Genome-wide association scan of trait depression. *Biological Psychiatry, 68*(9), 811–817.

51 Murakami, N., Kono, R., Nakahara, K., Ida, T., & Kuroda, H. (2000). Induction of unseasonable hibernation and involvement of serotonin in entrance into and maintenance of its hibernation of chipmunks T. asiaticus. *The Journal of Veterinary Medical Science, 62*(7), 763–766.

52 Bruder, G., Stewart, J., McGrath, G., Wexler, B., & Quitkin, F. (2002). Atypical depression: Enhanced right hemispheric dominance for perceiving emotional chimeric faces. *Journal of Abnormal Psychology, 111*(3), 446–454.

53 Burklund, L., Eisenberger, N., & Lieberman, M. (2007). The face of rejection: Rejection sensitivity moderates dorsal anterior cingulate activity to disapproving facial expressions. *Social Neuroscience, 2*(3–4), 238–253.

54 Masten, C. L., Eisenberger, N. I., Borofsky, L. A., Pfeifer, J. H., McNealy, K., Mazziotta, J. C., & Dapretto, M. (2009). Neural correlates of social exclusion during adolescence: Understanding the distress of peer rejection. *Social Cognitive and Affective Neuroscience, 4*(2), 143–57.

55 Farrow, T. F., Zheng, Y., Wilkinson, I. D., Spence, S. A., Deakin, J. F., Tarrier, N., et al. (2001). Investigating the functional anatomy of empathy and forgiveness. *Neuroreport, 12*(11), 2433–2438.

56 Masten, C., Eisenberger, N., Pfeifer, J., & Dapretto, M. (2010). Witnessing peer rejection during early adolescence: Neural correlates of empathy for experiences of social exclusion. *Social Neuroscience, 5*(5–6), 496–507.

57 Masten, C., Morelli, S., & Eisenberger, N. (2011). An fMRI investigation of empathy for 'social pain' and subsequent prosocial behavior. *NeuroImage, 55*(1), 381–388.

58 Willeit, M., Praschak-Rieder, N., Neumeister, A., Zill, P., Leisch, F., Stastny, J., et al. (2003). A polymorphism (5-HTTLPR) in the serotonin transporter promoter gene is

associated with DSM-IV depression subtypes in seasonal affective disorder. *Molecular Psychiatry, 8*(11), 942–946.

Chapter 6: Melancholic Depression

1 Boyle, P. A., Barnes, L. L., Buchman, A. S., & Bennett, D. A. (2009). Purpose in life is associated with mortality among community-dwelling older persons. *Psychosomatic Medicine, 71*(5), 574–579.

2 Gruenewald, T. L., Karlanamqla, A. S., Greendale, G. A., Singer, B. H., & Seeman, T. E. (2007). Feelings of usefulness to others, disability, and mortality in older adults: The MacArthur study of successful aging. *The Journals of Gerontology: Series B: Psychological Sciences and Social Sciences, 62*(1), P28–37.

3 Taylor, M. A., & Fink, M. (2006). *Melancholia: The diagnosis, pathophysiology, and treatment of depressive illness.* New York: Cambridge Univerity Press.

4 Fink, M., & Taylor, M. (2007). Resurrecting melancholia. *Acta Psychiatrica Scandinavica: Supplementum, 433,* 14–20.

5 Parker, G., Fink, M., Shorter, E., Taylor, M. A., Akiskal, H., Berrios, G., et al. (2010). Issues for DSM-5: Whither melancholia? The case for its classification as a distinct mood disorder. *American Journal of Psychiatry, 167*(7), 745–747.

6 Chessick, R. (1992). The death instinct revisited. *The Journal of the American Academy of Psychoanalysis, 20*(1), 3–28.

7 Tully, P., Winefield, H., Baker, R., Turnbull, D., & de Jonge, P. (2011). Confirmatory factor analysis of the Beck Depression Inventory-II and the association with cardiac morbidity and mortality after coronary revascularization. *Journal of Health Psychology, 16*(4), 584–595.

8 von Ammon Cavanaugh, S., Furlanetto, L., Creech, S., & Powell, L. (2001). Medical illness, past depression, and present depression: A predictive triad for in-hospital mortality. *The American Journal of Psychiatry, 158*(1), 43–48.

9 Covinsky, K. E., Kahana, E., Chin, M. H., Palmer, R. M., Fortinsky, R. H., & Landefeld, C. S. (1999). Depressive symptoms and 3-year mortality in older hospitalized medical patients. *Annals of Internal Medicine, 130*(7), 563–569.

10 Takeida, K., Nishi, M., & Miyake, H. (1997). Mental depression and death in elderly persons. *Journal of Epidemiology, 7*(4), 210–213.

11 Vythilingam, M., Chen, J., Bremner, J. D., Mazure, C. M., Maciejewski, P. K., & Nelson, J. C. (2003). Psychotic depression and mortality. *The American Journal of Psychiatry, 160*(3), 574–576..

12 Satin, J. R., Linden, W., & Phillips, M. J. (2009). Depression as a predictor of disease progression and mortality in cancer patients: A meta-analysis. *Cancer, 115*(22), 5349–5361.

13 Pinequart, M., & Duberstein, P. R. (2010). Depression and cancer mortality: A meta-analysis. *Psychological Medicine, 40*(11), 1797–1810.

14 Oldach, D. W., Richards, R. E., Borza, E. N., & Benitez, R. M. (1998). A mysterious death. *The New England Journal of Medicine, 338*(24), 1764–1769.

15 Greenberg, D. B. (2004). Barriers to the treatment of depression in cancer patients. *Journal of the Nationall Cancer Institute: Monographs, 32,* 127–135.

16 Mitchell, A. J., Vahabzadeh, A., & Magruder, K. (2011). Screening for distress and depression in cancer settings: 10 lessons from 40 years of primary-care research. *Psychooncology, 20*(6), 572–584.

17 Gutierrez, B. P. (1998). Variability in the serotonin transporter gene and increased risk for major depression with melancholia. *Human Genetics, 103*(3), 319–322.

18 Baune, B. T., Hohoff, C., Mortensen, L. S., Deckert, J., Arolt, V., & Domschke, K. (2008). Serotonin transporter polymorphism (5-HTTLPR) association with melancholic depression: a female specific effect? *Depression and Anxiety, 25*(11), 920–925.

19 Quinn, Q. R., Dobson-Stone, C., Outhred, T., Harris, A., & Kemp, A. H. (2012). The contribution of BDNF and 5-HTT polymorphisms and early life stress to the heterogeneity of major depressive disorder: A preliminary study. *Australia and New Zealand Journal of Psychiatry, 46*(1), 55–63.

20 McDonald, I. R., Lee, A. K., Than, K. A., & Martin, R. W. (1986). Failure of glucocorticoid feedback in males of a population of small marsupials (Antechinus swainsonii) during the period of mating. *The Journal of Endocrinology, 108*(1), 63–68.

21 Sapolsky, R. M. (2004). *Why zebras don't get ulcers.* New York: Holt.

22 Skulachev, V. P. (2002). Programmed death phenomena: From organelle to organism. *Annals of the New York Academy of Sciences, 959,* 214–237.

23 Pereira, A. M., Tiemensma, J., & Romijn, J. A. (2010). Neuropsychiatric disorders in Cushing's syndrome. *Neuroendocrinology, 92*(1), 65–70.

24 Fareau, G. G., & Vassilopoulou-Sellin, R. (2007). Hypercortisolemia and infection. *Infectious Disease Clinics of North America, 21*(3), 639–657.

25 Dantzer, R., O'Connor, J. C., Freund, G. G., Johnson, R. W., & Kelley, K. W. (2008). From inflammation to sickness and depression: When the immune system subjugates the brain. *Nature Reviews: Neuroscience, 9*(1), 46–56.

26 Harrison, N. A., Brydon, L., Walker, C., Gray, M. A., Steptoe, A., Dolan, R. J., & Critchley, H. D. (2009). Neural origins of human sickness in interoceptive responses to inflammation. *Biological Psychiatry, 66*(5), 415–422.

27 Harrison, N. A., Brydon, L., Walker, C., Gray, M. A., Steptoe, A., & Critchley, H. D. (2009). Inflammation causes mood changes through alterations in subgenual cingulate activity and mesolimbic connectivity. *Biological Psychiatry, 66*(5), 407–414.

28 Slavich, G. M., O'Donovan, A., Epel, E. S., & Kemeny, M. E. (2010). Black sheep get the blues: A psychobiological model of social rejection and depression. *Neuroscience and Biobehavioral Revews, 35*(1), 39–45.

29 Shorter, E., & Fink, M. (2010). *Endocrine psychiatry: Solving the riddle of melancholia.* New York: Oxford University Press.

30 Brown, R. P., Stoll, P. M., Stokes, P. E., Frances, A., Sweeney, J., Kocsis, J. H., & Mann, J. J. (1988). Adrenocortical hyperactivity in depression: Effects of agitation, delusions, melancholia, and other illness variables. *Psychiatry Research, 23*(2), 167–178.

31 Yerevanian, B. I., Feusner, J. D., Koek, R. J., & Mintz, J. (2004). The dexamethasone suppression test as a predictor of suicidal behavior in unipolar depression. *Journal of Affective Disorders, 83*(2–3), 103–108.

32 Meyers, B. S., Alpert, S., Gabriele, M., Kakuma, T., Kalayam, B., & Alexopoulos, G. S. (1993). State specificity of DST abnormalities in geriatric depression. *Biological Psychiatry, 34*(1–2), 108–114.

33 Jokinen, J., Nordstrom, A. L., & Nordstrom, P. (2008). ROC analysis of dexamethasone suppression test threshold in suicide prediction after attempted suicide. *Journal of Affective Disorders, 106*(1–2), 145–152.

34 Dwivedi, Y., Rizavi, H. S., & Pandey, G. N. (2006). Antidepressants reverse corticosterone-mediated decrease in brain-derived neurotrophic factor expression: Differential

regulation of specific exons by antidepressants and corticosterone. *Neuroscience, 139*(3), 1017–1029.

35 Pariante, C. M. (2009). Risk factors for development of depression and psychosis: Glucocorticoid receptors and pituitary implications for treatment with antidepressant and glucocorticoids. *Annals of the New York Academy of Sciences, 1179,* 144–152.

36 Wolkowitz, O. M., Reus, V. I., Manfredi, F., Ingbar, J., Brizendine, L., & Weingartner, H. (1993). Ketoconazole administration in hypercortisolemic depression. *The American Journal of Psychiatry, 150*(5), 810–812.

Chapter 7: Schizophrenia and Psychosis

1 Wrangham, R. (2009). *Catching fire: How cooking made us human.* New York: Basic Books.

2 Mercier, H., & Sperber, D. (2010). Why do humans reason? Arguments for an argumentative theory. *Behavioral and Brain Sciences, 34*(2), 57–74.

3 Anderson, E., Siegel, E. H., Bliss-Moreau, E., & Barrett, L. F. (2011). The visual impact of gossip. *Science, 332*(6036), 1446–1448.

4 Cortina, M., & Liotti, G. (2010). The intersubjective and cooperative origins of consciousness: An evolutionary-developmental approach. *Journal of the American Academy of Psychoanalytic and Dynamic Psychiatry, 38*(2), 291–314.

5 Schlegel, R. J., Hicks, J. A., King, L. A., & Arndt, J. (2011). Feeling like you know who you are: Perceived true self-knowledge and meaning in life. *Personality & Social Psychology Bulletin, 37*(6), 745–756.

6 Moskowitz, A., & Heim, G. (2011). Eugen Bleuler's dementia praecox or the group of schizophrenias (1911): A centenary appreciation and reconsideration. *Schizophrenia Bulletin, 37*(3), 471–479.

7 Burns, J. K. (2004). An evolutionary theory of schizophrenia: Cortical connectivity, metarepresentation, and the social brain. *The Behavioral and Brain Sciences, 27*(6), 831–855, 855–885.

8 Nesse, R. Quoted in Burns, J. K. (2004). An evolutionary theory of schizophrenia: Cortical connectivity, metarepresentation, and the social brain. *The Behavioral and Brain Sciences, 27*(6), 831–855, 855–885.

9 Gale, C. K., Wells, J. E., McGee, M. A., & Browne, M. A. (2011). A latent class analysis of psychosis-like experiences in the New Zealand Mental Health Survey. *Acta Psychiatrica Scandinavica, 124*(3), 205–213.

10 Seeman, P., Schwarz, J., Chen, J. F., Szechtman, H., Perreault, M., McKnight, G. S.,et al. (2006). Psychosis pathways converge via D2high dopamine receptors. *Synapse, 60*(4), 319–346.

11 Wise, R. A. (2008). Dopamine and reward: The anhedonia hypothesis 30 years on. *Neurotoxicity Research, 14*(2–3), 169–183.

12 Bressan, R. A., & Crippa, J. A. (2005). The role of dopamine in reward and pleasure behaviour: Review of data from preclinical research. *Acta Psychiatrica Scandinavica. Supplementum, 427,* 14–21.

13 Pani, L., & Gessa, G. L. (1997). Evolution of the dopaminergic system and its relationships with the psychopathology of pleasure. *International Journal of Clinical Pharmacology Research, 17*(2–3), 55–58.

14 Pani, L. (2000). Is there an evolutionary mismatch between the normal physiology of the human dopaminergic system and current environmental conditions in industrialized countries? *Molecular Psychiatry, 5*(5), 467–475.

15 Salimpoor, V. N., Benovoy, M., Larcher, K., Dagher, A., & Zatorre, R. J. (2011). Anatomically distinct dopamine release during anticipation and experience of peak emotion to music. *Nature Neuroscience, 14*(2), 257–262.

16 Menza, M. A., Golbe, L. I., Cody, R. A., & Forman, N. E. (1993). Dopamine-related personality traits in Parkinson's disease. *Neurology, 43*(3 Pt 1), 505–508.

17 Sharot, T., Shiner, T., Brown, A. C., Fan, J., & Dolan, R. J. (2009). Dopamine enhances expectation of pleasure in humans. *Current Biology, 19*(24), 2077–2080.

18 Bostwick, J. M., Hecksel, K. A., Stevens, S. R., Bower, J. H., & Ahlskog, J. E. (2009). Frequency of new-onset pathologic compulsive gambling or hypersexuality after drug treatment of idiopathic Parkinson disease. *Mayo Clinic Proceedings, 84*(4), 310–316.

19 Holman, A. J. (2009). Impulse control disorder behaviors associated with pramipexole used to treat fibromyalgia. *Journal of Gambling Studies, 25*(3), 425–431.

20 Voon, V., Fernagut, P. O., Wickens, J., Baunez, C., Rodriguez, M., Pavon, N., et al. (2009). Chronic dopaminergic stimulation in Parkinson's disease: From dyskinesias to impulse control disorders. *Lancet Neurology, 8*(12), 1140–1149.

21 Tomei, G., Capozzella A., Ciarrocca, M., Fiore, P., Rosati, M. V., Fiaschetti, M., et al. (2007). Plasma dopamine in workers exposed to urban stressor. *Toxicology and Industrial Health, 23*(7), 421–427.

22 Pezze, M. A., & Feldon, J. (2004). Mesolimbic dopaminergic pathways in fear conditioning. *Progress in Neurobiology, 74*(5), 301–3.

23 Schmidt, R., Morris, G., Hagen, E. H., Sullivan, R. J., Hammerstein, P., & Kempter, R. (2009). The dopamine puzzle. *Proceedings of the National Academy of Sciences of the United States of America, 106*(27), E75.

24 Huertas, E., Ponce, G., Koeneke, M. A., Poch, C., España-Serrano, L., Palomo, T., et al. (2010). The D2 dopamine receptor gene variant C957T affects human fear conditioning and aversive priming. *Genes, Brain, and Behavior, 9*(1), 103–109.

25 Lawrence, A. D., Goerendt, I. K., & Brooks, D. J. (2007). Impaired recognition of facial expressions of anger in Parkinson's disease patients acutely withdrawn from dopamine replacement therapy. *Neuropsychologia, 45*(1), 65–74.

26 Yoshimura, N., Kawamura, M., Masaoka, Y., & Homma, I. (2005). The amygdala of patients with Parkinson's disease is silent in response to fearful facial expressions. *Neuroscience, 131*(2), 523–534.

27 Overall, K. (2011). Personal Communication.

28 Doody, G. A., Götz, M., Johnstone, E. C., Frith, C. D., & Owens, D. G. (1998). Theory of mind and psychoses. *Psychological Medicine, 28*(2), 397–405.

29 Corcoran, R., Mercer, G. &, Frith, C. D. (1995). Schizophrenia, symptomatology and social inference: Investigating "theory of mind" in people with schizophrenia. *Schizophrenia Research, 17*(1), 5–13.

30 Frith, C. D., & Corcoran, R. (1996). Exploring 'theory of mind' in people with schizophrenia. *Psychological Medicine, 26*(3), 521–530.

31 Bora, E., Eryavuz, A., Kayahan, B., Sungu, G., & Veznedaroglu, B. (2006). Social functioning, theory of mind and neurocognition in outpatients with schizophrenia: Mental state decoding may be a better predictor of social functioning than mental state reasoning. *Psychiatry Research, 145*(2–3), 95–103.

32 Paulik, G., Badcock, J. C., & Maybery, M. T. (2007). Poor intentional inhibition in individuals predisposed to hallucinations. *Cognitive Neuropsychiatry, 12*(5), 457–470.

33 Simonsen, C., Sundet, K., Vaskinn, A., Birkenaes, A. B., Engh, J. A., Faerden, A., et al. (2011). Neurocognitive dysfunction in bipolar and schizophrenia spectrum disorders depends on history of psychosis rather than diagnostic group. *Schizophrenia Bulletin, 37*(1), 73–83.

34 Lera, G., Herrero, N., González, J., Aguilar, E., Sanjuán, J., & Leal, C. (2011). Insight among psychotic patients with auditory hallucinations. *Journal of Clinical Psychology, 67*(7), 701–708.

35 van der Meer, L., Groenewold, N., Nolen, W., & Aleman André. (2010). The neural basis of inhibiting one's own perspective in psychosis proneness: An fMRI study. *Early Psychoses: A Lifetime Perspective. Early Intervention in Psychiatry, 4*(1), 39.

36 Hooker, C. I., Aleman, A., van der Meer, L., & Modinos, G. (2010). Neural mechanisms of social and emotional processing in psychosis-prone populations. *Early Psychoses: A Lifetime Perspective. Early Intervention in Psychiatry, 4*(1), 39.

37 Paruch, J., Nikolaides, A., Klosterkötter, J., & Ruhrmann, S. (2010). Visual scan paths to affective facial expressions and relations to social functioning in individuals at risk. *Early Psychoses: A Lifetime Perspective. Early Intervention in Psychiatry, 4*(1), 41.

38 Stain, H. J., Hodne, S., Joa, I., ten Velden Hegelstad, W., Douglas, K. M., Langveld, J., et al. (2010). Story production and social functioning in first episode psychosis: Relationship to verbal learning and fluency. *Early Psychoses: A Lifetime Perspective. Early Intervention in Psychiatry, 4*(1), 77.

39 Nikolaides, A., Paruch, J., Klosterkötter, J., & Ruhrmann, S. (2010). Association of psychopathological measures and visual scanning behaviour of socially relevant material in individuals at high risk. *Early Psychoses: A Lifetime Perspective. Early Intervention in Psychiatry, 4*(1), 42.

40 Modinos, G., Renken, R., Shamay-Tsoory, S. G., Ormel, J., & Aleman, A. (2010). Neurobiological correlates of theory of mind in psychosis proneness. *Early Psychoses: A Lifetime Perspective. Early Intervention in Psychiatry, 4*(1), 38.

41 Lincoln, S. H. (2010). The process of simulation in individuals at clinical risk for psychosis. *Early Psychoses: A Lifetime Perspective. Early Intervention in Psychiatry, 4*(1), 40.

42 Havas, D. A., Glenberg, A. M., Gutowski, K. A., Lucarelli, M. J., & Davidson, R. J. (2010). Cosmetic use of botulinum toxin-a affects processing of emotional language. *Psychological Science, 21*(7), 895–900.

43 Davis, J. I., Senghas, A., Brandt, F., & Ochsner, K. N. (2010). The effects of BOTOX injections on emotional experience. *Emotion, 10*(3), 433–440.

44 Neal, D. T., & Chartrand, T. L. (2011). Embodied emotion perception: Amplifying and dampening facial feedback modulates emotion perception accuracy. *Social Psychological and Personality Science, 2*(6), 673–678.

45 Weinberger, D. R., & Berman, K. F. (1988). Speculation on the meaning of cerebral metabolic hypofrontality in schizophrenia. *Schizophrenia Bulletin, 14*(2), 157–168.

46 Rimol, L. M., Hartberg, C. B., Nesvåg, R., Fennema-Notestine, C., Hagler, D. J. Jr., Pung, C. J., et al. (2010). Cortical thickness and subcortical volumes in schizophrenia and bipolar disorder. *Biological Psychiatry, 68*(1), 41–50.

47 Cullen, A. E., De Brito, S., Gregory, S., Williams, S. C. R., Murray, R. M., Hodgins, S., & Laurens, K. R. (2010). Grey matter abnormalities in children aged 9–13 years presenting

antecedents of schizophrenia: a voxel-based morphometry study. *Early Psychoses: A Lifetime Perspective. Early Intervention in Psychiatry, 4*(1), 45.

48 Schulz, C. C., Koch, K., Wagner, G., Roebel, M., Schachtzabel, C., Gaser, C., et al. (2010). Reduced cortical thickness in first episode schizophrenia. *Schizophrenia Research, 116*(2–3), 204–209.

49 Buchy, L. A.-D. (2011). Cortical thickness is associated with poor insight in first-episode psychosis. *Journal of Psychiatric Research, 45*(6), 781–787.

50 Crespo-Facorro, B., Roiz-Santiáñez, R., Pérez-Iglesias, R., Rodriguez-Sanchez, J. M., Mata, I., Tordesillas-Gutierrez, D., et al. (2011). Global and regional cortical thinning in first-episode psychosis patients: Relationships with clinical and cognitive features. *Psychological Medicine, 41*(7), 1449–1460.

51 Nesse, R. M. (2009). Evolution at 150: Time for truly biological psychiatry. *The British Journal of Psychiatry: The Journal of Mental Science, 195*(6), 471–472.

52 Betcheva, E. T., Mushiroda, T., Takahashi, A., Kubo, M., Karanchanak, S. K., Zaharieva, I. T., et al. (2009). Case-control association study of 59 candidate genes reveals the DRD2 SNP rs6277 (C957T) as the only susceptibility factor for schizophrenia in the Bulgarian population. *Journal of Human Genetics, 54*(2), 98–107.

53 Hoenicka, J., Aragüés, M., Rodgríguez-Jiménez, R., Ponce, G., Martínez, I., Rubio, G. et al, Psychosis and Addictions Research Group (PARG). (2006). C957T DRD2 polymorphism is associated with schizophrenia in Spanish patients. *Acta Psychiatrica Scandinavica, 114*(6), 435–438.

54 Lawford, B. R., Young, R. M., Swagell, C. D., Barnes, M., Burton, S. C., Ward, W. K., et al. (2005). The C/C genotype of the C957T polymorphism of the dopamine D2 receptor is associated with schizophrenia. *Schizophrenia Research, 73*(1), 31–37.

55 Colzato, L. S., van den Wildenberg, W. P., Van der Does, A. J., & Hommel, B. (2010). Genetic markers of striatal dopamine predict individual differences in dysfunctional, but not functional impulsivity. *Neuroscience, 170*(3), 782–788.

56 Xu, H., Kellendonk, C. B., Simpson, E. H., Keilp, J. G., Bruder, G. E., Polan, H. J., et al. (2007). DRD2 C957T polymorphism interacts with the COMT Val158Met polymorphism in human working memory ability. *Schizophrenia Research, 90*(1–3), 104–107.

57 White, M. J., Lawford, B. R., Morris, C. P., & Young, R. M. (2009). Interaction between DRD2 C957T polymorphism and an acute psychosocial stressor on reward-related behavioral impulsivity. *Behavior Genetics, 39*(3), 285–295.

58 Colzato, L. S., Slagter, H. A., de Rover, M., & Hommel, B. (2011). Dopamine and the management of attentional resources: genetic markers of striatal d2 dopamine predict individual differences in the attentional blink. *Journal of Cognitive Neuroscience, 23*(11), 3576–3585.

59 Buonanno, A. (2010). The neuregulin signaling pathway and schizophrenia: From genes to synapses and neural circuits. *Brain Research Bulletin, 83*(3–4), 122–131.

60 Kéri, S. (2009). Genes for psychosis and creativity: A promoter polymorphism of the neuregulin 1 gene is related to creativity in people with high intellectual achievement. *Psychological Science, 20*(9), 1070–1073.

61 Esslinger, C., Walter, H., Kirsch, P., Erk, S., Schnell, K., Arnold, C., et al. (2009). Neural mechanisms of a genome-wide supported psychosis variant. *Science, 324*(5927), 605.

62 Mechelli, A., Viding, E., Pettersson-Yeo, W., Tognin, S., & McGuire, P. K. (2009). Genetic variation in neuregulin1 is associated with differences in prefrontal engagement in children. *Human Brain Mapping, 30*(12), 3934–3943.

63 Alaerts, M., Ceulemans, S., Forero, D., Moens, L. N., De Zutter, S., Heyrman, L., et al. (2009). Support for NRG1 as a susceptibility factor for schizophrenia in a northern Swedish isolated population. *Archives of General Psychiatry, 66*(8), 828–837.

64 Mill, J., Tang, T., Kaminsky, Z., Khare, T., Yazdanpanah, S., Bouchard, L., et al. (2008). Epigenomic profiling reveals DNA-methylation changes associated with major psychosis. *American Journal of Human Genetics, 82*(3), 696–711.

65 Rutten, B. P., & Mill, J. (2009). Epigenetic mediation of environmental influences in major psychotic disorders. *Schizophrenia Bulletin, 35*(6), 1045–1056.

66 Del Giudice, M. (2010). Reduced fertility in patients' families is consistent with the sexual selection model of schizophrenia and schizotypy. *PLoS One, 5*(12), e16040.

67 Kramer, P. F., Christensen C. H., Hazelwood, L. A., Dobi, A., Bock, R., Sibley, D. R., et al. (2011). Dopamine D2 receptor overexpression alters behavior and physiology in Drd2-EGFP mice. *The Journal of Neuroscience: The Official Journal of the Society for Neuroscience, 31*(1), 126–132.

68 DeMichele-Sweet, M. A., & Sweet, R. A. (2010). Genetics of psychosis in Alzheimer's disease: A review. *Journal of Alzheimer's Disease, 19*(3), 761–780.

69 Middle, F., Pritchard, A. L., Handoko, H., Hague, S., Holder, R., Bentham, P., & Lendon, C. L. (2010). No association between neuregulin 1 and psychotic symptoms in Alzheimer's disease patients. *Journal of Alzheimer's Disease, 20*(2), 561–567.

70 Fernández, M., Gobartt, A. L., Balaña, M., & COOPERA Study Group. (2010). Behavioural symptoms in patients with Alzheimer's disease and their association with cognitive impairment. *BMC Neurology, 10,* 87.

71 Ropacki, S. A., & Jeste, D. V. (2005). Epidemiology of and risk factors for psychosis of Alzheimer's disease: A review of 55 studies published from 1990 to 2003. *The American Journal of Psychiatry, 162*(11), 2022–2030.

72 Helsen, G. (2011). General paresis of the insane: A case with MR imaging. *Acta Neurologica Belgica, 111*(1), 69–71.

73 Lewis-Hanna, L. L., Hunter, M. D., Farrow, T. F., Wilkinson, I. D., & Woodruff, P. W. (2011). Enhanced cortical effects of auditory stimulation and auditory attention in healthy individuals prone to auditory hallucinations during partial wakefulness. *NeuroImage, 57*(3), 1154–1161.

74 Schmidt, R. E., & Gendolla, G. H. (2008). Dreaming of white bears: The return of the suppressed at sleep onset. *Consciousness and Cognition, 17*(3), 714–724.

75 Limosani, I., D'Agostino, A., Manzone, M. L., & Scarone, S. (2011). The dreaming brain/mind, consciousness and psychosis. *Consciousness and Cognition, 20*(4), 987–992.

76 Devillières, P., Opitz, M., Clervoy, P., & Stephany, J. (1996). Delusion and sleep deprivation. *L'Encéphale, 22*(3), 229–231.

77 Kahn-Greene, E. T., Killgore, D. B., Kamimori, G. H., Balkin, T. J., & Killgore, W. D. (2007). The effects of sleep deprivation on symptoms of psychopathology in healthy adults. *Sleep Medicine, 8*(3), 215–221.

78 Woodward, N. D., Cowan, R. L., Park, S., Ansari, M. S., Baldwin, R. M., Li, R., et al. (2011). Correlation of individual differences in schizotypal personality traits with amphetamine-induced dopamine release in striatal and extrastriatal brain regions. *The American Journal of Psychiatry, 168*(4), 418–426.

79 Domínguez, T., Vilagrà, R., Blanqué, J. M., Vainer, E., Berni, R., Montoro, M., et al. (2010). The association between relatives' expressed emotion with clinical and functional features of early-psychosis patients. *Early Psychoses: A Lifetime Perspective. Early Intervention in Psychiatry, 4*(1), 55.

80 Kéri, S., Kiss, I., Seres, I., & Kelemen, O. (2009). A polymorphism of the neuregulin 1 gene (SNP8NRG243177/rs6994992) affects reactivity to expressed emotion in schizophrenia. *American Journal of Medical Genetics. Part B, Neuropsychiatric genetics, 150B*(3), 418–420.

81 Monden, M. A. (2010). Development of first psychosis during travel. *Early Psychoses: A Lifetime Perspective. Early Intervention in Psychiatry, 4*(1), 69.

82 Kinoshita, Y., Kingdon, D., Kinoshita, K., Sarafudheen, S. Umadi, D., Dayson, D., et al. (2012). A semi-structured clinical interview for psychosis sub-groups (SCIPS): Development and psychometric properties. *Social Psychiatry and Psychiatric Epidemiology, 47*(4), 563–580.

83 Sim, M., Kim, J. H., Yim, S. J., Cho, S. J., & Kim, S. J. (2012). Increase in harm avoidance by genetic loading of schizophrenia. *Comprehensive Psychiatry, 53*(4), 372–378.

84 Buckley, P. F., Miller, B. J., Lehrer, D. S., & Castle, D. J. (2009). Psychiatric comorbidities and schizophrenia. *Schizophrenia Bulletin, 35*(2), 383–402.

85 Varghese, D., Scott, J., Welham, J., Bor, W., Naiman, J., O'Callaghan, M., et al. (2011). Psychotic-like experiences in major depression and anxiety disorders: A population-based survey in young adults. *Schizophrenia Bulletin, 37*(2), 389–393.

86 Ciapparelli, A., Paggini, R., Marazziti, D., Carmassi, C., Bianchi, M., Taponecco, C., et al. (2007). Comorbidity with axis I anxiety disorders in remitted psychotic patients 1 year after hospitalization. *CNS Spectrums, 12*(12), 913–919.

87 Baylé, F. J., Blanc, O., De Chazeron, I., Lesturgeon, J., Lancon, C., Caci, H., et al. (2011). Pharmacological management of anxiety in patients suffering from schizophrenia. *L'Encéphale, 37*(1), S83–89.

88 Savitz, A. J., Kahn, T. A., McGovern, K. E., & Kahn, J. P. (2011). Carbon dioxide induction of panic anxiety in schizophrenia with auditory hallucinations. *Psychiatry Research, 189*(1), 38–42.

89 Cassano, G. B., Pini, S., Saettoni, M., Rucci, P., & Dell'Osso, L. (1998). Occurrence and clinical correlates of psychiatric comorbidity in patients with psychotic disorders. *The Journal of Clinical Psychiatry, 59*(2), 60–68.

90 Roy, M.-A. (2010). Improving the detection of anxiety disorders in early psychosis. *Early Intervention in Psychiatry, 4*(1), 51..

91 Kahn, J. P., & Meyers, J. R. (2000). Treatment of comorbid panic disorder and schizophrenia: Evidence for a panic psychosis. *Psychiatric Annals, 30*(1), 29–33.

92 Kahn, J. P., Puertollano, M. A., Schane, M. D., & Klein, D. F. (1988). Adjunctive alprazolam for schizophrenia with panic anxiety: Clinical observation and pathogenetic implications. *The American Journal of Psychiatry, 145*(6), 742–744.

93 Pfleiderer, B., Zinkirciran, S., Michael, N., Hohoff, C., Kersting, A., Arolt, V., et al. (2010). Altered auditory processing in patients with panic disorder: A pilot study. *The World Journal of Biological Psychiatry, 11*(8), 945–955.

94 Lysaker, P. H., & Salyers, M. P. (2007). Anxiety symptoms in schizophrenia spectrum disorders: associations with social function, positive and negative symptoms, hope and trauma history. *Acta Psychiatrica Scandinavica, 116*(4), 290–298.

95 Smith, D. B. (2007). *Muses, madmen, and prophets.* New York: Penguin.

96 Bermanzohn, P. C., Porto, L., Arlow, P. B., Pollack, S., Stronger, R., & Siris, S. G. (2000). Hierarchical diagnosis in chronic schizophrenia: A clinical study of co-occurring syndromes. *Schizophrenia Bulletin, 26*(3), 517–525.

97 Kimhy, D., Goetz, R., Yale, S., Corcoran, C. & Malaspina, D. (2005). Delusions in individuals with schizophrenia: Factor structure, clinical correlates, and putative neurobiology. *Psychopathology, 38*(6), 338–344.

98 Nishimura, Y., Tanii, H., Hara, N., Inoue, K., Kaiya, H., Nishida, A., et al. (2009). Relationship between the prefrontal function during a cognitive task and the severity of the symptoms in patients with panic disorder: A multi-channel NIRS study. *Psychiatry Research, 172*(2), 168–172.

99 Maron, E., Nutt, D. J., Kuikka, J., & Tiihonen, J. (2010). Dopamine transporter binding in females with panic disorder may vary with clinical status. *Journal of Psychiatric Research, 44*(1), 56–59.

100 Kahn, J. P., Puertollano, M., Schane, M. D., & Klein, D. F. (1987). Schizophrenia, panic anxiety, and alprazolam. *The American Journal of Psychiatry, 144*(4), 527–528.

101 Guidotti, A., Auta, J., Davis, J. M., Dong, E., Grayson, D. R., Veldic, M., et al. (2005). GABAergic dysfunction in schizophrenia: New treatment strategies on the horizon. *Psychopharmacology, 180*(2), 191–205.

102 Mazeh, D., Bodner, E., Weizman, R., Delayahu, Y., Cholostov, A., Martin, T., & Barak, Y. (2009). Co-morbid social phobia in schizophrenia. *The International Journal of Social Psychiatry, 55*(3), 198–202.

103 Pallanti, S., Quercioli, L., & Hollander, E. (2004). Social anxiety in outpatients with schizophrenia: A relevant cause of disability. *The American Journal of Psychiatry, 161*(1), 53–58.

104 Pallanti, S., Quercioli, L., & Pazzagli A. (2000). Social anxiety and premorbid personality disorders in paranoid schizophrenic patients treated with clozapine. *CNS Spectrums, 5*(9), 29–43.

105 Tone, E. B., Goulding, S. M., & Compton, M. T. (2011). Associations among perceptual anomalies, social anxiety, and paranoia in a college student sample. *Psychiatry Research, 188*(2), 258–263.

106 Veras, A. B., do-Nascimento, J. S., Rodruigues, R. L., Guimarães, A. C., & Nardi, A. E. (2011). Psychotic symptoms in social anxiety disorder patients: Report of three cases. *International Archives of Medicine, 4*(1), 12.

107 Langdon, R., McGuire, J., Stevenson, R., & Catts, S. V. (2011). Clinical correlates of olfactory hallucinations in schizophrenia. *The British Journal of Clinical Psychology, 50*(2), 145–163.

108 Romm, K. L., Rossberg, J. I., Berg, A. O., Hansen, C. F. Andreassen, O. A., & Melle, I. (2011). Assessment of social anxiety in first episode psychosis using the Liebowitz Social Anxiety scale as a self-report measure. *European Psychiatry, 26*(2), 115–121.

109 Lysaker, P. H., Yanos, P. T., Outcalt, J., & Roe, D. (2010). Association of stigma, self-esteem, and symptoms with concurrent and prospective assessment of social anxiety in schizophrenia. *Clinical Schizophrenia & Related Psychoses, 4*(1), 41–48.

110 Lysaker, P. H., Davis, L. W., & Tsai, J. (2009). Suspiciousness and low self-esteem as predictors of misattributions of anger in schizophrenia spectrum disorders. *Psychiatry Research, 166*(2–3), 125–131.

111 Warman, D. M., Lysaker, P. H., Luedtke, B., & Martin, J. M. (2010). Self-esteem and delusion proneness. *The Journal of Nervous and Mental Disease, 198*(6), 455–457.

112 Kinoshita, Y., Kingdon, D., Kinoshita, K., Kinoshita, Y., Saka, K., Arisue, Y., et al. (2011). Fear of negative evaluation is associated with delusional ideation in non-clinical population and patients with schizophrenia. *Social Psychiatry and Psychiatric Epidemiology, 46*(8), 703–710.

113 Lysaker, P. H., Salvatore, G., Grant, M. L., Procacci, M., Olesek, K. L., Buck, K. D., et al. (2010). Deficits in theory of mind and social anxiety as independent paths to paranoid features in schizophrenia. *Schizophrenia Research, 124*(1–3), 81–85.

114 Kummer, A. Cardoso, F., & Texeira, A. L. (2008). Frequency of social phobia and psychometric properties of the Liebowitz social anxiety scale in Parkinson's disease. *Movement Disorders, 23*(12), 1739–1743.

115 Stefanis, N., Bozi, M., Christodoulou, C., Douzenis, A., Gasparinatos, G., Stamboulis, E., et al. (2010). Isolated delusional syndrome in Parkinson's Disease. *Parkinsonism & Related Disorders, 16*(8), 550–552.

116 Ecker, D., Unrath, A., Kassubek, J., & Sabolek, M. (2009). Dopamine agonists and their risk to induce psychotic episodes in Parkinson's disease: A case-control study. *BMC Neurology, 9*, 23.

117 Lysaker, P. H., & Whitney, K. A. (2009). Obsessive-compulsive symptoms in schizophrenia: Prevalence, correlates and treatment. *Expert Review of Neurotherapeutics, 9*(1), 99–107.

118 Owashi, T., Ota, A., Otsubo, T., Susa, Y., & Kamijima, K. (2010). Obsessive-compulsive disorder and obsessive-compulsive symptoms in Japanese inpatients with chronic schizophrenia: A possible schizophrenic subtype. *Psychiatry Research, 179*(3), 241–246.

119 Faragian, S., Pashinian, A., Fuchs, C., & Poyurovsky, M. (2009). Obsessive-compulsive symptom dimensions in schizophrenia patients with comorbid obsessive-compulsive disorder. *Progress in Neuro-Psychopharmacology & Biological Psychiatry, 33*(6), 1009–1012.

120 Van Dael, F., van Os, J., de Graaf, R., ten Have, M., & Myin-Germeys, I. (2010). Can obsessions drive you mad? Longitudinal evidence that obsessive-compulsive symptoms worsen the outcome of early psychotic experiences. *Early Psychoses: A Lifetime Perspective. Early Intervention in Psychiatry, 4*(1), 52.

121 Fontanelle, L., Lin, A., Pantelis, C., Wood, S., Nelson, B., & Yung, A. (2011). A longitudinal study of obsessive-compulsive disorder in individuals at ultra-high risk for psychosis. *Journal of Psychiatric Research, 45*(9), 1140–1145.

122 Bottas, A., Cooke, R. G., & Richter, M. A. (2005). Comorbidity and pathophysiology of obsessive-compulsive disorder in schizophrenia: Is there evidence for a schizo-obsessive subtype of schizophrenia? *Journal of Psychiatry & Neuroscience, 30*(3), 187–193.

123 Klemperer, F. (1996). Compulsions developing into command hallucinations. *Psychopathology, 29*(4), 249–251.

124 Fontanelle, L. F., Lopes, A. P., Borges, M. C., Pacheco, P. G., Nascimento, A. L., & Versiani, M. (2008). Auditory, visual, tactile, olfactory, and bodily hallucinations in patients with obsessive-compulsive disorder. *CNS Spectrums, 13*(2), 125–130.

125 Hermesh, H., Konas, S., Shiloh, R., Dar, R., Marom, S., Weizman, A., & Gross-Isseroff, R. (2004). Musical hallucinations: Prevalence in psychotic and nonpsychotic outpatients. *The Journal of Clinical Psychiatry, 65*(2), 191–197.

126 Sanchez, T. G., Rocha, S. C., Knobel, K. A., Kii, M. A., dos Santos, R. M., & Pereira, C. B. (2011). Musical hallucination associated with hearing loss. *Arquivos de Neuro-Psiquiatria, 69*(2B), 395–400.

127 Merabet, L. B., Maguire, D., Warde, A., Alterescu, K., Stickgold, R., & Pascual-Leone, A. (2004). Visual hallucinations during prolonged blindfolding in sighted subjects. *Journal of Neuro-Opthamology, 24*(2), 109–113.

128 Hylwa, S. A., Bury, J. E., Davis, M. D., Pittelkow M., & Bostwick, J. M. (2011). Delusional infestation, including delusions of parasitosis: Results of histologic examination of skin biopsy and patient-provided skin specimens. *Archives of Dermatology, 147*(9), 1041–1045.

129 Calikuşu, C., Yücel, B., Polat, A., & Baykal, C. (2003). The relation of psychogenic excoriation with psychiatric disorders: A comparative study. *Comprehensive Psychiatry,*
44(3), 256–261.

130 Engler, D. E. (2011). Personal Communication.

131 Pearson, M. L., Selby, J. V., Katz, K. A., Cantrell, V., Braden, C. R., Parise, M. E., et al.
(2012). Clinical, epidemiologic, histopathologic and molecular features of an unex-
plained dermopathy. *PLoS ONE, 7*(1), e29908.

132 Simonsen, H., Shand, A. J., Scott, N. W., & Eagles, J. M. (2011). Seasonal symptoms in
bipolar and primary care patients. *Journal of Affective Disorders, 132*(1–2), 200–208.

133 Rybakowski, J. K., Suwalska, A., Loiko, D., Rymanaszewska, J., & Kiejna, A. (2007).
Types of depression more frequent in bipolar than in unipolar affective illness: Results
of the Polish DEP-BI study. *Psychopathology, 40*(3), 153–158.

134 Blanco, C., Vesga-López, O., Stewart, J. W., Liu, S. M., Grant, B. F., & Hasin, D. S.
(2012). Epidemiology of major depression with atypical features: Results from the
National Epidemiologic Survey on Alcohol and Related Conditions (NESARC). *The*
Journal of Clinical Psychiatry, 73(2), 224–32.

135 Salvadore, G., Quiroz, J. A., Machado-Vieira, R., Henter, I. D., Manji, H. K., & Zarate
C. A., Jr. (2010). The neurobiology of the switch process in bipolar disorder: A review.
The Journal of Clinical Psychiatry, 71(11), 1488–1501.

136 Proudfoot, J., Doran, J., Manicavasagar, V., & Parker, G. (2011). The precipitants of
manic/hypomanic episodes in the context of bipolar disorder: A review. *Journal of*
Affective Disorders, 133(3), 381–387.

137 Hamilton, J. W. (2006). The critical effect of object loss in the development of episodic
manic illness. *The Journal of the American Academy of Psychoanalysis and Dynamic*
Psychiatry, 34(2), 333–348.

138 Pinsonneault, J. K., Han, D. D., Burdick, K. E., Kataki, M., Bertolino, A., Malhotra, A.
K., et al. (2011). Dopamine transporter gene variant affecting expression in human brain
is associated with bipolar disorder. *Neuropsychopharmacology, 36*(8), 1644–1655.

139 Adida, M., Clark, L., Pomietto, P., Kaladjian, A., Besnier, N., Azorin, J. M., et al. (2008).
Lack of insight may predict impaired decision making in manic patients. *Bipolar*
Disorders, 10(7), 829–837.

140 Adida, M., Jollant, F., Clark, L., Besnier, N., Guillaume, S., Kaladjian, A., et al. (2011).
Trait-related decision-making impairment in the three phases of bipolar disorder.
Biological Psychiatry, 70(4), 357–365..

141 Georgieva, L., Dimitrova, A., Ivanov, D., Nikolov, I., Williams, N. M., Grozeva, D.,
et al. (2008). Support for neuregulin 1 as a susceptibility gene for bipolar disorder and
schizophrenia. *Biological Psychiatry, 64*(5), 419–427.

142 Kupferschmidt, D. A., & Zakzanis, K. K. (2011). Toward a functional neuroanatomical
signature of bipolar disorder: Quantitative evidence from the neuroimaging literature.
Psychiatry Research, 193(2), 71–79.

143 Foland-Ross, L. C., Thompson, P. M., Sugar, C. A., Madsen, S. K., Shen, J. K., Penfold,
C., et al. (2011). Investigation of cortical thickness abnormalities in lithium-free adults
with bipolar I disorder using cortical pattern matching. *The American Journal of*
Psychiatry, 168(5), 530–539.

144 Ekman, C. J., Lind, J., Rydén, E., Ingvar, M., & Landén, M. (2010). Manic episodes
are associated with grey matter volume reduction: A voxel-based morphometry brain analysis. *Acta Psychiatrica Scandinavica, 122*(6), 507–515. doi: 10.1111/
j.1600–0447.2010.01586.x

145 Malhi, G. S., Lagopoulos, J., Das, P., Moss, K., Berk, M., & Coulston, C. M. (2008). A functional MRI study of theory of mind in euthymic bipolar disorder patients. *Bipolar Disorders, 10*(8), 943–956.

146 Foland, L. C., Altshuler, L. L., Bookheimer, S. Y., Eisenberger, N., Townsend, J., & Thompson, P. M. (2008). Evidence for deficient modulation of amygdala response by prefrontal cortex in bipolar mania. *Psychiatry Research, 162*(1), 27–37.

147 Green, M. J., Lino, B. J., Hwang, E. J., Sparks, A., James, C., & Mitchell, P. B. (2011). Cognitive regulation of emotion in bipolar I disorder and unaffected biological relatives. *Acta Psychiatrica Scandinavica, 124*(4), 307–316. doi: 10.1111/j.1600–0447.2011.01718.x.

148 Carrard, A., Salzmann, A., Malafosse, A., & Karege, F. (2011). Increased DNA methylation status of the serotonin receptor 5HTR1A gene promoter in schizophrenia and bipolar disorder. *Journal of Affective Disorders, 132*(3), 450–453.

149 Sobczak, S., Riedel, W. J., Booij, I., Aan Het Rot, M., Deutz, N. E., & Honig, A. (2002). Cognition following acute tryptophan depletion: Difference between first-degree relatives of bipolar disorder patients and matched healthy control volunteers. *Psychological Medicine, 32*(3), 503–515.

150 Daray, F. M., Thommi, S. B., & Ghaemi, S. N. (2010). The pharmacogenetics of antidepressant-induced mania: A systematic review and meta-analysis. *Bipolar Disorders, 12*(7), 702–706.

151 John, A. P., & Koloth, R. (2007). Severe serotonin toxicity and manic switch induced by combined use of tramadol and paroxetine. *The Australian and New Zealand Journal of Psychiatry, 41*(2), 192–193.

152 Yatham, L. N., Liddle, P. F., Erez, J., Kauer-Sant'Anna, M., Lam, R. W., Imperial, M., et al. (2010). Brain serotonin-2 receptors in acute mania. *The British Journal of Psychiatry, 196*(1), 47–51.

153 Griesinger, W. (1882). *Mental pathology and therapeutics.* (C. L. Robertson, Trans.) New York: William Wood. Retrieved from http://www.archive.org/details/mentalpathology00robegoog

154 Kim, D. R., Czarkowski, K. A., & Epperson, C. N. (2011). The relationship between bipolar disorder, seasonality, and premenstrual symptoms. *Current Psychiatry Reports, 13*(6), 500–503.

155 Conci Magris, D. M. (2009). Seasonal pattern in hospital admissions due to bipolar disorder in Santa María, Córdoba, Argentina. *Vertex, 20*(83), 10–15.

156 Ciarleglio, C. M., Resuehr, H. E., & McMahon, D. G. (2011). Interactions of the serotonin and circadian systems: Nature and nurture in rhythms and blues. *Neuroscience, 197*, 8–16.

157 Popova, N. K., & Voitenko, N. N. (1981). Brain serotonin metabolism in hibernation. *Pharmacology, Biochemistry, and Behavior, 14*(6), 773–777.

158 Naumenko, V. S., Tkachev, S. E., Kulikov, A. V., Semenova, T. P., Amerhanov, Z. G., Smirnova, N. P., & Popova, N. K. (2008). The brain 5-HT1A receptor gene expression in hibernation. *Genes, Brain, and Behavior, 7*(3), 300–305.

159 Moore, G. J., Cortese, B. M., Glitz, D. A., Zajac-Benitez, C., Quiroz, J. A., Uhde, T. W., et al. (2009). A longitudinal study of the effects of lithium treatment on prefrontal and subgenual prefrontal gray matter volume in treatment-responsive bipolar disorder patients. *The Journal of Clinical Psychiatry, 70*(5), 699–705.

160 Harrison-Read, P. E. (2009). Antimanic potency of typical neuroleptic drugs and affinity for dopamine D2 and serotonin 5-HT2A receptors – a new analysis of data

from the archives and implications for improved antimanic treatments. *Journal of Psychopharmacology, 23*(8), 899–907.

161 Applebaum, J., Bersudsky, Y., & Klein, E. (2007). Rapid tryptophan depletion as a treatment for acute mania: A double-blind, pilot-controlled study. *Bipolar Disorders, 9*(8), 884–887.

162 Milici, P. S. (1950). The involutional death reaction. *The Psychiatric Quarterly, 24*(4), 775–781.

163 Flint, A. J., Peasley-Miklus, C., Papademetriou, E., Meyers, B. S., Mulsant, B. H., Rothschild, A. J., Whyte, E. M., & STOP-PD Study Group. (2010). Effect of age on the frequency of anxiety disorders in major depression with psychotic features. *The American Journal of Geriatric Psychiatry, 18*(5), 404–412.

164 Carroll, B. J., Cassidy, F., Naftolowitz, D., Tatham, N. E., Wilson, W. H., Iranmanesh, A., et al. (2007). Pathophysiology of hypercortisolism in depression. *Acta Psychiatrica Scandinavica. Supplementum, 433*, 90–103.

165 Nelson, J. C., & Davis, J. M. (1997). DST studies in psychotic depression: A meta-analysis. *The American Journal of Psychiatry, 154*(11), 1497–1503.

166 Owasahi, T., Otsubo, T., Oshima, A., Nakagome, K., Higuchi, T., & Kamijima, K. (2008). Longitudinal neuroendocrine changes assessed by dexamethasone/CRH and growth hormone releasing hormone tests in psychotic depression. *Psychoneuroendocrinology, 33*(2), 152–161.

167 Blasey, C. M., Debattista, C., Roe, R., Block, T., & Belanoff, J. K. (2009). A multisite trial of mifepristone for the treatment of psychotic depression: A site-by-treatment interaction. *Contemporary Clinical Trials, 30*(4), 284–288.

168 Blasey, C. M., Block, T. S., Belanoff, J. K., & Roe, R. L. (2011). Efficacy and safety of mifepristone for the treatment of psychotic depression. *Journal of Clinical Psychopharmacology, 31*(4), 436–440.

169 Personal communication.

170 O'Tuathaigh, C. M., O'Connor, A. M., O'Sullivan, G. J., Lai, D., Harvey, R., Croke, D. T., & Waddington, J. L. (2008). Disruption to social dyadic interactions but not emotional/anxiety-related behaviour in mice with heterozygous 'knockout' of the schizophrenia risk gene neuregulin-1. *Progress in Neuropsychopharmacology & Biological Psychiatry, 32*(2), 462–466.

Chapter 8: Instinctive Herds and Primeval Ignorance

1 Ridley, M. (1996). *The origins of virtue: Human instincts and the evolution of cooperation.* New York: Penguin Books.

2 Lyko, F., Foret, S., Kucharski, R., Wolf, S., Falckenhayn, C., & Maleszka, R. (2010). The honey bee epigenomes: Differential methylation of brain DNA in queens and workers. *PLoS Biology, 8*(11), e1000506.

3 Seeley, T. D. (2010). *Honeybee democracy.* Princeton, NJ: Princeton Univeristy Press.

4 Miller, P. (2010). *The smart swarm: How understanding flocks, schools, and colonies can make us better at communicating, decision making, and getting things done.* New York: Avery.

5 Carrera, M., Herrán, A., Ramírez, M. L., Ayestaráran, A., Sierra-Biddle, D., Hoyuela, F., et al. (2006). Personality traits in early phases of panic disorder: Implications on the presence of agoraphobia, clinical severity and short-term outcome. *Acta Psychiatrica Scandinavica, 114*(6), 417–425.

6 Rosellini, A. J., & Brown, T. A. (2011). The NEO Five-Factor Inventory: Latent structure and relationships with dimensions of anxiety and depressive disorders in a large clinical sample. *Assessment, 18*(1), 27–38.

7 Stein, M. B., Schork, N. J., & Gelernter, J. (2004). A polymorphism of the beta1-adrenergic receptor is associated with low extraversion. *Biological Psychiatry, 56*(4), 217–224.

8 Goodwin, R. D., & Gotlib, I. H. (2004). Gender differences in depression: The role of personality factors. *Psychiatry Research, 126*(2), 135–142.

9 Kahn, J. P., & Sodikoff, C. (n.d.). Unpublished Data.

10 Berglas, S. (2002). The very real dangers of executive coaching. *Harvard Business Review, 80*(6), 86–92, 153.

11 McCrae, R. R., Scally, M., Terracciano, A., Abecasis, G. R., & Costa, P. T. Jr. (2010). An alternative to the search for single polymorphisms: Toward molecular personality scales for the five-factor model. *Journal of Personality and Social Psychology, 99*(6), 1014–1024.

12 Mahoney, C. J., Rohrer, J. D., Omar, R., Rossor, M. N., & Warren, J. D. (2011). Neuroanatomical profiles of personality change in frontotemporal lobar degeneration. *The British Journal of Psychiatry, 198*(5), 365–372.

13 DeYoung, C. G., Hirsh, J. B., Shane, M. S., Papdemetris, X., Rajeevan, N., & Gray, J. R. (2010). Testing predictions from personality neuroscience: Brain structure and the big five. *Psychological Science, 21*(6), 820–828.

14 Bastiaansen, L., Rossi, G., Schotte, C., & De Fruyt, F. (2011). The structure of personality disorders: Comparing the DSM-IV-TR Axis II classification with the five-factor model framework using structural equation modeling. *Journal of Personality Disorders, 25*(3), 378–396.

15 Weiss, A., King, J. E., & Hopkins, W. D. (2007). A cross-setting study of chimpanzee (Pan troglodytes) personality structure and development: Zoological parks and Yerkes National Primate Research Center. *American Journal of Primatology, 69*(11), 1264–1277.

16 Fulghum, R. (1993). *All I really need to know I learned in kindergarten: Uncommon thoughts on common things.* New York: Ballantine.

17 Diamond, J. (2005). *Guns, germs and steel: A short history of everybody for the last 13,000 years.* London: Vintage.

18 Darwin, C. (1995). *On the origin of species.* New York: Gramercy.

19 Gosling, S. D., Sandy, C. J., & Potter, J. (2010). Personalities of self-identified "dog people" and "cat people." *Anthrozoos: A Multidisciplinary Journal of The Interactions of People & Animals, 23*(3), 213–222.

20 Graham, J., Nosek, B. A., Haidt, J., Iyer, R., Koleva, S., & Ditto, P. H. (2011). Mapping the moral domain. *Journal of Personality and Social Psychology, 101*(2), 366–385.

21 Lewis, G. J., & Bates, T. C. (2011). From left to right: How the personality system allows basic traits to influence politics via characteristic moral adaptations. *British Journal of Psychology, 102*(3), 546–558.

22 Wright, J. C., & Baril, G. (2011). The role of cognitive resources in determining our moral intuitions: Are we all liberals at heart? *Journal of Experimental Social Psychology, 47*(5), 1007–1012.

23 *Follow my leader: A group's "intelligence" depends in part on its members' ignorance.* (2011, February 24). The Economist. Retrieved from: http://www.economist.com/node/18226831

24 Kahn, J. P., & Langlieb, A. M. (2003). *Mental health and productivity in the workplace: A handbook for organizations and clinicians.* New York: Jossey-Bass.

Chapter 9: The Rise of Reason and the Ascent of Angst

1 Pryor, K. W., Haag, R., & O'Reilly, J. (1969). The creative porpoise: Training for novel behavior. *Journal of the Experimental Analysis of Behavior, 12*(4), 653–661.

2 Schwartz, B. (1982). Failure to produce response variability with reinforcement. *Journal of the Experimental Analysis of Behavior, 37*(2), 171–181.

3 Mellars, P., & French, J. C. (2011). Tenfold population increase in Western Europe at the Neandertal-to-modern human transition. *Science, 333*(6042), 623–627.

4 Schwartz, C. E., Kunwar, P. S., Greve, D. N., Moran, L. R., Viner, J. C., Covino, J. M., et al. (2010). Structural differences in adult orbital and ventromedial prefrontal cortex predicted by infant temperament at 4 months of age. *Archives of General Psychiatry, 67*(1), 78–84.

5 Ghaemi, N. (2011). *A first-rate madness: Uncovering the links between leadership and mental illness.* New York: Penguin.

6 Moalic, J. M., Le Strat, Y., Lepagnol-Bestel, A. M., Ramoz, N., Loe-Mie, Y., Maussion, G., et al. (2010). Primate-accelerated evolutionary genes: Novel routes to drug discovery in psychiatric disorders. *Current Medicinal Chemistry, 17*(13), 1300–1316.

7 Kéri, S. (2009). Genes for psychosis and creativity: A promoter polymorphism of the neuregulin 1 gene is related to creativity in people with high intellectual achievement. *Psychological Science, 20*(9), 1070–1073.

8 Ludwig, A. M. (1994). Mental illness and creative activity in female writers. *The American Journal of Psychiatry, 151*(11), 1650–1656.

9 Cheney, D. L., & Seyfarth, R. M. (2007). *Baboon metaphysics: The evolution of a social mind.* Chicago: University of Chicago Press.

10 de Manzano, O., Cervenka, S., Karabanov, A., Farde, L., & Ullén, F. (2010). Thinking outside a less intact box: Thalamic dopamine D2 receptor densities are negatively related to psychometric creativity in healthy individuals. *PLoS One, 5*(5), e10670.

11 Takeuchi, H., Taki, Y., Sassa, Y., Hashizume, H., Sekiguchi, A., Fukushima, A., & Kawashima, R. (2010). Regional gray matter volume of dopaminergic system associate with creativity: Evidence from voxel-based morphometry. *NeuroImage, 51*(2), 578–585.

12 Kuhn, T. S. (1996). *The structure of scientific revolutions.* Chicago: University of Chicago Press.

13 Choi, C. Q. (2010, November 5). *Beer Lubricated the Rise of Civilization, Study Suggests.* LiveScience. Retrieved from http://www.livescience.com/10221-beer-lubricated-rise-civilization-study-suggests.html

14 Barnard, H., Dooley, A. N., Areshian, G., Gasparyan, B., & Faull, K. F. (2011). Chemical evidence for wine production around 4000 BCE in the Late Chalcolithic Near Eastern highlands. *Journal of Archaeological Science, 38*(5), 977–984.

15 Ait-Daoud, N., Roache, J. D., Dawes, M. A., Liu, L., Wang, X. Q., Javors, M. A., et al. (2009). Can serotonin transporter genotype predict craving in alcoholism? *Alcoholism, Clinical and Experimental Research, 33*(8), 1329–1335.

16 Johnson, B. A., Javors, M. A., Roache, J. D., Seneviratne, C., Bergeson, S. E., Ait-Daoud, N., et al. (2008). Can serotonin transporter genotype predict serotonergic function, chronicity, and severity of drinking? *Progress in Neuro-psychopharmacology & Biological Psychiatry, 32*(1), 209–216.

17 Oreland, S., Raudkivi, K., Oreland, L., Harro, J., Arborelius, L., & Nylander, I. (2011). Ethanol-induced effects on the dopamine and serotonin systems in adult Wistar rats are dependent on early-life experiences. *Brain Research, 1405,* 57–68.

18 Stevens, S., Rist, F., & Gerlach, A.L. (2009). Influence of alcohol on the processing of emotional facial expressions in individuals with social phobia. *The British Journal of Clinical Psychology, 48*(2), 125–140.

19 Buckner, J. D., Timpano, K. R., Zvolensky, M. J., Sachs-Ericsson, N., & Schmidt, N.B. (2008). Implications of comorbid alcohol dependence among individuals with social anxiety disorder. *Depression and Anxiety, 25*(12), 1028–1037.

20 Buckner, J. D., & Schmidt, N. B. (2009). Understanding social anxiety as a risk for alcohol use disorders: Fear of scrutiny, not social interaction fears, prospectively predicts alcohol use disorders. *Journal of Psychiatric Research, 43*(4), 477–483.

21 McGovern, P. E. (2009). *Uncorking the past: The quest for wine, beer, and other alcoholic beverages.* Berkeley, CA: University of California Press.

22 Goodwin, R. D. Lipsitz, J. D. Keyes, K. Galea, S., & Fyer, A. J. (2011). Family history of alcohol use disorders among adults with panic disorder in the community. *Journal of Psychiatric Research, 45*(8), 1123–1127.

23 Lê, A. D., Funk, D., Juzytsch, W., Coen, K., Navarre, B. M., Cifani, C., & Shaham, Y. (2011). Effect of prazosin and guanfacine on stress-induced reinstatement of alcohol and food seeking in rats. *Psychopharmacology, 218*(1), 89–99.

24 Squicciarini, M., & Swinnen, J. (2010). *AAWE Working Paper No.75: Economics: Women or Wine? Monogamy and Alcohol.* Retrieved from http://wine-economics.org/working-papers/AAWE_WP75.pdf

25 Kim, S. K., Lee, S. I., Shin, C. J., Son, J. W., & Ju, G. (2010). The genetic factors affecting drinking behaviors of Korean young adults with variant aldehyde dehydrogenase 2 genotype. *Psychiatry Investigation, 7*(4), 270–277.

26 Li, D., Zhao, H., & Gelernter, J. (2011). Strong association of the alcohol dehydrogenase 1B gene (ADH1B) with alcohol dependence and alcohol-induced medical diseases. *Biological Psychiatry, 70*(6), 504–512.

27 Hishimoto, A., Fukutake, M., Mouri, K., Nagasaki, Y., Asano, M., Ueno, Y., et al. (2010). Alcohol and aldehyde dehydrogenase polymorphisms and risk for suicide: A preliminary observation in the Japanese male population. *Genes, Brain and Behavior, 9*(5), 498–502.

28 Eng, M. Y., Luczak, S. E., & Wall, T. L. (2007). ALDH2, ADH1B, and ADH1C genotypes in Asians: A literature review. *Alcohol Research & Health, 30*(1), 22–27.

29 Hasin, D., Aharonovich, E., Liu, X., Mamman, Z., Matseoane, K., Carr, L. G., & Li, T. K. (2002). Alcohol dependence symptoms and alcohol dehydrogenase 2 polymorphism: Israeli Ashkenazis, Sephardics, and recent Russian immigrants. *Alcoholism, Clinical and Experimental Research, 26*(9), 1315–1321.

30 Mann, C. C. (2011, June). The birth of religion. *National Geographic.* Retrieved from http://ngm.nationalgeographic.com/2011/06/gobekli-tepe/mann-text

31 Harris, S., Kaplan, J. T., Curiel, A., Bookheimer, S. Y., Iacoboni, M., & Cohen, M. S. (2009). The neural correlates of religious and nonreligious belief. *PLoS One, 4*(10), e0007272.

32 Saroglou, V. (2010). Religiousness as a cultural adaptation of basic traits: A five-factor model perspective. *Personality and Social Psychology Review, 14*(1), 108–125.

33 Flannelly, K. J., Galek, K., Ellison, C. G., & Koenig, H. G. (2010). Beliefs about God, psychiatric symptoms, and evolutionary psychiatry. *Journal of Religion and Health, 49*(2), 246–261.

34 Schjoedt, U., Stødkilde-Jørgensen, H., Geertz, A. W., & Roepstorff, A. (2009). Highly religious participants recruit areas of social cognition in personal prayer. *Social Cognitive and Affective Neuroscience, 4*(2), 199–207.

35 Freud, S. (2010). *Civilization and its discontents.* Mansfield Centre, CT: Martino.

36 Abramowitz, J. S., Deacon, B. J., Woods, C. M., & Tolin, D.F. (2004). Association between Protestant religiosity and obsessive-compulsive symptoms and cognitions. *Depression and Anxiety, 20*(2), 70–76.

37 Decety, J., Michalska, K. J., & Kinzler, K. D. (2012). The contribution of emotion and cognition to moral sensitivity: A neurodevelopmental study. *Cererebral Cortex, 22*(1), 209–220.

38 Fenix, J. B., Cherlin, E. J., Prigerson, H. G., Johnson-Hurzeler, R., Kasl, S. V., & Bradley, E. H. (2006). Religiousness and major depression among bereaved family caregivers: A 13-month follow-up study. *Journal of Palliative Care, 22*(4), 286–292.

39 Kahn, T. A. (2010). *Cultural and social psychological analysis of the Torah.* Thesis, Wesleyan University.

40 Graham, J., Haidt, J., & Nosek, B. A. (2009). Liberals and conservatives rely on different sets of moral foundations. *Journal of Personality and Social Psychology, 96*(5), 1029–1046.

41 Pinker, S. (2011). *The better angels of our nature: Why violence has declined.* New York: Viking.

42 King, A. L., Valença, A. M., & Nardi, A. E. (2010). Nomophobia: The mobile phone in panic disorder with agoraphobia: Reducing phobias or worsening of dependence? *Cognitive and Behavioral Neurology, 23*(1), 52–54.

43 Stritzke, W. G. K., Nguyen, A., & Durkin, K. (2004). Shyness and computer-mediated communication: A self-presentational theory perspective. *Media Psychology, 6*(1), 1–22.

44 Lee, B. W., & Stapinski, L. A. (2012). Seeking safety on the internet: Relationship between social anxiety and problematic internet use. *Journal of Anxiety Disorders, 26*(1), 197–205.

45 Hernandez, D. (2011, August 6). *Too much Facebook time may be unhealthy for kids.* Los Angeles Times. Retrieved from http://articles.latimes.com/2011/aug/06/news/la-heb-facebook-teens-20110806

Chapter 10: Consciousness Has Consequences

1 Barnes, B. A., & Scott, C. M. (2011). A multilevel field investigation of emotional labor, affect, work withdrawal, and gender. *The Academy of Management Journal (AMJ), 54*(1), 116–136.

2 Koh, K. B., Kim, D. K., Kim, S. Y., Park, J. K., & Han, M. (2008). The relation between anger management style, mood and somatic symptoms in anxiety disorders and somatoform disorders. *Psychiatry Research, 160*(3), 372–379.

3 Berglas, S. (2002). The very real dangers of executive coaching. *Harvard Business Review, 80*(6), 86–92, 153.

4 Varki, N. M., Strobert, E., Dick, E. J., Jr., Benirschke, K., & Varki, A. (2011). Biomedical differences between human and nonhuman hominids: Potential roles for uniquely human aspects of sialic acid biology. *Annual Review of Pathology, 6*, 365–393.

5 Apicella, C. L., Marlowe, F. W., Fowler, J. H., & Christakis, N. A. (2012). Social networks and cooperation in hunter-gatherers. *Nature, 481*, 497–501.

6 Kahn, J., & Ad Hoc Committee of The Academy of Organizational and Occupational Psychiatry. (1997). Response to EEOC guidelines on reasonable accommodation for mental illness.

7 Gibbons, R. D., Brown, C. H., Hur, K., Marcus, S. M., Bhaumik, D. K., Erkens, J. A., et al. (2007). Early evidence on the effects of regulators' suicidality warnings on SSRI prescriptions and suicide in children and adolescents. *American Journal of Psychiatry, 164*(9), 1356–1363.

8 Gibbons, R. D., Brown, C. H., Hur, K., Marcus, S. M., Bhaumik, D. K., & Mann, J. J. (2007). Relationship between antidepressants and suicide attempts: An analysis of the Veterans Health Administration data sets. *The American Journal of Psychiatry, 164*(7), 1044–1049.

9 Mirza, S. K., & Deyo, R. A. (2007). Systematic review of randomized trials comparing lumbar fusion surgery to nonoperative care for treatment of chronic back pain. *Spine, 32*(7), 816–823.

10 Brox, J. I., Nygaard, Ø. P., Holm, I., Keller, A., Ingebrigtsen, T., & Reikerås, O. (2010). Four-year follow-up of surgical versus non-surgical therapy for chronic low back pain. *Annals of the Rheumatic Diseases, 69*(9), 1643–1648.

11 Kahn, J. P., Kornfeld, D. S., Blood, D. K., Lynn, R. B., Heller, S. S., & Frank, K. A. (1982). Type A behavior and the thallium stress test. *Psychosomatic Medicine, 44*(5), 431–436.

12 Katz, C., Yaseen, Z. S., Mojtabai, R., Cohen, L. J., & Galynker, I. I. (2011). Panic as an independent risk factor for suicide attempt in depressive illness: Findings from the National Epidemiological Survey on Alcohol and Related Conditions (NESARC). *The Journal of Clinical Psychiatry, 72*(12), 1628–1635.

13 Mittal, V., Brown, W. A., & Shorter, E. (2009). Are patients with depression at heightened risk of suicide as they begin to recover? *Psychiatric Services, 60*(3), 384–386.

14 Robinson, J., Sareen, J., Cox, B. J., & Bolton, J. M. (2011). Role of self-medication in the development of comorbid anxiety and substance use disorders: A longitudinal investigation. *Archives of General Psychiatry, 68*(8), 800–807.

15 Buckner, J. D., Timpano, K. R., Zvolensky, M. J., Sachs-Ericsson, N., & Schmidt, N.B. (2008). Implications of comorbid alcohol dependence among individuals with social anxiety disorder. *Depression and Anxiety, 25*(12), 1028–1037.

16 Schneier, F. R., Foose, T. E., Hasin, D. S., Heimberg, R. G., Liu, S. M., Grant, B. F., & Blanco, C. (2010). Social anxiety disorder and alcohol use disorder co-morbidity in the National Epidemiologic Survey on Alcohol and Related Conditions. *Psychological Medicine, 40*(6), 977–988.

17 Yoshimoto, K., McBride, W. J., Lumeng, L., & Li, T. K. (1992). Ethanol enhances the release of dopamine and serotonin in the nucleus accumbens of HAD and LAD lines of rats. *Alcoholism, Clinical and Experimental Research, 16*(4), 781–785.

18 Buckner, J. D., & Heimberg, R. G. (2010). Drinking behaviors in social situations account for alcohol-related problems among socially anxious individuals. *Psychology of Addictive Behaviors, 24*(4), 640–648.

19 Buckner, J. D., & Schmidt, N. B. (2009). Understanding social anxiety as a risk for alcohol use disorders: Fear of scrutiny, not social interaction fears, prospectively predicts alcohol use disorders. *Journal of Psychiatric Research, 43*(4), 477–483.

20 Terlecki, M. A., Buckner, J. D., Larimer, M. E., & Copeland, A. L. (2011). The role of social anxiety in a brief alcohol intervention for heavy-drinking college students. *Journal of Cognitive Psychotherapy, 25*(1), 7–21.

21 Goodwin, R. D., Lipsitz, J. D., Keyes, K., Galea, S., & Fyer, A. J. (2011). Family history of alcohol use disorders among adults with panic disorder in the community. *Journal of Psychiatric Research, 45*(8), 1123–1127.

22 Terracciano A., Löckenhoff, C. E., Crum, R. M., Bienvenu, O. J., & Costa, P. T., Jr. (2008). Five-factor model personality profiles of drug users. *BMC Psychiatry, 8,* 22.

23 McGovern, P. E. (2009). *Uncorking the past: The quest for wine, beer, and other alcoholic beverages.* Berkeley, CA: University of California Press.

24 Goodwin, R. D., & Hamilton, S. P. (2002). The early-onset fearful panic attack as a predictor of severe psychopathology. *Psychiatry Research, 109*(1), 71–79.

25 Tillfors, M., El-Khouri, B., Stein, M. B., & Trost, K. (2009). Relationships between social anxiety, depressive symptoms, and antisocial behaviors: Evidence from a prospective study of adolescent boys. *Journal of Anxiety Disorders, 23*(5), 718–724.

26 Marmorstein, N. R. (2006). Adult antisocial behaviour without conduct disorder: Demographic characteristics and risk for co-occurring psychopathology. *Canadian Journal of Psychiatry, 51*(4), 226–233.

27 Lacina, B., & Gleditsch, N. P. (2005). Monitoring trends in global combat: A new dataset of battle deaths. *European Journal of Population, 21,* 145–166.

28 Allam, A. H., Thompson, R. C., Wann, L. S., Miyamoto, M. I., Nur El-Din, Ael-H., et al. (2011). Atherosclerosis in ancient Egyptian mummies: The Horus study. *JACC Cardiovascular Imaging, 4*(4), 315–327.

29 Sapolsky, R. M. (2004). *Why zebras don't get ulcers.* New York: Holt.

30 Seldenrijk, A., Hamer, M., Lahiri, A., Penninx, B. W., & Steptoe, A. (2012). Psychological distress, cortisol stress response and subclinical coronary calcification. *Psychoneuroendocrinology, 37*(1), 48–55.

31 Scherrer, J. F., Chrusciel, T., Zeringue, A., Garfield, L. D., Hauptman, P. J., Lustman, P. J., et al. (2010). Anxiety disorders increase risk for incident myocardial infarction in depressed and nondepressed Veterans Administration patients. *American Heart Journal, 159*(5), 772–779.

32 Sardinha, A., Araújo, C. G., Soares-Filho, G. L., & Nardi, A.E. (2011). Anxiety, panic disorder and coronary artery disease: Issues concerning physical exercise and cognitive behavioral therapy. *Expert Review of Cardioivascular Therapy, 9*(2), 165–175.

33 Kahn, J. P., Drusin, R. E., & Klein, D. F. (1987). Idiopathic cardiomyopathy and panic disorder: Clinical association in cardiac transplant candidates. *The American Journal of Psychiatry, 144*(10), 1327–1330.

34 Pinderhughes, C. A., & Pearlman, C.A. (1969). Psychiatric aspects of idiopathic cardiomyopathy. *Psychosomatic Medicine, 31*(1), 57–67.

35 Kahn J. P., Gorman, J. M., King, D. L., Fyer, A. J., Liebowitz, M. R., & Klein, D. F. (1990). Cardiac left ventricular hypertrophy and chamber dilatation in panic disorder patients: Implications for idiopathic dilated cardiomyopathy. *Psychiatry Research, 32*(1), 55–61.

36 Yeragani, V. K., Balon, R., Pohl, R., Weinberg, P., & Thomas, S. (1992). Leftward shift of R-axis on electrocardiogram in patients with panic disorder and Depression. *Neuropsychobiology, 25*(2), 91–93.

37 Chen, Y. H., Tsai, S. Y., Lee, H. C., & Lin, H. C. (2009). Increased risk of acute myocardial infarction for patients with panic disorder: A nationwide population-based study. *Psychosomatic Medicine, 71*(7), 798–804.

38 George, D. T., Hibbeln, J. R., Ragan, P. W., Umhau, J. C., Phillips, M. J., Doty, L., et al. (2000). Lactate-induced rage and panic in a select group of subjects who perpetrate acts of domestic violence. *Biological Psychiatry, 47*(9), 804–812.

39 Kahn, J. P., Stevenson, E., Topol, P., & Klein, D. F. (1986). Agitated depression, alprazolam, and panic anxiety. *The American Journal of Psychiatry, 143*(9), 1172–1173.

40 Steptoe, A., Molloy, G. J., Messerli-Bürgy, N., Wikman, A., Randall, G., Perkins-Porras, L., & Kaski, J.C. (2011). Fear of dying and inflammation following acute coronary syndrome. *European Heart Journal, 32*(19), 2405–2411.

41 Bekoff, M., & Pierce, J. (2009). *Wild justice: The moral lives of animals.* Chicago: University of Chicago Press.

42 Yarnold, P. R., & Bryant, F. B. (1994). A measurement model for the Type A self-rating inventory. *Journal of Personality Assessment, 62*(1), 102–115.

43 Hausteiner, C., Klupsch, D., Emeny, R., Baumert, J., Ladwig, K. H., & KORA Investigators. (2010). Clustering of negative affectivity and social inhibition in the community: Prevalence of type D personality as a cardiovascular risk marker. *Psychosomatic Medicine, 72*(2), 163–171.

44 Bonaguidi, F. (2011). Anger predicts long-term mortality in patients with myocardial infarction. *European Society of Cardiology.* Retrieved from http://www.escardio.org/about/press/press-releases/esc11-paris/Pages/anger-predicts-mortality-mi.aspx

45 Chida, Y., & Steptoe, A. (2009). The association of anger and hostility with future coronary heart disease: A meta-analytic review of prospective evidence. *Journal of the American College of Cardiology, 53*(11), 936–946.

46 van Reedt Dortland, A. K., Giltay, E. J., van Veen, T., van Pelt, J., Zitman, F. G., & Penninx, B. W. (2010). Associations between serum lipids and major depressive disorder: Results from the Netherlands Study of Depression and Anxiety (NESDA). *The Journal of Clinical Psychiatry, 71*(6), 729–736.

47 Grant, N., Hamer, M., & Steptoe, A. (2009). Social isolation and stress-related cardiovascular, lipid, and cortisol responses. *Annals of Behavioral Medicine, 37*(1), 29–37.

48 Maseri, A., Beltrame, J. F., & Shimokawa, H. (2009). Role of coronary vasoconstriction in ischemic heart disease and search for novel therapeutic targets. *Circulation Journal, 73*(3), 394–403.

49 Mach, F. (2005). Inflammation is a crucial feature of atherosclerosis and a potential target to reduce cardiovascular events. *Handbook of Experimental Pharmacology, 170,* 697–722.

50 Kahn J. P., Perumal, A. S., Gully, R. J., Smith, T. M., Cooper, T. B., & Klein, D. F. (1987). Correlation of type A behaviour with adrenergic receptor density: Implications for coronary artery disease pathogenesis. *Lancet, 2*(8565), 937–939.

51 O'Donnell, K., Brydon, L., Wright, C. E., & Steptoe, A. (2008). Self-esteem levels and cardiovascular and inflammatory responses to acute stress. *Brain, Behavior, and Immunity, 22*(8), 1241–1247.

52 Slavich G. M., Way, B. M., Eisenberger, N. I., & Taylor, S. E. (2010). Neural sensitivity to social rejection is associated with inflammatory responses to social stress. *Proceedings of the National Academy of Sciences of the United States of America, 107*(33), 14817–14822.

53 Ellins, E., Halcox, J., Donald, A., Field, B., Brydon, L., Deanfield, J., & Steptoe, A. (2008). Arterial stiffness and inflammatory response to psychophysiological stress. *Brain, Behavior, and Immunity, 22*(6), 941–948.

54 Thorin, E., & Thorin-Trescases, N. (2009). Vascular endothelial ageing, heartbeat after heartbeat. *Cardiovascular Research, 84*(1), 24–32.

55 Polak, J. F., Pencina, M. J., Pencina, K. M., O'Donnell, C. J., Wolf, P. A., & D'Agostino, R. B., Sr. (2011). Carotid-wall intima-media thickness and cardiovascular events. *The New England Journal of Medicine, 365*(3), 213–221.

56 Egolf, B., Lasker, J., Wolf, S., & Potvin, L. (1992). The Roseto effect: A 50-year comparison of mortality rates. *The American Journal of Public Health, 82*(8), 1089–1092.

57 Wolf, S. (1992). Predictors of myocardial infarction over a span of 30 years in Roseto, Pennsylvania. *Integrative Physiological and Behavioral Science, 27*(3), 246–257.

58 Edston, E. (2006). The earlobe crease, coronary artery disease, and sudden cardiac death: An autopsy study of 520 individuals. *The American Journal of Forensic Medicine and Pathology, 27*(2), 129–133.

59 Buitrago-Lopez, A., Sanderson, J., Johnson, L., Warnakula, S., Wood, A., Di Angelantonio, E., & Franco, O. H. (2011). Chocolate consumption and cardiometabolic disorders: Systematic review and meta-analysis. *BMJ, 343*. doi: 10.1136/bmj.d4488

60 Kahneman, D., & Deaton, A. (2010). High income improves evaluation of life but not emotional well-being. *Proceedings of the National Academy of Sciences of the United States of America, 107*(38), 16489–16493.

61 Myhrvold, N. (2011, August 18). Descended from apes, acting like slime molds. *Bloomberg*. Retrieved from http://www.bloomberg.com/news/2011-08-18/descended-from-apes-acting-as-slime-molds-commentary-by-nathan-myhrvold.html

Chapter 11: How to Balance Your Reason and Instinct

1 Moore, A. S. (2010, November 7). Accomodation Angst. *The New York Times*, p. ED2.

2 Walker, I. (2007). Drivers overtaking bicyclists: Objective data on the effects of riding position, helmet use, vehicle type and apparent gender. *Accident Analysis and Prevention, 39(2)*, 417–425.

3 Flaherty, A. (2011). Brain illness and creativity: Mechanisms and treatment risks. *Canadian Journal of Psychiatry, 56(3)*, 129–131.

4 Merton, R. K. (1936). The unanticipated consequences of purposive social action. *American Sociological Review, 1*(6), 894–904.

5 Kahn, J. P., & Le Schack, P. (1995). Stress, distress and anxiety: Real causes and real solutions. *Newsweek (Health Supplement)*, A14–A17.

6 Kramer, P. D. (1993). *Listening to Prozac*. New York: Penguin.

7 Goleman, D., & Boyatis, R. (2008). Social intelligence and the biology of leadership. *Harvard Business Review, 86(9)*, 74–81, 136.

8 Kucera, S. (2012, Feb). Personal Communication.

9 Cochran, G., & Harpending, H. (2010). *The 10,000 year explosion: How civilization accelerated human evolution*. New York: Basic.

10 Chiao, J. Y., & Blizinsky, K. D. (2010). Culture-gene coevolution of individualism-collectivism and the serotonin transporter gene. *Proceedings. Biological Sciences/The Royal Society, 277*(1681), 529–537.

11 Way, B. M., & Lieberman, M. D. (2010). Is there a genetic contribution to cultural differences? Collectivism, individualism and genetic markers of social sensitivity. *Social Cognitive and Affective Neuroscience, 5*(2–3), 203–211.

12 Egusa, G., & Yamane, K. (2004). Lifestyle, serum lipids and coronary artery disease: Comparison of Japan with the United States. *Journal of Atherosclerosis and Thrombosis, 1(6)*, 304–312.

13 Alvergne A. J. M. (2010). Personality and reproductive success in a high-fertility human population. *Proceedings of the National Academy of Science U S A, 107*(26), 11745–11750.

14 Faulkner, W. (1975). *Requiem for a nun.* New York: Vintage.

BIBLIOGRAPHY

The books listed in this bibliography were essential sources for elaboration of the theory in this book or were about related subjects.

Adriaens, P. R., & De Block, A. (Eds.). (2011). *Maladapting minds: Philosophy, psychiatry, and evolutionary theory.* Oxford, England: Oxford University Press.

American Psychiatric Association. (2000). *Diagnostic and statistical manual of mental disorders DSM-IV-TR* (4th ed., Text Revision). Washington, DC: American Psychiatric Association.

Barrett, D. (2010). *Supernormal stimuli: How primal urges overran their evolutionary purpose.* New York: W. W. Norton.

Bekoff, M., & Pierce, J. (2009). *Wild justice: The moral lives of animals.* Chicago: University of Chicago Press.

Bowlby, J. (1973). *Separation: Anxiety and anger.* New York: Basic.

Brooks, D. (2011). *The social animal: The hidden soures of love, character, and achievement.* New York: Random House.

Brune, M. (2008). *Textbook of evolutionary psychiatry.* Oxford, England: Oxford University Press.

Burns, J. (2007). *The descent of madness: Evolutionary origins of psychosis and the social brain.* New York: Routledge.

Buss, D. M. (2008). *Evolutionary psychiatry: The new science of the mind.* Boston: Pearson/Allyn & Bacon.

Cheney, D. L., & Seyfarth, R. M. (2007). *Baboon metaphysics: The evolution of a social mind.* Chicago: University of Chicago Press.

Cochran, G., & Harpending, H. (2009). *The 10,000 year explosion: How civilization accelerated human evolution.* New York: Basic.

Darwin, C. (1995). *On the origin of species.* New York: Gramercy.

Darwin, C. (2007). *The expression of the emotions in man and animals.* Minneapolis, MN: Filiquarian.

Darwin, C. (2008). *The descent of man, and selection in relation to sex.* London: Folio Society.

Freud, S. (1987). *A phylogenetic fantasy.* Cambridge, MA: Belknap Press of Harvard University Press.

Freud, S. (2010). *Civilization and its discontents.* Mansfield Centre, CT: Martino.

Gilbert, P., & Bailey, K. G. (2000). *Genes on the couch: Explorations in evolutionary psychotherapy.* Philadelphia: Brunner-Routledge.

Horowitz, A. (2009). *Inside of a dog: What dogs see, smell, and know.* New York: Scribner.

Kahn, J. P., & Langlieb, A. M. (2003). *Mental health and productivity in the workplace: A handbook for organizations and clinicians.* New York: Jossey-Bass.

Kramer, P. D. (1997). *Listening to Prozac.* New York: Penguin.

Kuhn, T. S. (1996). *The structure of scientific revolutions.* Chicago: University of Chicago Press.

Kuijsten, M. (Ed.). (2006). *Reflections on the dawn of consciousness.* Henderson, NV: Julian Jaynes Society.

McGovern, P. E. (2009). *Uncorking the past: The quest for wine, beer, and other alcoholic beverages.* Berkeley, CA: University of California Press.

McGuire, M., & Troisi, A. (1998). *Darwinian psychiatry.* New York: Oxford University Press.

Miller, P. (2010). *The smart swarm: How understanding flocks, schools, and colonies can make us better at communicating, decision making, and getting things done.* New York: Avery.

Moalem, S. (2007). *Survival of the sickest: The surprising connections between disease and longevity.* New York: Harper Perennial.

Nesse, R. M., & Williams, G. C. (1994). *Why we get sick: The new science of Darwinian medicine.* New York: Vintage.

Pinker, S. (2011). *The better angels of our nature: Why violence has declined.* New York: Viking.

Ridley, M. (1996). *The origins of virtue: Human instincts and the evolution of cooperation.* New York: Penguin.

Sapolsky, R. M. (2004). *Why zebras don't get ulcers.* New York: Holt.

Seeley, T. D. (2010). *Honeybee democracy.* Princeton, NJ: Princeton Univeristy Press.

Shorter, E., & Fink, M. (2010). *Endocrine psychiatry: Solving the riddle of melancholia.* New York: Oxford University Press.

Smith, D. B. (2007). *Muses, madmen, and prophets.* New York: Penguin Group.

Standage, T. (2005). *A history of the world in 6 glasses.* New York: Walker.

Stevens, A. (1993). *The two million-year-old self.* College Station, TX: Texas A&M Press.

Stevens, A., & Price, J. (2000). *Evolutionary psychiatry: A new beginning.* New York: Routledge.

Taylor, M. A., & Fink, M. (2006). *Melancholia: The diagnosis, pathophysiology, and treatment of depressive illness.* New York: Cambridge Univerity Press.

Wilson, E. O. (1978). *On human nature.* Cambridge, MA: Harvard University Press.

Wilson, E. O. (2000). *Sociobiology: The new synthesis.* Cambridge, MA: Belknap Press of Harvard University Press.

Wrangham, R. (2009). *Catching fire: How cooking made us human.* New York: Basic.

INDEX